KEYS TO
Nursing
Success

Janet R. Katz, RN, MSN, RN,C

Carol Carter   Joyce Bishop   Sarah Lyman Kravits

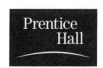

Prentice
Hall

Upper Saddle River, New Jersey 07458

Library of Congress Cataloging-in-Publication Data

Keys to nursing success / Janet R. Katz . . . [et al.].
    p.   ; cm.
    Includes bibliographical references and index.
    ISBN 0-13-019575-8
    1. Nursing.   2. Nursing—Study and teaching.   3. Nursing—Vocational guidance.   4.
Test-taking skills.   I. Title: Nursing success.   II. Katz, Janet R., 1953–
    [DNLM: 1. Nursing.   2. Career Choice.   3. Education, Nursing.   WY 16 K44 2001]
RT71 .K49 2001
610.73—dc21

00-040091

Acquisitions Editor: Sande Johnson
Assistant Editor: Michelle Williams
Production Editor: Holcomb Hathaway
Director of Manufacturing and Production: Bruce Johnson
Managing Editor: Mary Carnis
Manufacturing Manager: Ed O'Dougherty
Art Director: Marianne Frasco
Marketing Manager: Jeff McIlroy
Marketing Assistant: Barbara Rosenberg
Cover Design: Bruce Kenselaar
Cover Art: Paul Gourhan
Composition: Aerocraft Charter Art Service
Printing And Binding: Banta Book Group

Prentice-Hall International (UK) Limited, *London*
Prentice-Hall of Australia Pty. Limited, *Sydney*
Prentice-Hall Canada Inc., *Toronto*
Prentice-Hall Hispanoamericana, S.A., *Mexico*
Prentice-Hall of India Private Limited, *New Delhi*
Prentice-Hall of Japan, Inc., *Tokyo*
Pearson Education Singapore Pte. Ltd.
Editora Prentice-Hall do Brasil, Ltda., *Rio de Janeiro*

10 9 8 7 6 5 4 3 2 1
ISBN 0-13-019575-8

Brief Contents

Contents

CHAPTER 2
DISCOVERING NURSING   31

Exploring Your Options

CHAPTER 3
SELF-AWARENESS   55

Knowing Who You Are and How You Learn

CHAPTER 4
GOAL SETTING AND TIME MANAGEMENT   87
Mapping Your Course

CHAPTER 5
SCIENTIFIC INQUIRY   113
Critical and Creative Thinking in Nursing

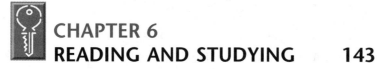

CHAPTER 6
READING AND STUDYING   143
Maximizing Written Resources

CHAPTER 7
NOTE-TAKING AND WRITING   173
Harnessing the Power of Words and Ideas

CHAPTER 8
LISTENING, MEMORY, AND TEST TAKING   205
Taking In, Retaining, and Demonstrating Knowledge

CHAPTER 9
WORKING IN THE LABORATORY   233

Safe Nursing in Action

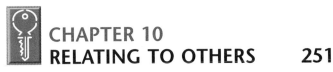

CHAPTER 10
RELATING TO OTHERS   251
Appreciating Your Diverse World

CHAPTER 11
MANAGING CAREER AND MONEY   281
Reality Resources

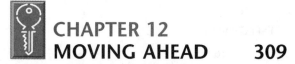

CHAPTER 12
MOVING AHEAD   309

Building a Smart Future

Preface

 KEYS TO NURSING SUCCESS
OWNER'S MANUAL

This book is to provide students having a current or potential nursing major with realistic and useful steps that will increase their chances for success in college and after college in the workplace. Some hints for *Success* in nursing follow.

THE ESSENTIALS FOR *SUCCESS*

Enjoy learning

See the importance of learning science and humanities

Understand ethical principles and responsibility in nursing

Continue learning after graduation

Use knowledge and skills responsibly

Graduate from college with a liberal arts education in addition to nursing

Complete an internship, perform extra work on special projects, or work in the clinical setting

Find a mentor

WHAT *SUCCESS* MAY INCLUDE (but not essential conditions)

High GPA

A career in nursing after graduation

Ability to have a secure career

Highly marketable degree

The Top Three Rules for *Success*

The top three rules for *success* are based on consistent behaviors that lead to gaining a healthy dose of knowledge and skill acquisition while you are in college. The top three rules you will need to follow to succeed as a nursing major are:

1. Go to class
2. Learn to study
3. Take school seriously (study)

As your authors, we have talked to students across the country. We've learned that you are concerned about your future, you want your education to serve a purpose, you are adjusting to constant life changes, and you want honest and direct guidance on how to achieve your goals. We designed the features of *Keys to Nursing Success* based on what you have told us about your needs.

The Contents of the Package: What's Included

We chose the topics in this book based on what you need to make the most of your educational experience. You need a strong sense of *self*, *learning style*, and *goals* in order to discover and pursue the best course of study. You need good *study skills* to take in and retain what you learn both in and out of class. You need to *manage your time*, *money*, and *relationships* so you can handle the changes life hands you. *Keys to Nursing Success* can guide you in all of these areas and more.

The distinguishing characteristics and sections of this book are designed to make your life easier by helping you take in and understand the material you read.

Lifelong learning. The ideas and strategies you learn that will help you succeed in school are the same ones that will bring you success in your career and in your personal life. Therefore, this book focuses on success strategies as they apply to *school*, *work*, and *life*, not just to the classroom or laboratory.

Thinking skills. Being able to remember facts and figures won't do you much good at school or beyond unless you can put that information to work through clear and competent thinking. This book has a chapter on *critical and creative thinking* that will help you explore your mind's actions and thinking processes.

Skill-building exercises. Today's graduates need to be effective thinkers, team players, writers, and strategic planners. The exercises at the end of the chapters will encourage you to develop these valuable career skills and to apply thinking processes to any topic or situation.

Diversity of voice. The world is becoming increasingly diverse in ethnicity, perspective, culture, lifestyle, race, choices, abilities, needs, and more. Every student, instructor, course, and school is unique. One point of view can't possibly apply to everyone. Therefore, many voices will speak to you from these pages. What you read will speak to your needs, offer ideas, and treat you with respect.

User-friendly features. The following features will make your life easier in small but significant ways.

- **Perforations.** Each page of this book is perforated so you can tear out exercises to hand in, take with you somewhere, or keep in your date book as a reference.
- **Exercises.** The exercises are together at the ends of the chapters, so if you want to hand them all in you can do so without also removing any of the text.
- **Definitions.** Selected words are defined in the margins of the text.
- **Long-term usefulness.** Yes, most people sell back some of the textbooks they use. If you take a good look at the material in *Keys to Nursing Success*, however, you may want to keep this book around. *Keys to Nursing Success* is a reference that you can return to over and over again as you work toward your goals in school, work, and life.

 ## TAKE ACTION: READ

You are responsible for your education, your growth, your knowledge, and your future. The best we can do is offer some great suggestions, strategies, ideas, and systems that can help. Ultimately, it's up to you to use whatever fits your particular self with all of its particular situations, needs, and wants, and make it your own. You've made a terrific start by choosing to pursue an education—take advantage of all it has to give you.

🔑 ACKNOWLEDGMENTS

This book has come about through a heroic group effort. We would like to take this opportunity to acknowledge the people who have made it happen. Many thanks to:

- Our student editors Michael Jackson and Aziza Davis.
- Student reviewers Sandi Armitage, Marisa Connell, Jennifer Moe, and Alex Toth.
- Our reviewers: Glenda Belote, Florida International University; John Bennett, Jr., University of Connecticut; Ann Bingham-Newman, California State University, L.A.; Mary Bixby, University of Missouri–Columbia; Barbara Blandford, Education Enhancement Center at Lawrenceville, NJ; Jerry Bouchie, St. Cloud State University; Mona Casady, SW Missouri State University; Janet Cutshall, Sussex County Community College; Valerie DeAngelis, Miami-Dade Community College; Rita Delude, NH Community Technical College; Judy Elsley, Weber State University (Ogden, UT); Gregg R. Godsey, Riverside High School (Washington); Sue Halter, Delgado Community College; Suzy Hampton, University of Montana; Maureen Hurley, University of Missouri–Kansas City; Karen Iversen, Heald Colleges; Kathryn Kelly, St. Cloud State University; Nancy Kosmicke, Mesa State College in Colorado; Frank T. Lyman, Jr., University of Maryland; Barnette Miller Moore, Indian River Community College in Florida; Rebecca Munro, Gonzaga University in Washington; Virginia Phares, DeVry of Atlanta; Brenda Prinzavalli, Beloit College in Wisconsin; Jacqueline Simon, Education Enhancement Center at Lawrenceville, NJ; Carolyn Smith, University of Southern Indiana; Joan Stottlemyer, Carroll College in Montana; Thomas Tyson, SUNY Stony Brook; Rose Wassman, DeAnza College; Michelle G. Wolf, Florida Southern College.
- The PRE 100 instructors at Baltimore City Community College, Liberty Campus, especially college President Dr. Jim Tschechtelin, Coordinator Jim Coleman, Rita Lenkin Hawkins, Sonia Lynch, Jack Taylor, and Peggy Winfield. Thanks also to Prentice Hall representative Alice Barr.
- The instructors at DeVry, especially Susan Chin and Carol Ozee.
- The instructors at Suffolk Community College and Prentice Hall representative Carol Abolafia.
- Our editorial consultant Rich Bucher, professor of sociology at Baltimore City Community College.
- Dr. Frank T. Lyman, inventor of the Thinktrix system.
- Professor Barbara Soloman, developer of the Learning Styles Inventory.
- The people who contributed their stories for Real World Perspectives: Anonymous, Clacy Albert, Laura Brinckerhoff, Brett Cross, Erica Epstein, Norma Espina, Jeff Felardeau, Edith Hall, Jacque Hall, Mike Jackson, Miriam Kapner, Karin Lounsbury, Matt Millard, Todd Montalbo, Carolyn Christina Moos, Carrie Nelson, Tan Pham, Chelsea

Phillips, Patti Reed-Zweiger, Raymond Reyes, Tim Short, Tom Smith, Janis M. Wignall, and Shirley Williamson.

- Kathleen Cole, assistant and student reviewer extraordinaire, and Giuseppe Morella.
- Our editor Sande Johnson.
- Our production team, especially Mary Carnis, Brian Hyland, Marianne Frasco, Steve Hartner, and Gay Pauley.
- The folks in our marketing department, especially Jeff McIlroy and Frank Mortimer, Jr.
- Jackie Fitzgerald, Beth Bollinger, Jennifer Collins, Amy Diehl, Byron Smith, Julie Wheeler, and Robin Diamond.
- The Prentice Hall representatives and the management team led by Gary June.
- Our families and friends.
- Cynthia Nordberg, interviewer for Real World Perspectives
- Judy Block, who contributed both editing suggestions and study skills text.

Finally, for their ideas, opinions, and stories, we would like to thank all of the students and professors with whom we work. We appreciate that, through reading this book, you give us the opportunity to learn and discover with you.

About the Authors

Janet R. Katz has practiced in cardiac rehabilitation, as well as acute and critical cardiac care. She is an instructor for Washington State University's College of Nursing and an adjunct instructor at Gonzaga University. Janet is the author of articles on nursing and medicine and the books *Majoring in Nursing* and *Keys to Science Success*. She is a contributor to the *Keys to Success in College Reader* on scientific research and health sciences careers. She is active in advancing the profession of nursing and its mission of disease prevention, health promotion, and health care advocacy for individuals, families, and communities, both locally and globally. After several careers that include a family planning counselor in central Massachusetts, research assistant at the University of Washington in Seattle, horseshoer in Palouse, Washington, and stage technician at Washington State University, she became a registered nurse. She lives in Spokane, Washington, with her husband, who teaches biology, and their two dogs.

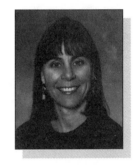

Carol Carter is Vice President and Director of Student Programs and Faculty Development at Prentice Hall. She has written *Majoring in the Rest of Your Life: College and Career Secrets for Students* and *Majoring in High School*. She has also co-authored *Graduating Into the Nineties, The Career Tool Kit, Keys to Career Success, Keys to Effective Learning*, and the first edition of *Keys to Success*. In 1992 Carol and other business people co-founded a nonprofit organization called LifeSkills, Inc., to help high school students explore their goals, their career options, and the real world through part-time employment and internships. LifeSkills is now part of the Tucson Unified School District and is featured in seventeen high schools in Tucson, Arizona.

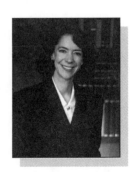

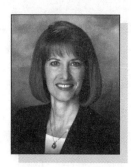

Joyce Bishop holds a Ph.D. in psychology and has taught for more than twenty years, receiving a number of honors, including Teacher of the Year. For the past four years she has been voted "favorite teacher" by the student body and Honor Society at Golden West College, Huntington Beach, California, where she has taught since 1986 and is a tenured professor. She is currently working with a federal grant to establish Learning Communities and Workplace Learning in her district, and has developed workshops and trained faculty in cooperative learning, active learning, multiple intelligences, workplace relevancy, learning styles, authentic assessment, team building, and the development of learning communities. She also co-authored *Keys to Effective Learning*.

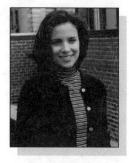

Sarah Lyman Kravits comes from a family of educators and has long cultivated an interest in educational development. She co-authored *The Career Tool Kit*, *Keys to Study Skills*, and the first edition of *Keys to Success* and has served as Program Director for LifeSkills, Inc., a nonprofit organization that aims to further the career and personal development of high school students. In that capacity she helped to formulate both curricular and organizational elements of the program, working closely with instructors, as well as members of the business community. She has also given faculty workshops in critical thinking, based on the Thinktrix critical thinking system. Sarah holds a B.A. in English and drama from the University of Virginia, where she was a Jefferson Scholar, and an M.F.A. from Catholic University.

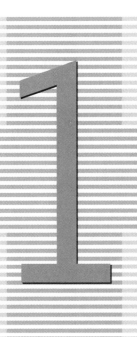

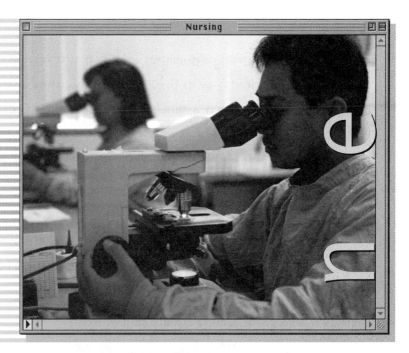

Nursing

Researching Your Nursing Education

Collecting the Basic Data

Welcome—or welcome back—to an education in nursing. Whether you are right out of high school, returning to student life after working for some years, or continuing on a current educational path, you are facing new challenges and changes. Every person has a right to seek the self-improvement, knowledge, and opportunity that an education can provide. By choosing to pursue nursing, you have given yourself a strong vote of confidence and the chance to improve your future.

This book will help you fulfill your potential as a nursing major by giving you keys—ideas, strategies, and skills—that can lead to success in school, on the job, and in life. Chapter 1 will give you an overview of the nursing education world. It will start by looking at today's nursing students—who they are and how they've changed—and at the connection between a nursing education and success. You will also discover in this chapter how various resources can help you deal with issues and problems and how teamwork plays a role in your success.

In this chapter, you will explore answers to the following questions:

- A BSN or an ADN?

- Why do you need to study a variety of arts and sciences?

- Who is pursuing nursing education today?

- How do science knowledge and skills promote success?

- Can graduate school help?

- What resources are available at your school?

- What barriers do men and minorities face in nursing?

- What is your role in a diverse world?

 ## A BSN OR AN ADN? THE DIFFERENCE BETWEEN A 2-YEAR AND A 4-YEAR DEGREE

You may take either of two routes to become a registered nurse. You may earn an associate's degree in nursing (ADN) in two years through a community college, or a bachelor's degree in nursing (BSN) in four years through a college or university. A few hospitals in some areas of the country still have three-year nursing diploma programs, a third option to becoming an RN.

The advantage to an ADN is that it takes less time to obtain, allowing you to join the work force sooner. Community colleges are also located in more areas than colleges and universities and they often cost less. An excellent cardiac nurse, Judy Meyers, said, "If it wasn't for community college I may have never become a nurse." Judy lived in a small town that was too far away from a university, but had a community college. Eventually, Judy moved, earned her bachelor's degree in nursing, then a master's degree, and just this last year, a Ph.D.

An ADN degree is an option if access and cost are issues, or if you need to get through school quickly in order to begin working right away. If this is the case, you should plan on returning to school at a later date to get your BSN. Many schools offer distance learning programs for RNs working toward a bachelor's degree. Some use video-taped courses, others teleconferencing and Web based programs. Or you may get a combination of all three.

The BSN degree is the preferred nursing degree. It is recommended by nursing professional organizations such as the National League for Nursing, The American Associations of Colleges of Nursing, and the American Nurses

Association. The importance of a four-year college education should become clearer to you as you read this book. In everyday practice, nurses need excellent communication skills, cultural understanding and experiences, in-depth knowledge of science and inquiry learning, as well as a combination of sociology, psychology, and philosophy. You will not learn everything needed to be an RN with the most employment opportunities in a two-year program. The better rounded your college education is, the more prepared you will be to meet the extraordinary challenges of a nursing career.

Another advantage to a BSN degree is that you are more competitive when it comes to finding a job. Most employers will choose a BSN over an ADN. And it is not uncommon to hear nursing experts propose graduate degrees in nursing as the most competitive degree in the marketplace. In order to go to graduate school you need a bachelor's degree.

If you have a choice, choose a bachelor's degree in nursing. If you don't, plan on earning it after you work as an ADN RN.

 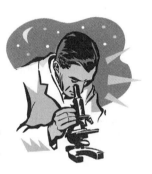

WHY DO YOU NEED TO STUDY A VARIETY OF ARTS AND SCIENCES?

You probably already know the reasons why a good science background is important: To keep up with rapid advances that affect daily life. With newspaper headlines announcing: "Scientists urge more prudent use of antibiotics" and magazine articles discussing robotics, DNA, and the "geometry lesson of the marching ants," it takes only basic observation to see that life is rapidly changing due to advances in science and technology. If you are 18 years old and just beginning college, think back ten years. What kind of computer did you have? What kind of treatments were available for HIV? If you are older and returning to school, the contrast is much more vivid. Do you remember a time when you didn't own a VCR? Did you have e-mail? Had you even heard of e-mail? Do you remember a time when no one talked about greenhouse gases or global warming? And almost everyone can remember a time when complex genetic engineering and cloning were not occurring.

Examples of how technology and science affects our lives abound, and it is for this reason that a knowledge of science and math is needed. You need this knowledge even if you do not pursue a nursing career; you need it to be an active citizen and a responsible family member. For instance, you must be able to understand the implications, both ethical and practical, of genetic testing and therapy, the spread of viruses, and of disappearing wetlands, rain forests, and other natural habitats. Can you understand the research presented in the articles you read? Can you discern fact from fiction, reality from sensationalism? If you read about a new study on exercise, engines, or equilibrium, can you put it to use?

All of us are called on to make political, social, and personal decisions regarding everything from healthcare to finances, from international foreign aid to environmental protection, and from genetically engineered tomatoes to gene therapy for a host of diseases. The decision to major in nursing is a good one and one that will be useful to you in many ways. Science and math knowledge and skills teach you critical thinking, creativity, teamwork, and all around good work habits; each one is essential to any kind of career you pursue.

Studying the humanities and arts gives you the needed knowledge to think in different ways and to understand new perspectives. For instance, think about studying art. Learning about the evolution of painting from Romantic Realism to Impressionism can help you understand how social changes affect human thinking and actions. If this seems far removed from nursing, consider health practices. In the past, people relied completely on physicians to tell them what to do. With today's technology and increased access to information people are assuming responsibility for their health. It is common now for people to work with their care providers to come to solutions rather than accepting what someone else tells them.

Technological and social changes affect human behavior and the health care system is evolving to meet these needs. People want more preventative care and disease prevention which is exactly what nurses provide. Nursing is the study of human beings and their response to health and illness. That response is based on many things, such as, culture, social learning, politics, and history. The more you learn in college the better prepared you'll be to work with all kinds of people.

> "A journey of a thousand miles must begin with a single step."
>
> LAO-TZU

A major purpose of going to college is to broaden your worldview by taking time to study subjects not specifically related to a major or career goal. The purpose of this book is to help you learn to succeed in nursing whether you remain in nursing your entire life or decide in your senior year to become an art major. And by the way, if this is the case, your science background will help you with painting (chemistry), sculpturing (physics and geometry), ceramics (chemistry and physics), and designing jewelry (metallurgy, physics, and anatomy). Remember, your goals may change as you go through college, but what you learn in the physical and life sciences, math, and humanities will help no matter what you decide.

WHO IS PURSUING NURSING EDUCATION TODAY?

In the late 1800s Florence Nightingale founded formal nursing education. Nightingale's work in the Crimea War greatly affected her views of health care and nursing. After making many reforms in how injured and sick British soldiers were treated, she set out to make major reforms in hospitals and nursing education. At that time, there were no formal training courses for nurses. So, along with reforms in the military system, Nightingale changed hospitals, instituted mandatory hand washing, and developed the first training of professional nurses.

In the United States, the first nursing school associated with a university was opened in 1909 at the University of Minnesota. However, most nursing education was based in hospitals, rather than universities, until the end of World War II. A severe nursing shortage along with the evolution of community colleges motivated the advent of two-year ADN programs where nurses could be quickly produced. Even at this time, nursing professionals debated the education needed to become an RN. Many believed, as they do today, that a 4-year BSN degree should be the minimum requirement for RN licensure, and were opposed to the ADN degree.

The Diverse Student Body

To give you an idea of who is going into nursing today, look at these interesting facts from the American Association of Colleges of Nursing:[1]

- Nursing students comprise more than half of all health professions' students.
- In 1980, 55 percent of registered nurses held a hospital diploma as their highest educational credential, 22 percent held the bachelor's degree, and 18 percent an associate degree.
- In 1996, a diploma was the highest educational credential for only 27 percent of RNs, while the number with bachelor's degrees had climbed to 31 percent, with 32 percent holding an associate degree.
- The number of diploma programs has declined to less than 10 percent of all RN education programs.
- In 1998, enrollment of RNs returning to school full-time to pursue the BSN degree was more than 7 percent above the previous year.
- The National Advisory Council on Nurse Education and Practice urges that at least two-thirds of nurses hold baccalaureate or higher degrees in nursing by 2010. Currently, only about 40 percent do.
- A 1995 report by the Pew Health Professions Commission recommended the closing of up to 20 percent of the nation's associate-degree and hospital-diploma nursing programs.
- Nursing schools estimate that an average of 77 percent of new BSN graduates had jobs waiting upon graduation between August 1997 and July 1998, 93 percent of master's-degree nursing graduates had jobs waiting.
- Less than 10 percent of all RNs are under 30 years old. The average age of an RN is 45 years old.[2]
- 5 percent of RNs are men.
- 90 percent of RNs are Caucasian.
- 4.2 percent are African–American.
- 3.4 percent are Asian/Pacific Islander.
- About 2 percent are Latino.
- Less than 1 percent are Native American.
- Twenty-three percent of college students were science majors in 1995. Of these, 6.9 percent majored in the health sciences; 4.8 percent in biological and life sciences; and 1.6 percent in physical sciences and science technologies. The remaining 10 percent studied computer science, engineering science, or mathematics.[3]
- Significantly more women than men students earned bachelor's degrees in health sciences. On the other hand, substantially more male than female students earned degrees in computer science, engineering science, or technology.[4]

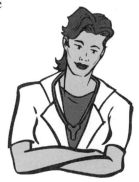

- Of the entire undergraduate population in the academic year 1995–96, 20 percent were supporting children. Among older students (entering as a freshman at the age of 20 or older), more than 40 percent were supporting children.[5]
- Almost 80 percent of undergraduates were employed at some time during their enrollment in the academic year 1995–96. Of students who worked, 26 percent worked full-time; 19 percent also attended school full-time.[6]
- Students are taking longer to get a degree. Of students graduating in 1995, 64.5 percent took more than four years to complete their degrees, and 25.6 percent took more than six years.[7]

Diversity in Degrees

Statistics from the National Center for Educational statistics paint a dramatic picture of the health science student population.

- The Bachelor of Science degree in nursing is the critical first step for a career in professional nursing.[8]
- Graduates can begin practice with an associate degree or hospital diploma, but the BSN degree is essential for nurses to practice as case-managers or supervisors in all clinical settings.[9]
- The BSN nurse is the only basic nursing graduate prepared to practice in all health care settings: critical care, ambulatory care, public health, and mental health, and thus has the greatest employment flexibility.[10]
- Patient care is now more complex, which has created an excess supply of associate degree and hospital diploma prepared nurses.[11]

The decision to take advantage of a nursing education is in your hands. You are responsible for seeking out opportunities and weaving school into the fabric of your life. You may face some of these challenges:

- Handling the responsibilities and stress of parenting children alone, without a spouse
- Returning to school as an older student and feeling out of your element
- Learning to adjust to the cultural and communication differences in the diverse student population
- Having a physical disability that presents challenges
- Having a learning disability such as dyslexia or attention-deficit hyperactivity disorder (ADHD)
- Balancing a school schedule with part-time or even full-time work
- Handling the enormous financial commitment college requires

Your school can help you work through these and other problems if you actively seek out solutions and help from available support systems around you. Explore some reasons why the hard work is worthwhile.

Men in Nursing

Nursing is predominantly a female profession, but that is changing. About 5 percent of RNs are men, but enrollment in nursing schools by men is creating a change. In 1996, 12 to 13 percent of students in nursing schools were men, and that was a considerable increase from the preceding few years. Surveys of college males suggest that they would be more likely to choose nursing if they had more information.

One group working to support and promote men in nursing is the American Assembly for Men in Nursing. The purpose of this organization is "to provide a framework for nurses, as a group, to meet, to discuss and influence factors, which affect men as nurses."[12] The following historical perspective is adapted from their website: www.aamn.org.

The first nursing school in the world was started in India in about 250 B.C. when only men became nurses. During the Byzantine Empire, nursing was also practiced primarily by men. In every plague that swept Europe, men risked their lives to provide nursing care. In 300 A.D., a group of men called the Parabolani, started a hospital and provided nursing care during the Black Plague epidemic. St. Alexis was a fifth century nurse and in the 1300s the Alexian Brothers were organized to provide nursing care for the victims of the Black Death.

Military, religious, and lay orders of men continued to provide nursing care throughout the Middle Ages. Some of the most famous of these were the Knights Hospitalers, the Teutonic Knights, the Tertiaries, the Knights of St. Lazarus, the Order of the Holy Spirit, and the Hospital Brothers of St. Anthony. St. John of God and St. Camillus de Lellis both started out as soldiers, and later turned to nursing. St. Camillus started the sign of the red cross which is still used today.

In the United States in 1783, James Derham, a black slave, worked as a nurse in New Orleans and saved the money to purchase his freedom. He later studied medicine and became a respected physician in Philadelphia (Benjamin Quarles, *The Negro in the Making of America*, 1987, p. 85). In 1808, Lazaro Orranti and Martin Ortega were two men employed as nurses at a hospital in San Antonio, Texas. The hospital employed only men as nurses. Prior to the Civil War, both male and female slaves were identified as "nurses." Victoria Clayton describes "Old Joe" who was "my husband's nurse in infancy" being entrusted with the care of the plantation, while the white men of the plantation were fighting in the Civil War. During the Civil War, both sides had military men serving as nurses. The Confederate Army designated thirty men per regiment to care for the wounded. The Union also had men in the military serving as nurses. Men, including Walt Whitman, served as volunteers.

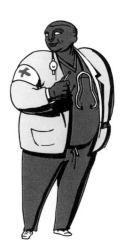

In 1901 the Army Nurse Corps were formed and only women could serve as nurses. The U.S. military nursing changed from being predominately male to being exclusively female. It was not until after the Korean War that men again served as nurses in the military.

Once men were again permitted into military nursing, the numbers also increased in civilian nursing. Nursing schools, which had denied admission to men, began to admit them. Gradually the numbers of men in nursing increased from less than 1 percent in 1966 to the 1996 figure of 5 percent.[13]

HOW DOES NURSING EDUCATION PROMOTE SUCCESS?

Nurses make up the majority of the nation's health care workers with 2.5 million registered nurses, yet misinformation from news stories, television, and other media continues to confuse the public with inaccurate images of nurses. As you plan an education in nursing, consider the following facts from the AACN:[14]

- The U.S. Bureau of Labor Statistics projects that employment for registered nurses will grow faster than the average for all occupations through 2008.

- Though often working collaboratively, nursing does not "assist" medicine or other fields.

- Nursing operates independent of, not auxiliary to, medicine and other disciplines.

- There are more than four times as many RNs in the United States as physicians.

- Nursing delivers all health care services, including primary and preventive care by advanced, independent nurse practitioners, in such clinical areas as pediatrics, family health, women's health, and gerontological care.

- Most health care services involve some form of care by nurses. Although 60 percent of all employed RNs work in hospitals, many are employed in a wide range of other settings, including private practices, public health agencies, primary care clinics, home health care, outpatient surgical centers, health maintenance organizations, nursing-school-operated nursing centers, insurance and managed care companies, nursing homes, schools, mental health agencies, hospices, the military, and industry.

- Nurses can be certified nurse–midwives and nurse–anesthetists, as well as, in cardiac, oncology, neonatal, neurological, obstetric/gynecological nursing, and other advanced clinical specialties.

Supporting the trend of a disastrous nursing shortage, the AACN projects the following statistics:

- If current trends continue, rising demand will outstrip the supply of RNs, beginning approximately 2010.

- By 2015, 114,000 jobs for full-time-equivalent RNs are expected to go unfilled nationwide, according to the Division of Nursing of the U.S. Department of Health and Human Services.

Other interesting information on nursing includes employment and salary data from the BLS:[15]

- In 1998, the average annual wage of workers in the most common health care occupations ranged from $18,970 for pharmacy technicians and aides to $102,020 for nurses, pharmacists, and doctors.
- Registered nurses averaged $42,071 per year.

And finally, the 1998–99 *Occupational Outlook Handbook* makes these significant points about registered nursing careers:

- It is the largest health care occupation, with over 1.9 million jobs.
- It is one of the five occupations projected to have the largest numbers of new jobs.
- Earnings are above average, particularly for advanced practice nurses who have additional education or training.

Education improves your quality of life and expands your self-concept. Income and employment get a boost from education. *The Digest of Education Statistics 1996* reports that income levels rise as educational levels rise. Figure 1-1 shows average income levels for different levels of educational attainment. Figure 1-2, also from a report in the *Digest*, shows how unemployment rates decrease as educational levels rise.

"Understanding is joyous."
CARL SAGAN

As you rise to the challenges of education, you will discover that your capacity for knowledge and personal growth is greater than you imagined. As your abilities grow, so do opportunities to learn and do more in class, on the job, and in your community.

All education increases your possibilities. Education gives you a *base of choices* and *increased power,* as shown in Figure 1-3. First, through different

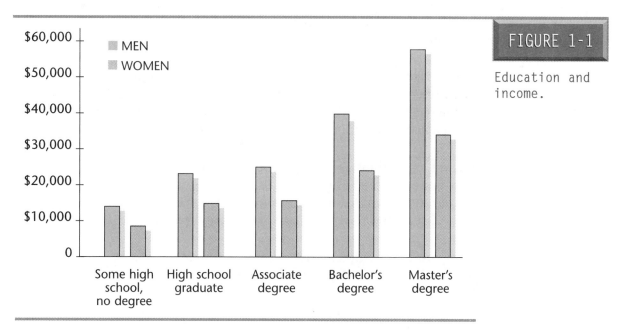

FIGURE 1-1

Education and income.

Source: U. S. Department of Commerce, Bureau of the Census, *Current Population Reports,* Series P-60, *Monthly Income of Households, Families, and Persons in the United States: 1994.*

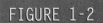

FIGURE 1-2

Education and employment.

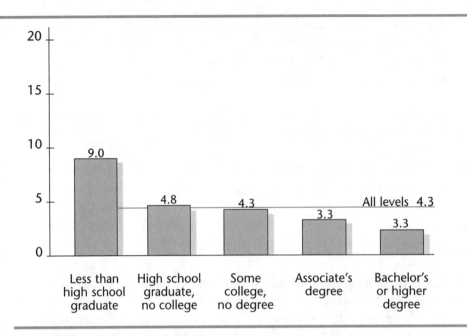

Source: U. S. Department of Commerce, Bureau of the Census, *Current Population Reports,* Series P-60, *Monthly Income of Households, Families, and Persons in the United States: 1994.*

courses of study, it introduces you to *more choices* of career and life goals. Second, through the different types of training you receive, it gives you *more power* to achieve the goals you choose. For example, while taking a writing class, you may learn about careers in journalism. This experience may lead you to take a class in journalistic writing that teaches you about science reporting. Down the road, you may decide to work on a newspaper as a science writer and to make science journalism your career. Looking back, you realize that two classes you took in college changed the course of your life.

A good science education improves your employability and earning potential. Learning additional skills raises your competency so you can fulfill the requirements of higher-level jobs. In addition, having a college degree in science makes an impression on potential employers.

Science education also makes you a well-rounded person as it widens your understanding about what is possible in the world. Science increases your awareness and appreciation of areas that affect and enrich human lives, such as music, art, literature, politics, and economics.

Your education affects both community involvement and personal health. Education helps to prepare individuals for community activism by helping them understand political, economic, and social conditions. Education also increases knowledge about health behaviors and preventive care. The more education you have, the more likely you are to practice healthy habits in your daily life and to make informed decisions.

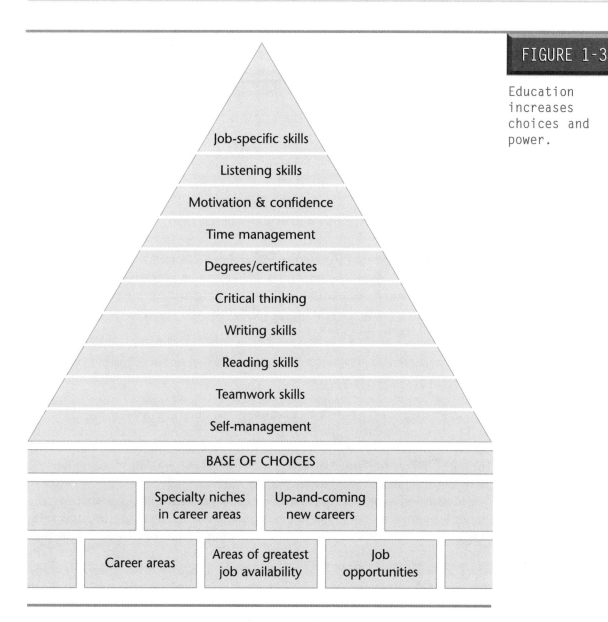

FIGURE 1-3

Education increases choices and power.

A science education is more than the process of going to school and earning a degree or certificate. It is a choice to improve your mind and your skills. Any program in science, no matter the length or the focus, is an opportunity to set and strive for goals. If you make the most of your mind, your time, and your educational opportunities, you will realize your potential. Using available resources is part of that process.

 ## CAN GRADUATE SCHOOL HELP?

The health system's increasing demand for front-line primary care, and the accelerating drive toward managed care, prevention, and cost-efficiency, are driving the nation's need for nurse practitioners, certified nurse–midwives, and other RNs with advanced practice skills.

Advanced Practice Nursing

The RN Population Study by the AACN says this about advanced practice nurses (those with master's degrees in a clinical specialty):

- Nurse practitioners and midwives average $55,014[16] per year.
- Clinical nurse specialists earned $52,532 per year in 1997.[17]
- The highest paying specialty area, nurse anesthetists earned an average salary of $86,319.[18]
- Mounting studies show that the quality of care by nurse practitioners and midwives is equal to, and at times better than, comparable services by physicians.[19]
- At the University of Rochester, researchers reported that intensive-care babies cared for by neonatal nurse practitioners averaged 2.4 fewer hospital days and more than $3,400 less in charges than those cared for by medical residents, despite the fact that the NPs' infants were younger and had significantly lower birthweight.[20]

What Do They Do?

Nurse Practitioners. Nurse Practitioners conduct physical exams; diagnose and treat common acute illnesses and injuries; provide immunizations; manage high blood pressure, diabetes, and other chronic problems; order and interpret X-rays and other lab tests; and counsel patients on adopting healthy lifestyles and health care options.

In addition to practicing in clinics and hospitals in metropolitan areas, the nation's estimated 71,000 nurse practitioners also deliver care in rural sites, inner cities, and other locations not adequately served by physicians, including other populations, such as children in schools and the elderly. Many NPs work in pediatrics, family health, women's health, and other specialties, and some have private practices. Nurse practitioners can prescribe medications in all states and the District of Columbia, while 18 states have given NPs authority to practice independently without physician collaboration or supervision.

Clinical Nurse Specialists. Clinical Nurse Specialists (CNSs) provide care in a range of specialty areas, such as cardiac, oncology, neonatal, and obstetric/gynecological nursing, as well as, pediatrics, neurological nursing, and psychiatric/mental health. Working in hospitals and other clinical sites, CNSs provide acute care and mental health services, develop quality assurance procedures, and serve as educators and consultants. An estimated 54,000 clinical nurse specialists are currently in practice nationwide.

Certified Nurse–Midwives. The nation's approximately 6,500 certified nurse–midwives (CNMs) provide prenatal and gynecological care to normal healthy women; deliver babies in hospitals, private homes, and birthing centers; and continue with follow-up postpartum care. In 1996, CNM deliveries accounted for 6.5 percent of all births in the U.S., up from 3.6 percent in 1989, according to the National Center for Health Statistics.[21]

Certified Registered Nurse Anesthetists. More than 30,000 certified registered nurse anesthetists (CRNAs) administer more than 65 percent of all anesthetics given to patients each year, and are the sole anesthesia providers in approximately one-third of U.S. hospitals, according to the American Association of Nurse Anesthetists (AANA). Of the 24 million anesthetics given annually, about 20 percent are administered by CRNAs practicing independently and 50 percent by CRNAs in collaboration with physician anesthesiologists, says AANA.[22] Working in the oldest of the advanced nursing specialties, CRNAs administer anesthesia for all types of surgery in settings ranging from operating rooms and dental offices to outpatient surgical centers.

WHAT RESOURCES ARE AVAILABLE AT YOUR SCHOOL?

Resources help you make the most of your education. As a student, you are investing money and time. Whether you complete your studies over the course of six months or sixty years, resources can help you get where you want to go.

Like any company that makes products or provides services, your school is a business. The goal of this particular business is the successful education of all who come through its doors. Table 1-1 offers a general summary of resources, most or all of which can be found at your school. Most schools offer a student orientation, near the beginning of your first semester, that will explain resources and other important information. Even if your school does not, you can orient yourself. The following sections will describe helpful resources—people, student services, organizations, and course catalogs and student handbooks.

People

Your school has an array of people who can help you make the most of your educational experience: instructors, administrative personnel, advisors and counselors, and teaching assistants. They're often busy with numerous responsibilities, but their assistance is provided as a standard part of your educational package. Take the opportunity to get to know them, and to let them get to know you. Together you can explore how they can help you achieve your goals.

Instructors are more than just sources of information during scheduled class time. Instructors can also become your mentors. Mentors are people who will help guide you as you develop yourself. Finding a mentor involves the following:

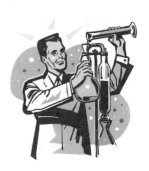

■ Get to know your instructors by working hard in labs and classes and by assisting in research projects. You can do this through work-study programs, teaching assistantships, or by volunteering. Read Bob Weinstein's book, *I'll Work for Free*, for other tips on finding such opportunities.

TABLE 1-1 How resources can help you.

RESOURCE	ACADEMIC ASSISTANCE	FINANCIAL ASSISTANCE	JOB/CAREER ASSISTANCE	PERSONAL ASSISTANCE
Instructors	Choosing classes, clarifying course material, help on assignments, dealing with study issues		Can tell you about their fields, may be a source of networking contacts	During office hours, are available to talk to you
Administrators	Academic problems, educational focus, problems with school services		Can be a source of valuable contacts	Can help you sort through personal problems with instructors or other school employees
Academic Advisors	Choosing, changing, or dropping courses; getting over academic hurdles; selecting/changing a major		Can advise you on what job opportunities may go along with your major or academic focus	
Personal Counselors	Can help when personal problems get in the way of academic success	Services may be free or offered on a "sliding scale" depending on what you can afford		Help with all kinds of personal problems
Financial Aid Office		Information and counseling on loans, grants, scholarships, financial planning, work-study programs	Information on job opportunities within your school environment (work-study program and others)	
Academic Centers	Help with what the center specializes in (reading, writing, math)		Perhaps an opportunity to work at the center	
Organizations and Clubs	If an academic club, can broaden your knowledge or experience in an area of study; can help you balance school with other enriching activities		Can help you develop skills, build knowledge, and make new contacts that may serve you in your working life	Depending on the club focus, can be an outlet for stress, a source of personal inspiration, a source of important friendships, an opportunity to help others
Fitness Center(s)		Usually free or low cost to enrolled students		Provides opportunity to build fitness and reduce stress; may have weight room, track, aerobic or dance classes, martial arts, team sports, exercise machines, etc.

(continued)

TABLE 1-1	*Continued.*

RESOURCE	ACADEMIC ASSISTANCE	FINANCIAL ASSISTANCE	JOB/CAREER ASSISTANCE	PERSONAL ASSISTANCE
Bulletin Boards	List academic events, class information, changes and additions to schedules, office hours, academic club meetings	List financial aid seminars, job opportunities, scholarship opportunities	List career forums, job sign-ups, and employment opportunities; offer a place for you to post a message if you are marketing a service	List support group meetings
Housing and Transportation Office		Can help find the most financially beneficial travel or housing plan		Can help commuters with parking, bus or train service, and permits; can help with finding on- or off-campus housing
Career Planning and Placement Office		Can help add to your income through job opportunities	Job listings, help with résumés and interviews, possible interview appointments, factual information about the workplace (job trends, salaries, etc.)	
Tutors	One-on-one help with academic subjects; assistance with specific assignments		If you decide to become a tutor, a chance to find out if teaching and working with people is for you	
Student Health Office		May provide low-cost or no-cost health care to enrolled students; may offer reduced-cost prescription plan		Wellness care (regular examinations), illness care, hospital and specialist referrals, and prescriptions
Adult Education Center	Academic help tailored to the returning adult student	May have specific financial-aid advice	May have job listings or other help with coordinating work and classes	May offer child-care assistance and opportunities to get to know other returning adults
Support Groups and Hotlines	If school-related, they offer a chance to hear how others have both stumbled and succeeded in school— and a chance to share your story			Personal help with whatever the hotline or support group specializes in; a chance to talk to someone whose job is to listen
School Publications	Academic news and course changes	News about financial aid opportunities or work-study programs	Job listings, information about the workplace and the job market	Articles and announcements about topics that may help you

- Get hands-on experience in healthcare. This is crucial to understanding what the field is all about. It may include volunteering in your community at a food bank, crisis clinic, or for hospice, doing library reference work for a professor, or helping at a local nursing organization. Whatever it takes, do this kind of work to get to know your instructors, practicing nurses, and your community's needs.

- Work hard to show that you have an interest. You can help clarify your interest in that field and at the same time develop a relationship with an expert.

The value of a mentor extends beyond finding someone to help guide you while you are in school. A mentor can help you with job and graduate school recommendations through connections they have around the country.

In this book the term "instructor" is used for simplicity's sake, but instructors have official titles that show their rank. From lowest to highest, these include lecturer, instructor, assistant professor, associate professor, and full professor (often just called professor).

Instructors have many time-draining responsibilities outside of teaching. However, you can gain access to your instructors while still respecting the demands on their time. Most instructors keep office hours, and they will tell you the location and times. You are responsible for seeking out your instructor during office hours. If your schedule makes this impossible, let your instructor know. Perhaps you and your instructor can get together at another time. Electronic mail (e-mail) systems allow you to communicate with your instructor using e-mail.

Teaching assistants are people who help an instructor with a course. You may or may not have teaching assistants in your courses. Often they are studying to be instructors themselves. Sometimes they teach the smaller discussion sections that accompany a large group lecture. They can be a great resource when your instructor is too swamped to talk to you.

Your school's *administrative personnel* have the responsibility of delivering to you—the student consumer—a first-rate product. That product is the sum total of your education, comprising facilities, instructors, materials, and courses. Schedule a meeting with your dean, the chair of a particular department, or other school administrator if you have an issue to discuss, such as a conflict with an instructor, an inability to get into a class you need, or a school regulation that causes a problem for you. Although administrators don't interact with students as often as instructors do, it is their business to know how the school is serving you.

Nursing advisors and counselors can help with both the educational and personal sides of being a student. They provide information, advice, referrals, and other sources of help. Generally, students are assigned academic advisors with whom they meet at least once a semester. Your academic advisor will help you find out about classes, choose a schedule, and help you apply to nursing school. Visit your academic advisor more than once a semester if you have questions or want to make changes.

Counselors, although not usually assigned, are available to you at any time, usually through student services. Don't hesitate to seek a counselor's help if you have something on your mind. The ups and downs of your personal life greatly influence the quality of your work in school. If you put some effort into working through personal problems, you will be more able to do your work well and hand it in on time. Occasionally, an illness or family difficulty may interfere with your schoolwork enough to call for special provisions for the completion of your classes. Most colleges are more than happy to assist you during challenging times.

Student Services

Your school has a variety of services aimed at helping students. Basic services offered by almost every school include the following:

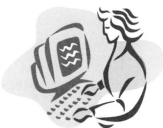

- academic advising and personal counseling
- student health/wellness
- career planning and placement
- tutoring

    Depending on your school, you may also find other services:

- child care
- housing and transportation
- adult education services (for adults returning to school)
- disabled student services
- various support groups
- school publications that help keep you informed of developments that affect you

    Often a school will have special services for specific populations. For example, at a school where most of the students commute, there may be a transportation office that helps students locate bus schedules and routes, find parking and sign up for permits, or track down car pools. Similarly, at a school where many students are parents, a child-care center may provide day care during class time and also refer students to outside babysitters. You will find additional details about school services in Table 1-1. They can help you earn the maximum benefit from your educational experience.

Organizations

No matter what your needs or interests are, your school probably has an organization that would interest you or can help you. Some organizations are sponsored by the school (academic clubs), some are independent but have a branch at the school (government ROTC programs), and some are student-run organizations (Latino Student Association). Some organizations focus on courses of study (Nursing Club), some are primarily social (fraternities and sororities), some are artistic (Chamber Orchestra), and some are geared toward a hobby or activity (Runner's Club). Some you join in order to help others (Big Brothers or Big Sisters), and some offer help to you (Overeaters Anonymous).

When you consider adding a new activity to your life, weigh the positive effects against the negative effects. Positive effects could be new friends, fun activities, help, a break from schoolwork, stress relief, improved academic performance, increased teamwork and leadership skills, aid to others, and experience that can broaden your horizons. On the negative side, there may be a heavy time commitment, dues, inconvenient location or meeting times, or too much responsibility. Explore any club carefully to see if it makes sense for you. As you make your decision, consider this: Studies have shown that students who join organizations tend to persist in their educational goals more than those who don't branch out.

To find out about organizations at your school, consult your student handbook, ask friends and instructors, or check the activities office or center if your school has one. Some schools, on registration days, have an area where organizations set up tables and make themselves available to talk to interested students. Some organizations seek you out based on your academic achievements. Find out as much as you can. Ask what is expected in terms of time, responsibility, and any necessary financial commitment. Talk to students who are currently involved. Perhaps give an organization a test run to see if you like it.

If you try out an organization, make a commitment that you will stay for the right reasons. Don't be afraid of being labeled a "dropout"; if something becomes more than you can handle, bow out gracefully. In the best of all possible worlds, your involvement in organizations will enrich your life, expand your network of acquaintances, boost your time management skills, and help you achieve goals.

Nursing Student Organizations

Depending on your school, there will be nursing student organization chapters on or off campus. The National Student Nurses Association may be contacted to find your local chapter. But, the simplest method for locating student nurse organizations is to contact your school's nursing advisor. The advisor will know of, or help you contact, other students involved in your local group. These groups will support you in finding and getting into a nursing program of your choice, provide information on all phases of being a student nurse, and, finally, be a great resource for finding jobs after you graduate. They also provide opportunities for experiences in leadership within your school.

The following is an excerpt from an article by Diane J. Mancino, the executive director of the NSNA, describing the benefits of the organization.[23]

> ...While much has changed since NSNA began 47 years ago, the NSNA remains the training ground, the "boot camp," of leadership development for the nursing profession. With 30,000 members in 1,200 nursing programs and 600 constituent chapters, NSNA has given many of the profession's current leaders a strong head start in their successful careers.
>
> In an effort to strengthen its commitment to leadership development, the 1998–99 NSNA Board of Directors established the NSNA

"Leadership U." Over the next three years, the NSNA Leadership U will:

■ provide a structure through which NSNA members may meet the learning objectives of leadership and management courses in nursing education programs

■ provide tools to validate the leadership and management competencies that students learn and practice through participation in NSNA's many programs and activities

■ offer a formal mentor-protégé program

■ track professional careers of NSNA leaders through the "Follow the Leader" longitudinal study

■ provide formal recognition through the presentation of NSNA Leadership U certificates upon graduation from nursing school.

To accelerate the transition of graduating NSNA members into active members of professional nursing organizations, NSNA recently published Recruiting New Graduates Into Professional Nursing Organizations.[*]

[*]"Recruiting New Graduates into Professional Nursing Organizations" is available at www.nsna.org. The publication is also available for $10 from: NSNA, 555 West 57th St., Suite 1327, New York, NY 10019 (212) 581-2211; FAX (212) 581-2368.

College Catalogs and Student Handbooks

Navigating through your school's course offerings, the departments and resource offices, and even the layout of the campus can seem overwhelming. There are two publications that can help you find your way—the college catalog and the student handbook. Most schools provide these materials as a standard part of their enrollment information.

The *college catalog* is your school's academic directory. It lists every department and course available at the school. Each course name will generally have two parts. Take "EN101" or "CHEM205," for example. The first part is one or more letters indicating department and subject matter, and the second part is a number indicating course level (lower numbers for introductory courses and higher numbers for more advanced ones). The catalog groups courses according to subject matter and lists them from the lowest-level courses up to the most advanced, indicating the number of credits earned for each class. See Figure 1-4 for a segment of an actual college catalog from Gonzaga University.[24] A course book released prior to each semester will indicate details such as the instructor, the days the course meets, the time of day, the location (building and room), and the maximum number of students who can take the course.

Your college catalog contains a wealth of other information. It may give general school policies such as admissions requirements, the registration process, and withdrawal procedures. It may list the departments to show the range of subjects you may study. It may outline instructional programs, detailing core requirements as well as requirements for various majors, degrees, and

| FIGURE 1-4 | Segment of Gonzaga University catalog. |

■NURSING – 73

The program for the Family Nurse Practitioner Post-Master's Certificate consists of 28 semester credits and provides both theoretical and clinical application components. In some instances, depending on the learner's background, additional credits may be encouraged or required. The goal of the program is to prepare practitioners to provide primary care to families; including adolescents, pregnant women, adults, and the aged; and to meet the health care needs of underserved populations in a wide variety or urban, rural, and frontier settings. Graduates are qualified to take the American Nurses Credentialing Center's and the American Academy of Nurse Practitioners' certification examinations for FNPs. National certification is a credential needed in many states to obtain advanced practice licensure.

Distinctive features of the Family Nurse Practitioner Post-Master's Certificate program are graduate level academic credits; integration of MSN/FNP and certificate FNP learners in most courses; emphasis on Jesuit inspired values of knowledge, sensitivity, integrity, excellence, and justice; pursuit of humanistic and ethical alternatives to solve contemporary nursing and health care problems; critical reasoning vital to professional judgement and ethical decision making; study of health care ethics from the perspectives of both an individual and an organization; on-campus and distance learning formats; course load and timeline adjusted to personal circumstances; and maximization of career mobility.

Admission

Application packets may be obtained from the Department of Nursing. In special circumstances, individuals applying for admission may be permitted to take courses for one semester while the admission process is completed. The designated fee must accompany the application form. Admission decisions are based upon the applicant's total profile and space available. Application deadlines are April 1 for summer or fall semester and November 15 for spring semester.

Each applicant must submit the following materials to the Graduate School:
(1) A completed application form (see appendix) and non-refundable fee;
(2) Typewritten statement (maximum 500 words) which describes the applicant's:
  (a) interest in the FNP Post-Master's Certificate program and what he/she hopes to gain from the certificate;
  (b) professional goals;
  (c) personal and professional strengths; and
  (d) professional experiences;
(3) Two letters of recommendation from individuals who can evaluate the applicant's leadership, interpersonal skills, critical thinking and judgement, and professional practice (e.g., employer, professional colleague, professor) sent directly to the Graduate School Dean using the confidential recommendation forms (see appendix);
(4) Current professional vita (format provided in application packet);
(5) Copy of current RN license; and
(6) Two official transcripts from each college or university attended for graduate study, including documentation of an earned master's degree with a major in nursing.

Prerequisites

A master's degree with a major in nursing from an accredited college or university is required.

Program Outline (28 credits)

Nurse Leadership Core - 6 credits
Nurs 500 Foundations for Advanced Practice	1 credit
Nurs 510P Leadership Foundations for Nurse Practitioners	2 credits
Phi 555 Leadership and Health Care Ethics	3 credits

Nursing Practice Core - 22 credits
Nurs 533 Cellular Pathophysiology/ Pharmacology	3 credits
Nurs 601P Advanced Nursing Practice I	5 credits
Nurs 602P Advanced Nursing Practice II	4 credits
Nurs 603P Advanced Nursing Practice III	4-5 credits
Nurs 604P Advanced Nursing Practice IV	4-6 credits
Nurs 614P Advanced Nursing Practice*	2 credits

*completed if Nurs 603P and Nurs 604P taken 4 credits each

Nursing Leadership Core

NURS 500 Foundations for Advanced Practice   1 credit
Analysis of the concept of leadership in advanced nursing practice including theories of leadership and identification of a personalized model for leadership in nursing. *Fall, Spring, Summer.*

NURS 501 Leadership in Clinical Nursing Practice   3 credits
Analysis of selected leadership theories and models applicable to nursing practice. Examination of nursing theories and other theories utilized in nursing practice, the domain of nursing, nursing care delivery models, and issues affecting nursing practice including ethical, legal, political, and economic considerations. Prerequisite: NURS 500 or concurrent. *Fall, Spring.*

NURS 502 Leadership in Nursing Education   3 credits
Examination of selected leadership theories and models applicable to nursing education. Analysis of learning and instructional theories, variables affecting learning and instruction, and curriculum design and development. Application of concepts in informal and formal teaching situations encountered in nursing practice with diverse target learners. Prerequisite: NURS 500 or concurrent. *Spring, Summer.*

NURS 503 Leadership in Nursing Management   3 credits
Examination of selected leadership theories and models applicable to nursing management. Analysis of organizational and management theories and concepts, health care policies, and systems with integration into nursing practice. Prerequisite: NURS 500 or concurrent. Summer, *Fall.*

NURS 504 Leadership in Nursing Consultation   3 credits
Analysis of selected leadership theories and models applicable to nursing consultation. Examination of consultation and change theories, interpersonal relationships, group dynamics, intra and interdisciplinary relationships, intra and interagency relationships, and principles of community assessment. Application of concepts to nursing practice. Prerequisite: NURS 500 or concurrent. *Fall, Spring.*

NURS 510P Leadership Foundations for Nurse Practitioners   2credits
Examination of selected leadership theories and models applicable to FNP practice. Analysis of selected nursing theories and other theories used in nursing practice, the domain of nursing, learning and instructional theories, organizational and management theories, consultation theories and models, group dynamics, community assessment strategies. Application of concepts to nursing practice. Prerequisite: Enrollment in Certificate program. *Fall, Spring, Summer (when demand).*

FIGURE 1-4   Continued.

74 – NURSING

NURS 505 Research Strategies in Nursing   3 credits
Study of the research process emphasizing designs, methodologies, principles of measurement, and strategies for data analysis appropriate in the investigation of nursing problems. Prerequisite: Foundational research course, statistics. *Spring, Summer.*

PHI 555 Leadership and Health Care Ethics   3 credits
This required ethics course is designed to consider health care issues from both an individual and organizational perspective.

Nursing Practice Core
Practitioner Option (PO)

NURS 533 Cellular Pathophysiology/Pharmacology 3credits
Examination of advanced physiological, pathophysiological, and pharmacological concepts, emphasizing cellular and biochemical processes. Stresses utilization of advanced concepts to understand pathophysiology of disease and rationale for pharmacological treatment and as basis for critical thinking and decision making. (Required in PO option). *Summer, Fall.*

NURS 601P Advanced Nursing Practice I   5 credits
Analysis of selected assessment and management strategies for common and acute health problems encountered in primary care settings. Emphasizes physiological processes of selected common and acute health problems across life span. Stresses laboratory and advanced physical assessment techniques as well as pharmacological and nonpharmacological intervention strategies. Application of concepts in primary care clinical practice (120 contact hours). Prerequisite: NURS 500, 501, 533, 504 or concurrent. Competency in health assessment*. *Fall, Spring.*
> * Competency may be established in 1 of 2 ways: successful completion of NURS 600 or by competency examination. NURS 600 does not fulfill elective requirement for PO option.

NURS 602P Advanced Nursing Practice II   4 credits
Analysis of health promotion assessment and management strategies for individuals and families throughout the life span. Analysis of theories salient to health promotion and health protection incorporating a developmental perspective. Assessment and intervention strategies for pharmacological and nonpharmacological management of well child, well adult, well older person, and pregnant and post partal woman in the context of family. Application of concepts in primary care clinical practice (120 contact hours). Prerequisite: NURS 601P, NURS 502 or concurrent. *Spring, Summer.*

NURS 603P Advanced Nursing Practice III   4-5 credits
Analysis of selected assessment and management strategies including pharmacological and nonpharmacological interventions for conditions affecting human structure, mobility, and perception. Application of concepts in primary care clinical practice (120-180 contact hours). Prerequisite: All 500-level courses and NURS 602P. *Summer, Fall.*

NURS 604P Advanced Nursing Practice IV   4-6 credits
Analysis of selected assessment and management strategies including pharmacological and nonpharmacological interventions for clients with chronic and complex disease. Examination of primary care practice management in various settings. Application of concepts in primary care clinical practice (120-240 contact hours). Prerequisite: NURS 603P. *Fall, Spring.*

NURS 614P Advanced Nursing Practice   2 credits
Application of primary care concepts in clinical practice in primary care (120 contact hours). Prerequisite: NURS 603P. Fall, Spring, Summer. (Taken if NURS 603P and NURS 604P taken for 4 credits each).

Individualized Option (IO)

NURS 601I Advanced Nursing Practice I   4 credits
Provides theoretical and experiential basis for practice of nursing in clinical specialty of choice. Application of concepts in clinical practice (45 contact hours). Prerequisite: NURS 500, 501 or concurrent. *Fall, Spring, Summer.*

NURS 602I Advanced Nursing Practice I   4 credits
Continuation of NURS 601I with incorporation of functional role development. Application of concepts in clinical practice (90 contact hours). Prerequisite: *NURS 601I. Fall, Spring, Summer.*

NURS 603I Advanced Nursing Practice III   5 credits
Continuation of NURS 602I with refinement and extension of functional role development. Application of concepts in clinical practice (135 contact hours). Prerequisite: All 500-level courses and NURS 602I. *Fall, Spring, Summer.*

NURS 604I Advanced Nursing Practice IV   6 credits
Synthesis and application of clinical specialty and functional role knowledge and skills in select area of practice. Application of concepts in clinical practice (180 contact hours). Prerequisite: NURS 603I. *Fall, Spring, Summer.*

Both Options

NURS 675 Research Proposal Seminar   1 credit
Development of thesis proposal. Credit is granted at completion of successful defense of proposal. Prerequisite: NURS 505 or concurrent. *Fall, Spring, Summer.*

NURS 676 Thesis   1 credit
Individual guidance in conduct of study and preparation of report. Credit is granted at completion and acceptance of final report of thesis. Prerequisite: NURS 505 and 675. *Fall, Spring, Summer.*

NURS 677 Thesis   1 credit
Individual guidance in conduct of study and preparation of report. Credit is granted at completion and acceptance of final report of thesis. Prerequisite: NURS 505 and 675. *Fall, Spring, Summer.*

Nursing Electives

NURS 523 Pathophysiology   2-3 credits
In-depth analysis of selected pathophysiological problems with emphasis on current research. Stresses application of knowledge to nursing problems.

NURS 525 Nutrition in Health and Disease   2-3 credits
Examines basis for rational decision making and recommendations about the role of nutrition in health and disease. Reviews biochemical properties and physiological function of nutrients. Analyzes specific claims for nutrients and food supplements. Explores basis for nutritional prescriptions as part of a therapeutic modality.

NURS 530 Dying with Dignity   2-3 credits
Emphasizes psychological, spiritual, and socio-cultural aspects of death and dying in various situations encountered by nurses. Considers variations across the age span and perspectives in caring for individuals, families, and groups. Stresses identification of own values, attitudes, and feelings regarding death and dying to prepare self to assist others.

NURS 533 Cellular Pathophysiology and
**   Pharmacology**   3 credits
Examination of advanced physiological, pathophysiological, and pharmacological concepts, emphasizing cellular and biochemical processes. Stresses utilization of advanced concepts to understand pathophysiology of disease and rationale for pharmacological treatment and as basis for critical thinking and decision making. (Required in PO option). Summer, Fall.

certificates. It may also list administrative personnel as well as faculty and staff for each department. The college catalog is an important resource in planning your academic career. When you have a question, consult the catalog first before you spend time and energy looking elsewhere.

Your *student handbook* describes important policies such as how to add or drop a class, what the grading system means, campus rules, drug and alcohol policies, what kinds of records your school keeps, safety tips, and more. Keep your student handbook where you can find it easily, in your study area at home or someplace safe at school. The information it gives you can save you a lot of trouble when you need to find out information about a resource or service. If you call for locations and hours before you visit a particular office, you'll avoid the frustration of dropping by when the office is closed.

Your student handbook also looks beyond specific courses to the big picture, helping you to navigate student life. In it you will find some or all of the following, and maybe more: information on available housing (for on-campus residents) and on parking and driving (for commuters); overviews of the support offices for students, such as academic advising, counseling, career planning and placement, student health, disabled student services, child care, financial aid, and individual centers for academic subject areas such as writing or math; descriptions of special-interest clubs; and details about library and computer services. It may also list hours, locations, phone numbers, and addresses for all offices, clubs, and organizations.

Making the most of your resources is one way to adjust to your new environment. Interacting with people around you is another.

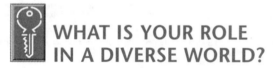

WHAT IS YOUR ROLE IN A DIVERSE WORLD?

It is not news that we are moving toward a global economy, nor that life is becoming increasingly complex. The turn of the century heralds predictions of vast change as we move from the industrial age of the past 200 years to the knowledge, or information, age. Science and technology have significantly contributed to these changes with advances in computers, communications, and transportation systems. What in the past affected only small regional groups of people, now affects us all. For example, war and civil unrest in the Sudan affects politics throughout the world. Japan's or Russia's economic problems cause fluctuations in the U. S. stock market.

Diversity Is Real in Nursing

What this means for you as a nursing student is that you will be a part of a global structure. As a nurse of any kind, you will not be working in a vacuum; you will have contact with a variety of people, even if you work in a small clinic miles from anyone or anything. You will still need to write grants, present your findings, and communicate to get supplies. Furthermore, the people you contact will not always be from the same culture as you. This is not a choice anymore, but a reality. Part of your education is learning about diversity and, more importantly, participating in it. You can accomplish this by

- Meeting and working with other students in your classes that are from different ethnic or cultural backgrounds than you are.
- Taking courses on multiculturalism.
- Traveling to other countries to study or to visit.
- Reading books, fiction and nonfiction, that describe the perspectives of people that have grown up in different circumstances than you.
- Watching foreign movies or those made by minority groups (e.g., *Smoke Signals*, 1998, is an award-wining movie produced, directed, written, and acted by American Indians).
- Keeping up with international news.
- Learning a foreign language.

Ethnocentrism

When groups of people believe that their way of thinking is the only way, or a better way than anyone else's, they are being ethnocentric. Ethnocentrism creates an opinion that one's particular group is better than anyone else's. It's important to be proud of your identity, but it's one thing to think your group is terrific and another thing to think that your group is superior to all other groups.

A group can be organized around any sort of uniqueness—the same skin color, accent, country of origin, ideas, interests, religion, traditions, and much more. The problem arises when celebrating your own uniqueness leads to putting down someone else's. One example is thinking that when someone speaks with an accent, he or she doesn't know as much as you do. Another example is thinking that it is disrespectful for someone not to look you in the eye during a conversation. In certain other cultures, it is considered rude to look people in the eye, especially if that person happens to be an authority.

Ethnocentrism has many negative effects. It can get in the way of effective communication, as you will see in more detail when you read Chapter 10. It can prevent you from getting to know people from different backgrounds. It can result in people being shut out and denied opportunities that all people deserve. It limits you and your potential because it denies you exposure to new ideas that could help you grow and learn. Finally, it can hinder your ability to work with others, which can cause problems for you both at school and on the job.

TERMS

Ethnocentrism
The condition of thinking that one's particular ethnic group is superior to others.

Diversity and Teamwork

Much of what nurses accomplish relies on teamwork. Think of the path of your accomplishments, and you will find that other people had roles in your success. When you earn a degree, complete a project, or raise a family, you don't do it alone. You are part of many hard-working teams. As the African proverb goes, it takes an entire village to raise a child.

Your success at school and at work depends on your ability to cooperate in a team setting. At school you will work with study groups, complete group projects, interact with instructors and administrators, and perhaps live with a

EIKO KAWAIDE

Senior, Elmira Nursing College, Elmira, New York

I started my nursing education in Tokyo, Japan, which is where I come from. For a short while, I worked in a hospital there, too. Although I liked the work, I realized that, though working one-on-one with patients can be very satisfying, I wanted to do more. There are many fields of study in the nursing profession, and I wasn't sure what to choose until I took a course in community health. From this class I discovered that I might be able to use my education to affect entire populations of people. One day I hope to help improve community health in a developing country.

I started learning English a few years ago in order to someday work as a community health nurse in the third world. Through studying English at an English school, I got a chance to go to the U.S. by winning a scholarship to Elmira College. I saw this as a great chance for me to both master English and deepen my knowledge of medicine and nursing. I was sure that studying in the U.S. would help me to achieve my life goals.

In this branch of nursing, I would be able to involve myself in many exciting issues. Maybe I could support public policy to better serve the

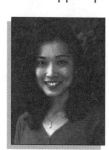

health care needs of third-world countries. One problem that needs addressing is how to plan and implement primary health care effectively. I am also interested in helping child survival in underprivileged countries and communities. I recently read a book about child survival. Just giving medicine or food doesn't help much, unless we focus on the context of poverty and underdevelopment. Many children are suffering from hunger and disease, and they are less resistant to disease because of lack of adequate nutrition. I

really want to deal with such kinds of problems and help to decrease infant and under-five mortality rates.

Global programs like WHO's "Health for All by the Year 2000" are very intriguing to me. I also think about the possibilities of improving connections between Japan and developing countries to help more people who are suffering from health problems. I know these are big dreams, but I've heard that nursing care is moving out of the hospitals and into the community—including the international community. What can I do to prepare myself for the future?

MARGRETTA MADDEN STYLES

Immediate Past President, International Council of Nurses, Geneva, Switzerland

Nurses have always played a very active role in public health, liberally applying their commitment and expertise throughout the world. Public health

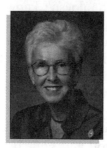

focuses on health promotion and prevention and involves all members of the community. Therefore, it offers the most for your investment.

Indeed, nursing has been moving out of hospitals for many decades, more so in some countries than in others. In many developing nations, where resources are scant, public health and community nursing has long been the primary mode of health care.

How can you best prepare for the future? There are four keys to developing a career in nursing, as well as other professions. *Education, education, education* is the number one factor. So you are headed in the right direction.

Mentors and linkages are the second and third keys. As an aspiring professional, you will need the support and advice of persons who are successful and well-recognized in your field. They will share with you the wisdom of their experiences and guide you toward the achievement of your own goals. Good mentors will also assist you in connecting with individuals, organizations, and other resources essential to the development of your career.

In order to achieve your goals relating to international public health, you should pursue linkages through three major sectors:

- **School to school linkages.** Inquire at your university about institutional relationships with schools in other nations. Is this a route available to you to hook up with nurses in their "sister" schools?

- **Health sector linkages.** Are your governmental health authorities able and willing to introduce you to nurses within your WHO region or with the WHO itself?

- **The world network of nurses associations.** This may be the best linkage of all. In this you are very fortunate. The Japanese Nurses Association is the largest in the world, with connections through the International Council of Nurses to counterparts, such as, the American Nurses Association, in 120 nations. The JNA is well-known for its assistance to and work with other nations. The president of JNA is a world leader in the profession.

Focused expertise is the fourth key to professional success. Define your specialty. What particular expertise do you want to develop and practice throughout your career? Focus! Then through education, mentors, and linkages make yourself one of the most informed, scholarly, and well-recognized authorities within your specialty. Be the best in your field.

You are well on your way. Just continue down the path you have chosen.

roommate. At work you will regularly team up with coworkers to achieve goals. At home you work with family or housemates to manage the tasks and responsibilities of daily life. Your achievements depend on how you communicate, share tasks, and develop a common vision.

Any team will gain strength from the diversity of its members. In fact, diversity is an asset in a team. Consider a five-person basketball team, composed of a center, a power forward, a small forward, a shooting guard, and a point guard. Each person has a different role and a different style of play, but only by combining their abilities can they achieve success. The more diverse the team members, the greater the chance that new ideas and solutions will find their way to the table, increasing the chances of solving any problem. As a member of any team, use these three strategies to maximize team success.

1. Open your mind and accept that different team members have valuable roles.
2. Consider the new information and ideas that others offer.
3. Evaluate contributions based on how they help solve the problem or achieve the goal instead of based on the identity of the person who had the idea. Successful teams use what works.
4. Reflect on your own views and realize they are just one way of seeing things. The way you communicate may be different from someone else's style. Yours in not right or wrong and neither is theirs.

Living Your Role

It's not always easy to open your mind to differences. However, doing so can benefit both you and others around you. You may consider actions like these as you define your role in the diverse world:

- To accept diversity as a fact of life. The world will only continue to diversify. The more you adapt to and appreciate this diversity, the more enriched your life will be. Diversity is an asset, not a deficiency.

"Nourish your-
self with
love of truth,
goodness,
righteousness,
with reverence
and admiration
for wisdom,
beauty, order,
wherever such
attributes are
made manifest."

FLORENCE
NIGHTINGALE,
1852

- To explore differences. Open your mind and learn about what is unfamiliar around you.

- To celebrate your own uniqueness as well as that of others. It's natural to think that your own way is the best way. Expand your horizons by considering your way as one good way and seeking out different and useful ways to which other people can introduce you.

- To consider new perspectives. The wide variety of ideas and perspectives brought by people from all different groups and situations creates a wealth of thought from which the world can find solutions to tough and complex problems.

- To continue to learn. Education is one of the most productive ways to combat discrimination and become more open-minded about differences. Classes such as sociology and ethics can increase your awareness of the lives, choices, and values of people in other cultures. Even though your personal beliefs may be challenged in the process, facing how you feel about others is a positive step toward harmony among people.

Throughout this book you will find references to a diverse mixture of people in different life circumstances. Chapter 10 will go into more detail about communicating across lines of difference and addressing the problems that arise when people have trouble accepting each other's differences. Diversity is not a subject that you study at one point in the semester and then leave behind. It is a theme that touches every chapter in this book and every part of your life. Note especially the "Real World Perspective" feature in some chapters, which often highlights people from different backgrounds who are striving to learn about themselves and their world.

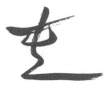

In Chinese writing, this character has two meanings: One is "chaos"; the other is "opportunity." The character communicates the belief that every challenging, chaotic, demanding situation in life also presents an opportunity. By responding to challenges in a positive and active way, you can discover the opportunity that lies within the chaos.

Let this concept reassure you as you begin college. You may feel that you are going through a time of chaos and change. Remember that no matter how difficult the obstacles, you have the ability to persevere. You can create opportunities for yourself to learn, grow, and improve.

Applications Chapter 1

KEY INTO YOUR LIFE
Opportunities to Apply What You Learn

 Internet Exercise

You will be using the Internet as you progress in school, and if you don't feel comfortable using it now, you will soon! This exercise is intended to introduce you to a few of the many Internet sites, including one on how to evaluate Internet resources.

Step 1. Get together with a group of two to four other students and go to the library or computer lab.

Step 2. Once you get on the Internet go to the following site:

http://www.hitiweb.mitretek.org/docs/criteria.html

Scroll down to "2. Quality Criteria for Evaluation of Health Information" and write down the information under criteria "C1 Credibility." Use these five criteria to evaluate a science or nursing Internet source.

Step 3. To find a science or nursing Internet source, use the link at the top of the page and go to "Agency for Health Care Policy Research."

Step 4. From here go to "Research Findings," and pick a topic.

Step 5. Using the criteria listed from the evaluation site (the criteria is for health information but may be used in other cases), apply it to the information you found. Is it credible? How do you know?

Step 6. Are there links to any other nursing or health websites of interest to you?

 *Skills Analysis, or
"I'll never forget the time . . ."*

One method for discovering what skills and important interests you have is by telling a story from your life. Start thinking of a time you did something that was fascinating, significant, or in any way particularly memorable. It doesn't have to be anything that seems connected to nursing. Begin with the statement: "I'll never forget the time I . . ." and fill in the rest. You can tell another person your story or write it down. Ask yourself the following questions:

- What was so important to you about this event?
- What underlying feelings and thoughts were associated with it?
- What skills, such as observation, reaction, communication, caution, or humor, did you use?

Write down the answers to these questions, and explore ways they might be connected to a health care field of study like nursing.

Career Analysis, or "My three top careers would be . . ."

This is another complete-the-sentence exercise to help loosen up your brain and get your thoughts going (often referred to as brainstorming).

1. List the name of one person you can think of in a nursing career. If you can't think of anyone, write down someone you think could help find such a person, for instance, a mentor, a parent, a reference librarian, or a teacher.

   _____

   _____

   _____

2. Find out how to contact this person either using a phone book or an Internet search. Many people in nursing work for universities, so you can find a way to contact them through the school's website, or if they are well known, use a search engine.

   _____

   _____

   _____

3. Call or e-mail the person, and set up an appointment to meet with them in person, or via e-mail, if that is more convenient for them.

4. Ask them the following questions and add some of your own:
   - What is the most interesting part of your work?
   - The least interesting?
   - If I wanted to pursue this area, what advice would you give?
   - What skills should I be working on in school?
   - How can I get more information?

KEY TO SELF-EXPRESSION
Discovery Through Journal Writing

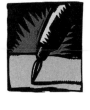

To record your thoughts, use a separate journal or the lined page at the end of the chapter.

Writing a journal requires a high level of reflection that goes way beyond a "Dear diary" approach. Reflection is an essential element of nursing and critical thinking. The ability to observe yourself and your thoughts and feelings is a valuable step toward learning to observe the world around you. Observation is one of the most important skills in nursing. Thinking about your thoughts, feelings, and the events that occur each day will assist you in developing an observant mind as well as sharpen your imagination and creativity, which is required to understand and work in nursing.

Start the journal process by writing a detailed description of your environment. You can go into the backyard, into the kitchen, or onto your front porch. Take as long as you need to do this exercise. Minimum: 10 minutes of continuous writing; maximum: several days, or weeks, if that helps you get all the details as precise as possible. (If you need help, consider the following question as a starting point: What do you see, smell, hear, feel?)

Journal

Name _____ Date _____

2

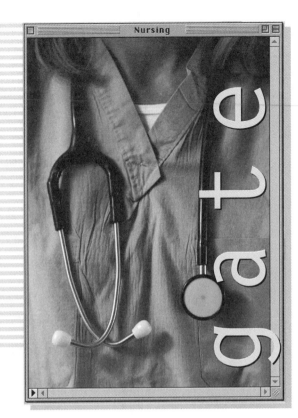

Discovering Nursing

Exploring Your Options

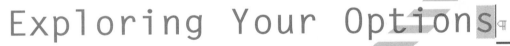

Countless opportunities are available in the profession of nursing. In this chapter you will learn what skills you already possess and what skills you need to develop to succeed in completing a nursing education. Different health science careers will be discussed so that you can compare them with nursing. Specific specialty areas within nursing will also be explored to see if one captures your interest. Remember, consider your values as well as your professional goals as you read this chapter. Many nurses integrate their values into their work, making a career in nursing meaningful beyond finding and maintaining a job. Mariah A. Taylor, RN, MSN, CPNP, and founder of the North Portland Nurse Practitioner Community Health Clinic in Oregon puts it like this:

I base my life on a single principle—love for humanity. My love and service stretches to include all segments of humanity—all colors, all creeds, all shapes and sizes, but especially humanity's children. I treat all children, from birth to 21 years, with the highest quality of care, compassion, and respect possible. I truly believe health care is a right, and not a privilege, especially for the underprivileged.[1]

In this chapter, you will explore answers to the following questions:

- Do you realize the opportunities?

- What skills do you already have to succeed in nursing?

- What skills do you need to develop to succeed in nursing?

- What are some of the practice areas and career options?

- How can you begin to choose a nursing or pre-nursing major?

 DO YOU REALIZE THE OPPORTUNITIES?

If you are choosing nursing as a career, be it as a first, second, or even third career, you need to be aware of the intense drive by nursing organizations and health care specialists to increase recruitment of younger people and minorities, including men, into nursing. While part of this is motivated by the critical need to increase diversity in nursing, another reason is the growing alarm over a nursing shortage.

Peter Buerhaus, director of the Harvard Nursing Research Institute, and others, have predicted significant shortages of RNs to begin in 2007.[2] Reasons for the shortage include:

> "Tell me to what you pay attention and I will tell you who you are."
>
> JOSE ORTEGA Y GASSETT

- An aging nursing population. The average age of today's working RN is 45. Less than 10 percent of nurses are under age 30. If fewer nurses come into the profession and as older nurses begin to retire, the shortage is expected to worsen, escalating to 2010.[3]

- Attempts to cut health care costs. Although health care has increased in complexity due to new technologies and treatments, the health care industry is cutting costs by replacing RNs with lower paid unlicensed technicians. The result? Many nurses, experiencing increased stress, are leaving the profession, or moving into less stressful work situations.[4]

- Declining enrollments in BSN programs. Again, the problem of attracting minorities and men into the profession adds to a decline in the numbers of students choosing to go into nursing. Traditionally, nurses have been women, but as career opportunities expand for women, fewer are going into nursing. Uncertainty over RN earnings and advancement opportunities also influence young student's career decisions. It is important to analyze your reasons for wanting to go into nursing. There are many misconceptions about what nurses do and how much money they make. Hopefully, this book will help you gain a realistic picture of nursing.[5]

■ The demand for nurses will be greater than the supply. It is projected that over the next 5 to 10 years the number of RNs leaving the job market will exceed those coming into it.[6]

Health care trends are requiring more RNs than ever. Changes in the US population, such as people living longer, is one reason. Longer life span means that more people will be living with chronic illnesses. Another reason more RNs will be needed is that people want to stay as active as possible and will need good case management to keep them vital and healthy as long as possible. And nurses are the experts on health promotion in the health care field.[7]

Over half of Americans believe that the quality of health care is affected by a shortage of nurses.[8] According to a recent Harris poll, people trust nurses and expect to be cared for by them. Nancy Dickenson-Hazard, RN, MSN, FAAN, Executive Officer of Sigma Theta Tau International said: "This poll reaffirms what we already know: that nurses are the critical difference in today's health care system and that they are well trusted by the general public. We feel it is crucial to promote nursing as a scientific profession with multiple career opportunities."[9]

Nursing holds many career options, which is a plus in terms of employment opportunity, scholarships and grants to attend school, and encouragement from nursing organizations. At the same time, as a professional nurse, you will be faced with many challenges and difficulties in trying to meet the needs of society. But, take heart, opportunities abound, options are abundant, and a life of meaningful work is within your grasp.

> "A 1993 Gallup survey indicated that 86 percent of Americans would be willing to have a nurse practitioner manage their care."
>
> AMERICAN NURSES ASSOCIATION

The Nursing Shortage

Talking Points From the American Nurses Association (July, 1999)[10]

QUESTION: *How do we know there is a nursing shortage?*

A FEW OF THE ANSWERS: Nursefinder, a temporary help agency with 119 offices in 36 states, has 8,000 nurses in hospitals, but cannot keep up with the demand (*The New York Times*, March 23, 1999).

Hospitals are taking measures to entice nurses: $500 or more as a bonus to employees who refer a new employee; $1,500 to $8,000 relocation allowances to a new employee; $500 to $5,000 sign-on bonuses (*Modern Healthcare*, Dec. 14, 1998).

Newsweek magazine is filled with advertisements for nurses. "Want to make an easy $4,000?" asks an ad for a hospital in Los Angeles, which offered a sign-on bonus to qualified RNs (*Sacramento Bee*, Jan. 17, 1998).

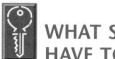

WHAT SKILLS DO YOU ALREADY HAVE TO SUCCEED IN NURSING?

Science and Humanities

If you love science and are good at it, you have it made. If you like, or love, science and are fair at it, you also have it made, although perhaps you will need to work harder. If you like, or love, science but have a hard time with it, or if it's been so long since you took a science class that you don't remember much about it anymore, don't give up. Two things will help you succeed: determination and a tutor. Determination is your job and a tutor is your school's. Free tutoring is available because almost all graduate students work in this role as part of their education and training.

Nancy Hoffman, nursing advisor at Washington State University, confided that when she decided to return to school as a science major after raising her two children, the thought of taking chemistry terrified her. All she could think of was how much she had hated high school chemistry. When she returned to school, the first class she took was biology. Her grade was a C. She said, "I thanked God every day for that C."

She knew that if she was to continue in school with any success, she would have to find a way to get through chemistry. She explained, "Chemistry was like traveling to a foreign land where the people spoke a foreign language. I couldn't understand any of it." So she went to her school's learning center and found a tutor who was a graduate student in chemistry. For the first two months of the semester, she met with him after every class to review the material. Her final grade in organic chemistry? An A.

Now she knew how to review on her own, or with other students, and received A's in all her science classes. She advises all students to visit their school's learning center to find out who, or what, can help them. She explained, "Don't let embarrassment keep you from asking for help."[11]

Interest in Health Care and People

Another thing you have going for you is that you want to do something that involves working with other people, or at the very least, you want to contribute in some way to the health and well being of someone somewhere. A

How to Find a Tutor

This book will help you become a better student, which will go a long way toward ensuring your success as a nursing major, but part of succeeding is knowing when to ask for help. Tutors are an excellent source of help with any class. Contact your school's Academic Office, adult education center, or ask your advisor, teaching assistant, or instructor to help you find one. The people at your school want to help you succeed in college, and they will likely bend over backward to assist you. It's possible they are sitting in their offices right now, waiting for you to come see them.

background in the liberal arts will help you achieve this. Whatever you read in literature courses, view or hear in art courses, and read and write about in sociology and psychology, will help you be a better nursing student. All these areas help you understand human nature in all its various forms. Your ability to talk to others is enhanced by your knowledge of different subjects and talking to others is a key to success in nursing. Communication is one of the most important skills to develop as you go on your way.

An interest in doing something that helps people is a very good start toward a career in nursing. It is also very likely that unless you have already worked in a health care setting with nurses or have family members who are nurses and who talk about their work, you do not have a realistic image of what nurses do. If your source about nurses is television or movies, you definitely have a confused image of nursing. Television shows, such as, ER and Chicago Hope, have some positive images of nurses, but fail to take into consideration the complexity and responsibility involved in being a nurse.

In one survey, college students gave seven reasons for wanting to become a nurse.[12] One reason was the desire to help and care for other people; to work with people who have illnesses. Other reasons included the many professional opportunities, job security, a love of science, and the perception that nursing has many personal benefits. All these reasons are good ones for wanting to become a nurse.

WHAT SKILLS DO YOU NEED TO DEVELOP TO SUCCEED IN NURSING?

To answer this question consider a survey of thousands of oncology (cancer) nurses. The nurses were asked to give three words that they thought most accurately described a good oncology nurse. The top five were caring, compassion, knowledge, dedication, and professional.[13]

Caring

What does caring mean to you? Caring is a term that is so strongly associated with nursing that it is usually the first thing people think or mention about being a nurse. Care is the heart and soul of nursing. Caring means taking the time for actively listening, advocating for those in need, valuing and respecting all individuals, being able to examine your own biases and reflect on your thoughts and actions, and it means such things as making pain relief a priority, and the healing process an act of body, mind, and spirit.

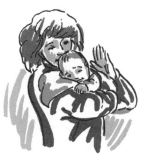

Compassion

Compassion is the ability to be considerate, humane, merciful, and kind. Consideration of another's needs despite your own beliefs, acting with respect and concern for another's well being, and the ability to assist others towards a full development of their potential in any given circumstance is what compassion is about.

Knowledge

Understanding the theories used in nursing, including scientific theories, those related to health behaviors, and especially nursing theories and diagnoses, is essential. Knowledge includes the ability to put theory and research into practice using the types of critical thinking and inquiry skills as discussed in Chapter 5.

Dedication

Commitment with diligence is essential in nursing practice. Sticking with a project, despite initial or repeated problems is especially important in research, in your studies, and in nursing practice. Attention to detail and careful analysis and execution of procedures can be developed in science classes and, later, in nursing school.

Professionalism

Professional behavior is developed through belonging to, supporting, and participating in nursing organizations. These organizations, such as, the American Nurses Association, work on many levels to promote nursing practice, health and welfare of the public, and health policy through social and political action. Professional actions include respect for others at all times, acting with integrity and for the best of your clients and fellow nursing colleagues.

Other important skills to develop include the following:

Advocacy

To advocate for yourself, another individual, or for a community means that you use your expertise as an RN to protect human rights. RNs may do this by helping others make informed decisions, by acting as a mediator between a client and a doctor, family members, or even the legal system. To advocate is to inform and support a person, provide desired information, and present information in a way that it can be understood. It also means understanding that someone may not want information. Advocacy means that an individual's or group's needs are your main concern. It requires you to be assertive, convey concern, understand different communication styles, and practice good working relationships.

Creativity

Many discoveries and solutions to problems come from creativity, or from a mind that can see things just a little bit differently from others. Having a broad education and experience in literature, philosophy, and politics will help you develop the ability to view problems in fresh new ways. Each field of study has its ways of viewing and understanding the world. The more of these you learn, the more flexible and adaptable you will be in your ability and skills as a nursing student and as a nurse.

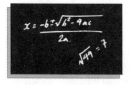

Mathematics

You've no doubt heard people freely admit that they have a problem with math, or a "math block." Have you ever heard anyone freely admit they can't read? Admission of this problem is perceived as shameful, yet saying the same of math is acceptable. What does this say of our view of math skills? The ability to use math is essential in nursing. Most schools of nursing require you to take a math test of medication calculations before you can proceed in your course work. You will also need statistics to learn about nursing research. Math skills are not optional in the information age of the 21st century.

Observation

Observation is a skill that many nurses would tell you is their greatest asset as a nurse. The ability to study people and nature, see patterns, and notice things that others may not notice, requires astute observational skills. All nursing endeavors demand the ability to see, hear, smell, and touch. Observation skills can be enhanced in many ways, such as, taking a plant identification course to learn how to identity plants and trees. Anatomy, microbiology, even art courses, allow you plenty of opportunity to practice observing attributes of things you may not have noticed before. Observation is a skill that is developed over time and one that is crucial to the assessment process: a huge part of being a nurse.

WHAT ARE SOME OF THE PRACTICE AREAS AND CAREER OPTIONS?

Nursing is divided into specialty areas based on either the setting of the practice or by the population served. Most of these areas overlap. For instance, you may want to be a pediatric nurse, which is one of the nursing specialty areas based on the population served—children. But, will the practice setting be in a hospital, in an outpatient clinic, in home health, or a clinic for homeless children? The areas described below are intended to give you an idea of the many options available in nursing. It does not by any means represent a comprehensive list. Suggestions for websites to visit to obtain more information are given at the end of the chapter.

Practice Setting

Nearly all health care services involve care by nurses and approximately 60 percent of that care occurs in hospitals. But the number of RNs working in other settings is increasing as changes in health care systems lean toward shorter hospital stays and more preventive health care. A sample of practice settings includes:

- Hospital
    - acute care or critical care
- Ambulatory Care
    - primary care clinics
    - family health clinics

- private practices
- other specialty clinics
- outpatient surgical centers
- Extended Stay Facility
  - nursing home
  - rehabilitation center
- Colleges and Universities
- Nursing Professional Organizations
- Research Science
- Government and Politics
- Computers
- Law

Populations and Services Provided

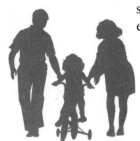

Nurses work with all kinds of people in all stages of development, and in all places around the world. The list below is categorized by developmental stages, but other population categories could include people at high risk for strokes, people with diabetes, hypertension, asthma, or those with heart disease. An example of some of the populations served by nurses include:

newborns	adolescents	men
infants	pediatrics	elders
children	families	geriatric
maternity	women	hospice

What Is the Overall Job Outlook?

Nursing is the largest health care occupation, with over 1.9 million jobs. It is one of five occupations that is expected to grow the fastest. According to the Bureau of Labor Statistics (BLS), the outlook is excellent! The following is the BLS opinion on the matter:[14]

Employment of registered nurses is expected to grow faster than the average for all occupations through the year 2006 and, because the occupation is large, many new jobs will result. As nursing school enrollments level off or decline, as they have on a cyclical basis in the past, the number of qualified applicants will fall, reducing reported competition for jobs. There will always be a need for traditional hospital nurses, but a large number of new nurses will be employed in home health, long-term, and ambulatory care.

Faster than average growth will be driven by technological advances in patient care, which permit a greater number of medical problems to be treated, and increasing emphasis on primary care. In addition, the number of older people, who are much more likely than younger people to need medical care, is projected to grow very rapidly. Many job openings also will result from the need to replace experienced nurses who leave the occupation, especially as the average age of the registered nurse population continues to rise.

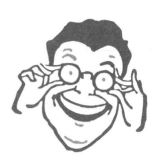

Employment in home health care is expected to grow the fastest. This is in response to a growing number of older persons with functional disabilities, consumer preference for care in the home, and technological advances that make it possible to bring increasingly complex treatments into the home. The type of care demanded will require nurses who are able to perform complex procedures.

Employment in nursing homes is expected to grow much faster-than-average due to increases in the number of people in their eighties and nineties, many of whom will require long-term care. In addition, the financial pressure on hospitals to release patients as soon as possible should produce more nursing home admissions. Growth in units to provide specialized long-term rehabilitation for stroke and head injury patients or to treat Alzheimer's victims will also increase employment.

An increasing proportion of sophisticated procedures, which once were performed only in hospitals, are being performed in physicians' offices and clinics, including HMOs, ambulatory surgical centers, and emergency medical centers. Accordingly, employment is expected to grow faster than average in these places as health care in general expands.

In evolving integrated health care networks, nurses may rotate among employment settings. Since jobs in traditional hospital nursing positions are no longer the only option, RNs will need to be flexible. Opportunities will be best for nurses with advanced education and training, such as, nurse practitioners.

Sources of Additional Information

The National League for Nursing (NLN) publishes a variety of nursing and nursing education materials, including a list of nursing programs and information on student financial aid. For a complete list of NLN publications, write for a career information brochure. Send your request to:

Communications Department, National League for Nursing, 350 Hudson St., New York, NY 10014. FAX: (212) 989-2272, or go to www.nln.org.

For a list of BSN. and graduate programs, write to:

American Association of Colleges of Nursing, 1 Dupont Circle NW, Suite 530, Washington, DC 20036. FAX: (202) 785-8320, or go to www.aacn.org.

Information on registered nurses is also available from:

American Nurses Association, 600 Maryland Ave. SW., Washington, DC 20024-2571, or go to www.nursingworld.org.

What Is the Earning Potential?

Earnings for nurses, according to the 1998–99 Occupational Outlook Handbook, are above average. According to the Bureau of Labor Statistics (1997) and the Health Resources Services Administration (1996), the average annual salary for an employed RN was $42,017. Nurse practitioners and midwifes earned an average of $54,182. College professors earned an average of $66,132 in 1998. Overall in 1996 (the most recent government statistics) the average salary of all working nurses across all settings was $42,071. The average CRNA (nurse anesthetist) earned $86,319 in 1996.

What Kind of Work Do Nurses Do?

This is a difficult question to answer as the work of nurses covers so many areas. But to summarize: nurses promote health, prevent disease, and help patients cope with illness. They act as advocates and health educators for patients, families, and communities, as well as, provide direct patient care by observing, assessing, and recording symptoms, reactions, and progress. RNs work with physicians and advanced practice nurses and manage client care through nursing care plans. The following sections are intended to give you an idea of a few areas within nursing, where it is practiced, what the roles are, and what educational preparation is involved.

What Is Hospital Nursing?

Hospital nurses form the largest group of nurses. Many are staff nurses, providing patient care management and bedside or direct nursing care. They also supervise licensed practical nurses, aides, and unlicensed assistive personnel. Hospital nurses usually choose one area such as surgery, maternity, pediatrics, emergency room, intensive care, or treatment of cancer patients, or they may rotate among departments.

The practice settings. *Hospital Departments and Units*

intensive care	air ambulance
step down or acute care	home health
outpatient	hospice
operating room	research
post operative recovery room	chemical dependency
labor and delivery	psychiatric
emergency	

The roles. Hospital nurses work as staff nurses on units or in departments, as managers and administrators, as educators for current and new staff, as computer specialists, and in quality management and infection control.

Educational preparation. Many new graduates of both ADN and BSN programs are hired by hospitals. Depending on the hospital size, specialty area, and where you want to work, your degree will matter. Most departments prefer to hire a BSN nurse because they will have the greatest ability to advance. Critical care and other specialty units like the emergency department may require several years experience in other nursing units. A master's degree in nursing (MSN) is required in most areas, such as, management, education, or case management.

What Is Ambulatory Care Nursing?

Ambulatory care nursing takes place in clinics or environments where patients come to be evaluated and treated.

The practice settings.

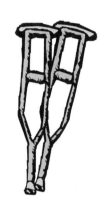

outpatient departments	nurse-managed centers
physician or nurse practitioner group practices	health maintenance organizations (HMOs)

The roles. The definition that best captures the work of ambulatory care nursing is one that defines the role, rather than the practice site. The American Academy of Ambulatory Care Nursing (AAACN) provides core values to define the practice. In summary these values include: shared responsibility of care among patients, families, and members of the health care team; providing education to help patients and families make informed decisions (remember the definition of advocacy mentioned earlier in this chapter); giving continuity of care; providing care that balances quality, patient needs, cost, and resource use.[15]

Educational preparation. Most nurses working in ambulatory care have many years experience in nursing. Many of these nurses also have less than a BSN degree which has become a concern of the AAACN. The expansion of the role requires increasing coordination and management in the health care network and community. Continuing education is an ongoing challenge. New graduates may be hired if they have school experience in ambulatory settings.

What Is Community Nursing?

Community nursing in the United States and other countries around the world has been the backbone of health care for millions of people. The World Health Organization called nurses "indispensable" contributors to world wide national health programs.[16] Changes in health care are influencing community nursing by increasing the need for more nurses who can assess entire populations (rather than just individual clients); determine areas of the greatest need for services; provide cost-effective care in teams; and evaluate future trends and practices that save money and maintain high quality. If that sounds like a big job—it is!

Public health nurses work in government and private agencies and clinics, schools, retirement communities, and other community settings. They focus on populations, working with individuals, groups, and families to improve the overall health of communities. They also work as partners with communities to plan and implement programs. Public health nurses instruct individuals, families, and other groups in health education, disease prevention, nutrition, and child care. They arrange for immunizations, blood pressure testing, and other health screening. These nurses also work with community leaders, teachers, parents, and physicians in community health education.

The practice settings. *Community and Public Health*

hospice	occupational health/industry
home health	nursing-school-operated nursing centers
mental health	insurance and managed care companies
rural health	health maintenance organizations
schools	the military

The roles. To understand the roles you must think about factors that influence community health. According to Carole A. Gutt (1997) they are the following: illiteracy, unemployment, poverty, homelessness, substance abuse, the return of infectious diseases, such as, tuberculosis, chronic illnesses, women's health, violence, teen pregnancy, sexually transmitted diseases, HIV/AIDS, and well child care.[17] Community health nurses cannot rectify these problems alone, but through their practice they can educate, enact policy reforms, and care for the public from birth to death.

Educational preparation. Many community health nurses think that education in politics must accompany nursing education. From the list of areas that influence community health nursing, it is easy to see why understanding health policy and politics is necessary. About 23 percent of community nurses have diplomas; 33 percent ADNs; 33 percent BSNs; about 10 percent MSNs; and less than 0.5 percent Ph.D.s.[18] As with ambulatory nursing and other types of nursing, an increase in the health care system's complexity and client needs means a demand for many more BSN nurses. The area of greatest growth in community and public health nursing is likely to be for community nurse specialists and other advanced practice nurses with MSN degrees.

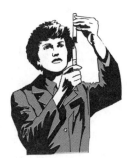

What Are Advanced Practice Nurses?

At the advanced level, nurse practitioners provide an example. Nurse practitioners (NPs) provide basic primary health care. They diagnose and treat common acute illnesses and injuries. Nurse practitioners can prescribe medications in most states. Other advanced practice nurses (ARNPs) include clinical nurse specialists (CNS), certified registered nurse anesthetists (CRNAs), and certified nurse–midwives (CNM).

The practice settings.

Primary Care Settings	Nursing Homes
■ physician offices	Schools
■ health maintenance organizations	Colleges
■ community and public health clinics	Industrial Settings
Hospitals: all units, including emergency and critical care	Home Health Agencies

The roles. Advanced practice nurses often work in a specialty area, such as, pediatrics, cardiology, or geriatrics, to name a few. Nurse practitioners perform many functions, including primary care interventions, health assessment, risk appraisal, health education and counseling, diagnosis and management of acute minor illnesses and injuries, and management of chronic conditions.

Another role for advanced practice nurses is as clinical nurse specialist (CNS). These nurses work with patients and families in addition to acting as consultants for other nursing staff. Many serve on university teaching faculty. CNS roles may include clinical research, teaching, consultation, leadership, and administration.

Along with nurse practitioners and clinical nurse specialists, there are nurse midwives and nurse anesthetists. See Figure 2-1 for more information on these types of nursing practice.

| FIGURE 2-1 | Specialty areas for advanced practice nurses, including what they do, where they do it, and who they work with. In light of the anticipated shortage of advanced practice nurses, obtaining your APN degree is a wise career path to consider. |

ADVANCED PRACTICE NURSES	APPLICATION OF ADVANCED KNOWLEDGE & SKILLS	PATIENT POPULATION SERVED	PRACTICE SETTINGS
Certified Nurse–Midwives	Well-women health care: management of pregnancy, childbirth, antepartum, and postpartum care, health promotion	Childbearing women	Homes, hospitals, birthing centers, ambulatory care
Clinical Nurse Practitioner (Specialist)	Management of complex patient health care problems in various clinical specialty areas through direct care, consultation, research, education, and administration	Individuals with physical or psychiatric illness and disability, maternal, and child heath problems	Hospitals, ambulatory care, community care, home health, rehabilitation
Nurse Anesthetist	Pre-operative assessment, administration of anesthesia, recovery	Individuals in all age groups undergoing surgical procedures	Hospital, operating rooms, ambulatory care, surgical settings
Nurse Practitioner	Management of a wide range of health problems through physical examination, diagnosis, treatment, and family/patient education and counseling; primary care and health promotion	Individuals and families women, infants, children, elderly, adults, and others	Primary care, long-term care, ambulatory and community care, hospitals

From the American Association of Colleges of Nursing, 1996.[19]

Other Advanced Nursing Roles

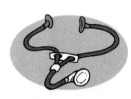

Advanced nursing roles include those of college educators, case managers, health policy and government workers, nurse entrepreneurs, parish nursing, nursing informatics, researchers, executives, and international leaders. You should be able to see that nursing is not without opportunity for just about any interest you may have. The career field is growing in all directions and the only limit is your imagination, education, and experience. All three can be improved with graduate education, motivation, and persistence.

Educational preparation. Advanced practice nurses have met higher educational and clinical practice requirements beyond the basic nursing education and licensing required of all RNs. This requires a master's degree in nursing (MSN) which usually takes 2 to 3 years to earn. It also includes special licensing and certification examinations, depending on the specialty area.

What Is International Nursing?

The International Council of Nurses (ICN) and the World Health Organization (WHO) are two organizations that play big roles in international health and international nursing. The ICN's goals are to influence health, social policy, and professional and socioeconomic standards worldwide; and to empower national nursing associations to act on behalf of nurses and the public.[20] The WHO stands on a belief that the enjoyment of the highest attainable standard of health is the fundamental right of every individual without distinction of race, religion, political belief, or social condition.[21] (Refer to the beginning of this chapter to see how Nurse Practitioner Mariah Taylor's values mirror WHO commitments.)

These are important goals, but unless you are an international student, especially from a non-industrialized country, you may wonder how these goals pertain to you. International health is as important to citizens in the U.S. as it is to those in Gambia. With global travel, economies, and technologies, what happens in one place on the globe affects us all. A disease in one country can more easily find its way to another than ever before.

Many schools and colleges of nursing are using international exchanges as a method for educating nursing students about important global issues. If you have an opportunity to do an exchange, take advantage of it. Even an experience within the U.S. where poverty and poor health care access are rampant will be extremely beneficial.

Resources

For further information on international nursing opportunities, begin with the following:

International Nursing Center, www.ana.org/anf/inc. This site has links to the WHO and the PHO (Pan American Health Organization), the National Council for International Health, and International Council of Nurses. Under "Links of Interest" you will find international links leading to information on jobs.

Nursing Around the World, www.nurse-dk.com. This site is from Denmark and provides links to employment opportunities around the world.

International Nursing Jobs, www.imc-la.com/nursingjob.htm. A page for the International Medical Corps.

Sites of Interest to Nursing Students, www2.csn.net/-tbracket/html. htm#Student Resources. This site has links to just about everything, including overseas job opportunities.

Further Information on Other Nursing Specialties

The following sources will provide valuable information about other nursing specialties.

> Critical Care Nursing: American Association of Critical Care Nursing, (800) 899-2226 or www.aacn.org
>
> Emergency Nursing: Emergency Nursing Association, (800) 2GET-ENA or www. ena.org
>
> Intravenous Nursing: The Intravenous Nurses Society, www.insl.org
>
> Nurse Anesthesia: American Association of Nurse Anesthetists, www.aana.com
>
> Orthopedic Nursing: National Association of Orthopaedic Nurses, www.naon.iNurse.com
>
> Perioperative Nursing: Association of Perioperative Registered Nurses, (800) 755-2676 or www.aorn.org
>
> Psychiatric-mental health nursing: American Psychiatric Nurses Association, www.apna.org
>
> Rehabilitation Nursing: Association of Rehabilitation Nurses, (800) 229-7530 or www.rehabnurse.org
>
> School Nursing: National Association of School Nurses, www.nasn.org

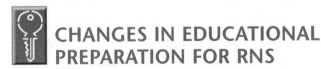 ## CHANGES IN EDUCATIONAL PREPARATION FOR RNS

For many years attempts have been made to raise the educational requirements for the initial RN license, or entry into practice, to a bachelor's degree and, possibly, to create new job titles. These changes, should they occur, have to be made through state legislation. Changes in licensing requirements will not affect RNs currently licensed with diplomas, or associate degrees, who would be "grandfathered" into the new laws.

The BLS (1999) says on this matter that "Individuals considering nursing should carefully weigh the pros and cons of enrolling in a BSN. program, since their advancement opportunities are broader. In fact, some career paths are open only to nurses with bachelor's or advanced degrees. A bachelor's degree is generally necessary for administrative positions, and is a prerequisite for admission to graduate nursing programs in research, consulting, teaching, or a clinical specialization."[22]

MARK MCINTYRE

Senior, Jacksonville State University,
Jacksonville, Alabama

Nursing school has exposed me to many wonderful opportunities to explore my interests. I recently completed an internship for a senior adult day program, and I've also worked for a local mental health clinic. From these experiences, as well as my classes, I've discovered that I love psychiatric nursing. I found out that I prefer to work with people who suffer from pathological disorders rather than behavioral problems. I also liked the senior population because they are very appreciative and you can see that they benefit so much from the attention and therapy they receive.

Even though I have a strong sense of what I like to do, I'm not sure what direction to take next. Throughout my clinicals, I've felt a little unsure about the setting I want to work in. The work environments in the smaller, local clinics don't appeal to me because most of their

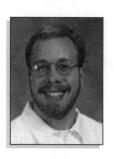

patients seem to exhibit conduct and substance-related disorders rather than clinical illnesses such as schizophrenia, which is my main interest. I've also heard that there's a high degree of burnout among staff. I don't think I want to work in hospitals, either, but I wonder if that will hinder my nursing career.

Presently I'm working part-time as a pharmacy technician for a mental health clinic, and I'm enjoying it. Many people tell me that the field of pharmaceutical sales is wide open and is hiring BSNs right out of college, but I fear that such a position may take me away from patient contact. Since I'm a senior and will be graduating soon, I'm hoping to find my niche. Given my education, what are my options in psychiatric nursing?

LAUREL BRINK

Graduate student, Gonzaga University,
Spokane, Washington

In her book, *From Novice to Expert,* Patricia Benner (1984), describes the transitions nurses make from one level of knowledge and competency to another. She says that the gift of being a novice is that it offers a tremendous opportunity for growth and professional development. The challenge is to discover, often by trial and error, strategies that develop the dimensions of psychiatric nursing needed for expertise. It is vital to read professional journals, attend seminars, and join and volunteer in professional psychiatric nursing and mental health organiza-

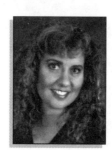

tions in order to network and form mentor relationships. These relationships can provide invaluable input about this multifaceted field.

In setting realistic goals as a new graduate, I recommend working for at least one year as a community mental health nurse. This can be instrumental in understanding the system all the way from payer sources to direct client services, referral resources, and creating partnerships and connections. Every mental illness has physiological and behavioral components. Schizophrenic clients may have substance abuse problems as well. Hospital experience is difficult to replace. It is in this setting that the schizophrenic client resides when decompensation occurs. In either in-patient or out-patient settings, the psychiatric nurse is the best therapeutic tool for modeling healthy behavior. It is also important to check with your State Nurse Practice Act to see what standards and parameters for practice a Bachelor of Science Registered Nurse degree allows.

With breadth of knowledge and experience, psychiatric nurses can serve as client advocates in a special way. Social activism on behalf of this vulnerable, high-risk population is a truly important societal need. Nurses grounded in holistic health, the integration of body, mind, and spirit can expand and evolve models of psychiatric care. Graduate school preparation will further increase your capacity to develop knowledge, expertise, and credibility that can be translated into action. The importance of education and training throughout one's professional career cannot be stressed enough.

Competence in nursing develops over time. The key to prevention of burn-out is setting limits and maintaining principles of self-care. And remember, when you feel overwhelmed and discouraged, staying grounded in your purpose and passion for becoming a nurse will help you endure these growth-producing times. In order to determine what you want to be, it is important to know who you want to become. Writing a personal mission statement will help you reflect on and define your deepest values, talents, and sense of mission needed to guide your professional development. To stimulate thinking along these lines, I highly recommend Barbara M. Dossey's book, *Florence Nightingale: Mystic, Visionary, Healer*, Springhouse Corp (2000), Springhouse, PA. Our challenge is to continue to grow and take initiative in order to stimulate positive change in our own lives, as well as, work with integrity in the healthcare institutions we serve. The proud history of nursing provides strength for the journey.

NURSING EDUCATION IN A NUTSHELL

To end this section and to preview what you can expect once you get into nursing school, look at what the *Occupational Outlook Handbook* for 1998–1999 says about what happens once you are accepted and enroll in a school or college of nursing:

> Nursing education includes classroom instruction and supervised clinical experience in hospitals and other health facilities. Students take courses in anatomy, physiology, microbiology, chemistry, nutrition, psychology and other behavioral sciences, and nursing. Course work also includes liberal arts classes. Supervised clinical experience is provided in hospital departments, such as, pediatrics, psychiatry, maternity, and surgery. A growing number of programs include clinical experience in nursing homes, public health departments, home health agencies, and ambulatory clinics.[23]

HOW CAN YOU BEGIN TO CHOOSE A NURSING OR PRE-NURSING MAJOR?

While many students come to college knowing what they want to study, many do not. That's completely normal. College is a perfect time to begin exploring your different interests. In the process, you may discover talents and strengths you never realized you had. For example, taking an environmental class may teach you that you have a passion for finding solutions to pollution problems.

While some of your explorations may take you down paths that don't resonate with your personality and interests, each experience will help to clarify who you really are and what you want to do with your life. Thinking about

TERMS

Major
A subject of
academic knowl-
edge chosen as a
field of spe-
cialization,
requiring a
specific course
of study.

choosing a major involves exploring potential majors, being open to changing majors, and linking majors to career areas.

Exploring Potential Majors

Here are some steps to help you explore majors that may interest you.

Take a variety of classes. Although you will generally have core requirements to fulfill, use your electives to branch out. Try to take at least one class in each area that sparks your interest.

Don't rule out subject areas that aren't classified as "safe." Friends or parents may have warned you against pursuing certain careers, encouraging you to stay with "safe" careers that pay well. Even though financial stability is important, following your heart's dreams and desires is equally important. Choosing between the "safe" path and the path of the heart can be challenging. Only you can decide which is best for you.

Letting your misconceptions and stereotypes of nursing as a profession for women only can limit your opportunity for a satisfying career. More men than ever are going into nursing. They see career flexibility in schedules, the ability to work anywhere in the world, a secure income, endless opportunities for change of work setting over time, and opportunities to do work that is challenging, satisfying, and rewarding, while allowing for a personal life with time and energy for others.

Spend time getting to know yourself, your interests, and your abilities. The more you know about yourself, the more ability you will have to focus on areas that make the most of who you are and what you can do. Pay close attention to which areas inspire you to greater heights and which areas seem to weaken your initiative.

Work closely with your advisor. Begin discussing your major early on with your advisor, even if you don't intend to declare a major right away. For any given major, your advisor may be able to tell you about both the corresponding department at your school and the possibilities in related career areas. You may also discuss with your advisor the possibility of a double major (completing the requirements for two different majors) or designing your own major, if your school offers an opportunity to do so.

Changing Majors

Some people may change their minds several times before honing in on a major that fits. Although this may add to the time you spend in college, being happy with your decision is important. For example, a student majoring in science education may begin student teaching only to discover that he really doesn't feel comfortable in front of students.

If this happens to you, don't be discouraged. You're certainly not alone. Changing a major is much like changing a job. Skills and experiences from one job will assist you in your next position, and some of the courses from your first major may apply—or even transfer as credits—to your next major. Talk with your academic advisor about any desire to change majors. Sometimes an advisor can speak to department heads in order to get the maximum number of credits transferred to your new major.

Whatever you decide, realize that you do have the right to change your mind. Continual self-discovery is part of the journey. No matter how many detours you make, each interesting class you take along the way helps to point you toward a major that feels like home.

Linking Majors to Careers

The point of declaring and pursuing a major is to help you reach a significant level of knowledge in one area in preparation for a career. Before you discard a major as not practical enough, consider where it might be able to take you. Thinking through the possibilities may open doors that you never knew existed. Besides finding an exciting path, you may discover highly marketable and beneficial to humankind as well.

For each major there are many career options that aren't obvious right away. For example, a student working toward a nursing degree doesn't have to work in a hospital. This student could develop health policy, act as a consultant for business, develop an online health education service, work overseas for the Peace Corps, or create a public television program. The sky's the limit: flight nursing, for example.

Explore the educational requirements of any area that interests you. Your choice of a school may be more or less crucial depending on the career area. For example, pursuing a career in nursing education requires a major in nursing and a graduate degree in nursing.

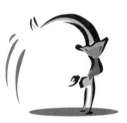

Joie de Vivre

The French have a phrase that has become commonly used in the English language as well: *joie de vivre*, which literally means "joy of living." A person with *joie de vivre* is one who finds joy and optimism in all parts of life, who is able to enjoy life's pleasures and find something positive in its struggles. Without experiencing difficult and sometimes painful challenges, people might have a hard time recognizing and experiencing happiness and satisfaction.

Think of this concept as you examine your level of personal wellness. If your focus on what is positive about yourself, that attitude can affect all other areas of your life. Give yourself the gift of self-respect so that you can nourish your body and mind every day, in every situation. Through both stressful obstacles and happy successes, you can find the joy of living.

Applications   **Chapter 2**

KEY INTO YOUR LIFE
Opportunities to Apply What You Learn

 Learning from Others

TOOLS TO USE:

> College catalog
> Other students
> Instructors and professors
> Career center
> Student organization members
> Faculty websites

Using any or all of the tools above, choose one person who works in a nursing practice area of interest to you. Base your decision on the recommendations of others or from information from faculty web pages. This person may also have research experience. They should be available to you, that is, have on-campus office hours. Call them and request a meeting.

Ask them the following questions and add any of your own:

1. What is your educational background?

_____

2. How did you decide on this area?

_____

_____

_____

3. Was it hard to find work in the area and how did you go about it?

_____

_____

_____

4. What areas are there that are related to this work?

_____

_____

5. Do you ever have students work with you? _____

6. Can I contact you later if I have more questions? _____

 ## *Alertness to Real World Research in the News*

To be a success in nursing, you must study all aspects of it, including what is in the news. Pay attention to what appears in the popular press (newspapers, magazines, television news) and in scientific journals.

1. For one week, review a local newspaper and the local television news. Keep notes on the health news presented.

2. In class, divide into small groups and discuss your notes, looking for common threads between the newsworthy information and other social or political trends.

3. In small groups, discuss whether there is a great deal of information about nurses, or very little. Discuss why or why not.

 ## *Alertness to Nursing Images on TV and in the Movies*

Nurses on TV or in the movies are fictional characters meant to make simulations of supposed real life emergencies realistic and, at least, dramatic. The purpose of this exercise is to discover images that are positive and those that are negative. Remember, absence of nurses in situations where nurses would normally be present is a negative image. It makes nursing work invisible and unimportant, or to imply that others do the work of nurses.

1. Write down your image of a nurse, using as much description of who, what, why, and where that you can think of.

_____

_____

_____

2. List a movie or television show you have seen that you think shows what nurses do in their practice. Describe the nurse you see in this situation.

_____

_____

_____

3. Compare answers from question nos. 1 and 2. How do they differ? How are they the same? What do they tell you about how you see the career of nursing? What would you like to do as a nurse?

_____

_____

_____

 ## Interests, Majors, and Careers

On a separate sheet, write for 5 to 10 minutes on the following and then share in small groups: What in your view is the most important thing that influenced you to think about a career in nursing? Write a story about that situation or idea. Be as specific as you can, using sights, smells, feelings, places, times. In the small group, talk about why you think your story was influential in your career decision.

Prepare to write by listing activities and subjects you like.

1. _____
2. _____
3. _____
4. _____
5. _____
6. _____

Name three practice areas that might relate to your interests and help you achieve your career goals.

1. _____
2. _____
3. _____

For each area, name someone in that area you could contact. Use the website (Sigma Theta Tau).

1. _____
2. _____
3. _____

For more information on careers, check the Sigma Theta Tau International Nursing Honor Society website, www.nursingsociety.org/career/main.html. You will find helpful profiles from nurses working in the following areas:

Community nursing
Pediatrics
Nurse practitioner
Trauma/emergency
Parish nursing
Mother and baby
Intensive Care
Government
Correctional facilities

Transplants
Psychiatric nursing
Geriatrics
Military
Oncology
Cardiac
Adolescent health and counseling
Research

Choose one or two areas of interest and go to the website to read about a nurse working in that area. Write down three points that make this nurse's career area of special interest to you. Write down one question you have for that nurse and email it to him or her.

KEY TO SELF-EXPRESSION
Discovery Through Journal Writing

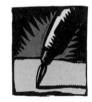

To record your thoughts, use a separate journal or the lined page at the end of the chapter.

Observing What You Already Observed

Return to your first journal entry and read it through. Next, return to the initial observation site and begin observing it again. Record all new observations in your journal. You should spend a minimum of 10 minutes of continuous, uninterrupted writing. When you are finished, read what you wrote. Think about how your first and second observations differed and how they were the same. Reflect on this observation process and write your thoughts, or feelings about it.

Journal

Name _____   Date _____

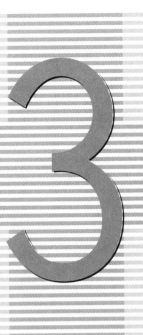

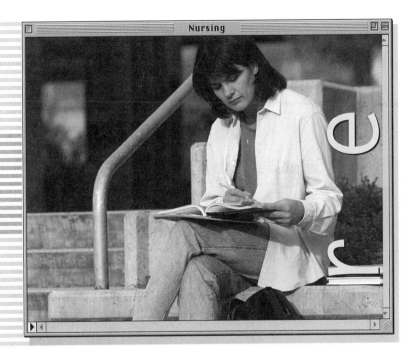

Nursing

3

Self-Awareness

Knowing Who You Are and How You Learn

L earning is not something you do just in college. Throughout your life, learning can help you keep up with the rapid pace at which the world is changing.

Technology, for example, is changing so fast that you cannot learn today about all of the computer operations that will be commonplace five years from now. However, you can learn how to be an effective learner in school and in the workplace so that you can keep pace with changes as they occur. In this chapter, you will learn what recent studies show about the math and science abilities of students in the United States and how you can learn to be a better science learner—and nursing student. You will also become aware of your learning style by completing three different learning style assessments. Each assessment will add a different dimension to the picture you are forming of yourself. You will then explore other important elements of self: your self-perception, your preferences, your habits, your abilities, and your attitudes.

In this chapter, you will explore answers to the following questions:

■ How well did your school prepare you for college science?

■ Is there one best way to learn?

■ How can you discover your learning styles?

■ What are the benefits of knowing your learning styles?

■ How do you explore who you are?

WHY DO YOU NEED SCIENCE AND MATH TO BE A NURSE?

Lacking a realistic view of what nurses do makes this a question you might be asking. For instance, as a prenursing student you may be taking chemistry and math. Perhaps you understand the need for chemistry because you understand that chemical reactions underlie physiological reactions. The kidneys, for instance, spend most of their time regulating ions. Or, you may know that medications interact with receptors on cells to set off various chemical processes that can cause both positive and negative effects and that muscle cells are regulated by the inflow and outflow of calcium, sodium, and potassium. But, you might wonder, what is the purpose of math and other science courses that seem less obviously related to health and illness? Let the following example illustrate the reason math skills as well as science are important.

Matt is an emergency nurse in a large urban hospital. He is taking care of a 23-year-old who has been in a motor vehicle accident. The patient is very badly hurt and needs immediate surgery for internal trauma. Matt needs to give her antibiotics, along with other medications, before she goes to surgery. Matt will be giving the antibiotics intravenously (into a vein with a needle).

In the pharmacy, the antibiotic, powder or solution, is mixed with a specific volume of fluid and sent to Matt. Matt gets the antibiotics premixed and on the IV medication bag the rate of administration is written to give the correct dose. Matt is having a hectic day, another big trauma case is coming through the doors, and so he decides to hang the medications right away.

Unfortunately, Matt administered the medication without checking the original order or the pharmacy math calculations and gave the young patient the wrong dose. Luckily, he caught the error and corrected it before the patient went to surgery with either too little antibiotic (no therapeutic effect) or too much antibiotic (potential harmful effect).

In school Matt took math and science prerequisites and in nursing school he learned how to calculate medication dosages. Therefore, he could have easily figured the rate the intravenous antibiotic needed to run in order to give the correct dose. If only he had used those skills. After this last experience, and while he is filling out the incident report, he vows to check each medication every time. Matt also knew from biochemistry that a chemical reaction of the antibiotic occurred in the kidneys. It was important to be very careful because giving the drug incorrectly could cause kidney damage.

Next time Matt receives a drug from the pharmacy he checks it by recalculating the equations. Noticing a mistake, he calls the pharmacy and they also recheck it. The medication is corrected before it is sent to the emergency department. Matt rechecks it a second time before he gives it. He is also thinking about possible side affects and what he needs to monitor while the patient is under his care.

This example is not intended to imply that pharmacists often make mistakes. But, everyone can make mistakes. A nurse's job, along with the rest of the health care team, is to do the very best to prevent them. This is the most dramatic reason a strong background in science and math is crucial to being a nurse. Science gives you the skills you need to provide safe, rational, and effective nursing care. Just as an air traffic controller must understand trajectories and math, or where the planes are going in the air, so nurses need to understand what keeps people going. Both have people's lives in their hands.

Science and math also teach you how to think critically (for more on critical thinking, see Chapter 5) and how to observe; how to reason and how to problem solve. Nurses use reasoning and problem-solving skills everyday. Understanding how to do this requires knowing why you do this. Understanding about chemicals and cell receptors, and about numbers of milliliters an IV needs to run to give a certain number of micrograms are essential keys to success in nursing. Remember, too, nurses work with the whole person. They take care of bodies and minds, and science teaches you about how the mind works, too. This can help you problem solve questions about why a person behaves the way they do. For instance, why does your patient continue to drink alcohol even though his liver is shot? Why doesn't a client with diabetes take her medicine?

On the other hand, if you deal with psychiatric problems, you need science to help you understand treatments, and to think about things, such as what effect sleep deprivation or poor nutrition have on a patient's behavior.

This is what nurses do. They apply the knowledge learned in school, on the job, and in continuing education classes, to real-life situations. If you want to do safe, high quality work you must be well educated. Theory and its connecting principles are key to being a good nurse in your area of practice. And don't let anyone tell you otherwise!

HOW WELL DID YOUR SCHOOL PREPARE YOU FOR COLLEGE SCIENCE?

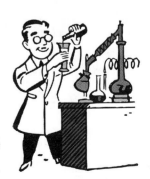

In recent years, you may have seen headlines like *Newsweek's*, "An 'F' in World Competition," that emphasize the poor science and math abilities of U. S. students. The media have focused on test scores, especially in relation to other countries, but those scores do not necessarily represent the entire picture. The United States has students in many states with high scores when compared to other nations of the world, despite the fact that, as a whole, the United States falls behind other countries.[1]

Secretary of Education Richard W. Riley made the following points about high school education at a recent conference of mathematicians and math educators[2]:

- U. S. students scored among the lowest in the world in mathematics and science, general knowledge; physics; and advanced mathematics.

- U. S. fourth graders scored as well as or better than fourth graders in many other countries did in math and science.

- U. S. eighth graders showed a decline in science and math performance.

- U. S. twelfth graders performed below the international average of the 21 countries tested.

There has been controversy among educators about the interpretation of international testing scores, but everyone seems to agree that U. S. schools need to be graduating students who are far better prepared in math and science than is currently the case.

Within the United States, there is great variation among high school students' scores, often depending on the state they live in. If you come from Iowa or Utah, your high school is doing very well in preparing you in math and science. Or you may live in a state where students had poorer scores; if so, your high school may not have prepared you to meet the challenge of pre-nursing and nursing courses. You will have some catching up to do, but that's not an impossible feat. Students have been attending college and graduating with nursing honors from every state in the union. And you can, too.

 ## IS THERE ONE BEST WAY TO LEARN?

Your mind is the most powerful tool you will ever possess. You are accomplished at many skills and can process all kinds of information. However, when you have trouble accomplishing a particular task, you may become convinced that you can't learn how to do anything new. You may feel that those who can do what you can't have the "right" kind of ability. Not only is this perception incorrect, it can also damage your belief in yourself.

There is no one "best" way to learn. Instead, there are many different learning styles, and different styles are suited to different situations. Your individual learning profile is made up of a combination of learning styles. Each person's profile is unique. Just like personality traits, learning styles are part of your personal characteristics. Knowing how you learn is one of the first steps in discovering who you are.

Discovering your favorite learning style will help you to develop study plans that work best for you, but you must learn to use all the learning styles. The next section will help you find out your preferred style, but that style will not be the only one you will need to succeed in the sciences and

TERMS

Learning style
A particular way
in which the
mind receives
and processes
information.

in nursing courses. To be successful, you must become adept at all methods of learning.

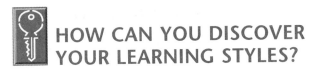

HOW CAN YOU DISCOVER YOUR LEARNING STYLES?

Your brain is so complex that one inventory cannot give you all the information you need to maximize your learning skills. You will learn about and complete three assessments: the *Learning Styles Inventory*, the *Pathways to Learning* inventory based on the Multiple Intelligences Theory, and the *Personality Spectrum*. Each of these assessments evaluates your mind's abilities in a different way, although they often have related ideas. Your results will combine to form your learning styles profile, consisting of the styles and types that best fit the ways that you learn and interact with others. After you complete the various learning styles inventories, you will read about strategies that can help you make the most of particular styles and types, both in school and beyond. Your learning styles profile will help you to improve your understanding of yourself, how you learn, and how you may function as a learner in the workplace.

Learning Styles Inventory

One of the first instruments to measure psychological types, the Myers–Briggs Type Indicator (MBTI), was designed by Katharine Briggs and her daughter, Isabel Briggs Myers. Later David Keirsey and Marilyn Bates combined the sixteen Myers-Briggs types into four temperaments. Barbara Soloman, Associate Director of the University Undesignated Student Program at North Carolina State University, has developed the following learning styles inventory based on these theories and on her work with thousands of students.[3]

"Students learn in many ways," says Professor Soloman. "Mismatches often exist between common learning styles and standard teaching styles. Therefore, students often do poorly and get discouraged. Some students doubt themselves and doubt their ability to succeed in the curriculum of their choice. Some settle for low grades and even leave school. If students understand how they learn most effectively, they can tailor their studying to their own needs."

"Learning effectively" and "tailoring studying to your own needs" mean choosing study techniques that help you learn. For example, if a student responds more to visual images than to words, he or she may want to construct notes in a more visual way. Or, if a student learns better when talking to people than when studying alone, he or she may want to study primarily in pairs or groups.

Science and nursing courses use a variety of teaching methods. For instance, in one course you may be doing a great deal of reading, while in another you will do hands-on work in a laboratory or a clinical setting. Most instructors use a variety of teaching methods to appeal to their students' different learning styles. Variety usually means good teaching because it helps keep your attention and also helps you learn other styles by practicing them.

"Nurses are the best value in health care. More than a decade of research shows that nurse staffing levels and skill mix make a difference in the outcomes of hospitalized patients. Studies show that when there are more nurses, there are lower mortality rates, shorter lengths of stay, lower costs, and fewer complications."
BEVERLY MALONE, PH.D., RN, FAAN.

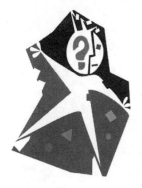

The Dimensions of Learning

The Learning Styles Inventory has four "dimensions," within each of which are two opposing styles. At the end of the inventory, you will have two scores in each of the four dimensions. The difference between your two scores in any dimension tells you which of the two styles in that dimension is dominant for you. A few people will score right in between the two styles, indicating that they have fairly equal parts of both styles. Following are brief descriptions of the four dimensions. You will learn more about them in the section on study strategies, after you complete all three assessments.

Active/Reflective. *Active* learners learn best by experiencing knowledge through their own actions. *Reflective* learners understand information best when they have had time to reflect on it on their own.

Factual/Theoretical. *Factual* learners learn best through specific facts, data, and detailed experimentation. *Theoretical* learners are more comfortable with big-picture ideas, symbols, and new concepts.

Visual/Verbal. *Visual* learners remember best what they see: diagrams, flowcharts, time lines, films, and demonstrations. *Verbal* learners gain the most learning from reading, hearing spoken words, participating in discussion, and explaining things to others.

Holistic
Relating to the wholes of complete systems rather than the analysis of parts.

Linear/Holistic. *Linear* learners find it easiest to learn material presented step by step in a logical, ordered progression. *Holistic* learners progress in fits and starts, perhaps feeling lost for a while, but eventually seeing the big picture in a clear and creative way.

Please complete this inventory by circling **a** or **b** to indicate your answer to each question. Answer every question and choose only one answer for each question. If both answers seem to apply to you, choose the answer that applies more often.

1. I study best
   a. in a study group.
   b. alone or with a partner.

2. I would rather be considered
   a. realistic.
   b. imaginative.

3. When I recall what I did yesterday, I am most likely to think in terms of
   a. pictures/images.
   b. words/verbal descriptions.

4. I usually think new material is
   a. easier at the beginning and then harder as it becomes more complicated.
   b. often confusing at the beginning but easier as I start to understand what the whole subject is about.

5. When given a new activity to learn, I would rather first
   a. try it out.
   b. think about how I'm going to do it.

6. If I were an instructor, I would rather teach a course
   a. that deals with real-life situations and what to do about them.
   b. that deals with ideas and encourages students to think about them.

7. I prefer to receive new information in the form of
   a. pictures, diagrams, graphs, or maps.
   b. written directions or verbal information.

8. I learn
   a. at a fairly regular pace. If I study hard, I'll "get it" and then move on.
   b. in fits and starts. I might be totally confused and then suddenly it all "clicks."

9. I understand something better after
   a. I attempt to do it myself.
   b. I give myself time to think about how it works.

10. I find it easier
    a. to learn facts.
    b. to learn ideas/concepts.

11. In a book with lots of pictures and charts, I am likely to
    a. look over the pictures and charts carefully.
    b. focus on the written text.

12. It's easier for me to memorize facts from
    a. a list.
    b. a whole story/essay with the facts embedded in it.

13. I will more easily remember
    a. something I have done myself.
    b. something I have thought or read about.

14. I am usually
    a. aware of my surroundings. I remember people and places and usually recall where I put things.
    b. unaware of my surroundings. I forget people and places. I frequently misplace things.

15. I like instructors
    a. who put a lot of diagrams on the board.
    b. who spend a lot of time explaining.

16. Once I understand
    a. all the parts, I understand the whole thing.
    b. the whole thing, I see how the parts fit.

17. When I am learning something new, I would rather
    a. talk about it.
    b. think about it.

18. I am good at
    a. being careful about the details of my work.
    b. having creative ideas about how to do my work.

19. I remember best
    a. what I see.
    b. what I hear.

20. When I solve problems that involve some math, I usually
    a. work my way to the solutions one step at a time.
    b. see the solutions but then have to struggle to figure out the steps to get to them.

21. In a lecture class, I would prefer occasional in-class
    a. discussions or group problem-solving sessions.
    b. pauses that give opportunities to think or write about ideas presented in the lecture.

22. On a multiple-choice test, I am more likely to
    a. run out of time.
    b. lose points because of not reading carefully or making careless errors.

23. When I get directions to a new place, I prefer
    a. a map.
    b. written instructions.

24. When I'm thinking about something I've read,
    a. I remember the incidents and try to put them together to figure out the themes.
    b. I just know what the themes are when I finish reading and then I have to back up and find the incidents that demonstrate them.

25. When I get a new computer or VCR, I tend to
    a. plug it in and start punching buttons.
    b. read the manual and follow instructions.

26. In reading for pleasure, I prefer
    a. something that teaches me new facts or tells me how to do something.
    b. something that gives me new ideas to think about.

27. When I see a diagram or sketch in class, I am most likely to remember
    a. the picture.
    b. what the instructor said about it.

28. It is more important to me that an instructor
    a. lay out the material in clear, sequential steps.
    b. give me an overall picture and relate the material to other subjects.

SCORING SHEET

Use Table 3-1 to enter your scores.

1. Put 1s in the boxes that reflect your answers (e.g., if you answered **a** to Question 3, put a **1** in the column headed **a** next to the number **3**).
2. Total the 1s in the columns and write the totals in the indicated spaces at the base of the columns.

TABLE 3-1   Learning styles inventory scores.

Active/Reflective			Factual/Theoretical			Visual/Verbal			Linear/Holistic		
Q#	a	b	Q#	a	b	Q#	a	b	Q#	a	b
1			2			3			4		
5			6			7			8		
9			10			11			12		
13			14			15			16		
17			18			19			20		
21			22			23			24		
25			26			27			28		
Total			Total			Total			Total		

3. For each of the four dimensions, circle your two scores on the bar scale and then fill in the bar between the scores. For example, if under "ACTV/REFL" you had 2 a and 5 b responses, you would fill in the bar between those two scores, as this sample shows:

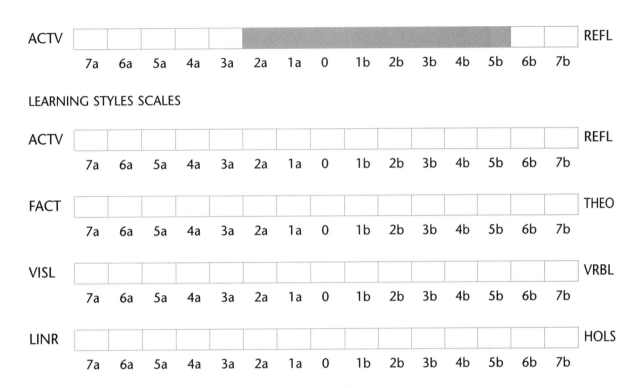

LEARNING STYLES SCALES

If your filled-in bar has the 0 close to its center, you are well balanced on the two dimensions of that scale. If your bar is drawn mainly to one side, you have a strong preference for that one dimension and may have difficulty learning in the other dimension.

Continue on to the next assessment. After you complete all three, the next section of the chapter will help you understand and make use of your results from each assessment.

Multiple Intelligences Theory

Howard Gardner, a Harvard University professor, has developed a theory called Multiple Intelligences. He believes there are at least eight distinct intelligences possessed by all people, and that every person has developed some intelligences more fully than others. Most people have experienced a time when they learned something very quickly and comfortably. Most have also had the opposite experience when, no matter how hard they tried, something they wanted to learn just would not sink in. According to the Multiple Intelligences Theory, when you find a task or subject easy, you are probably using a more fully developed intelligence; when you have more trouble, you may be using a less-developed intelligence.[4]

Following are brief descriptions of the focus of each of the intelligences. Study skills that reinforce each intelligence will be described later in the chapter.

TERMS

Intelligence
As defined by H. Gardner, an ability to solve problems or fashion products that are useful in a particular cultural setting or community.

- Verbal-Linguistic Intelligence—ability to communicate through language (listening, reading, writing, speaking)

- Logical-Mathematical Intelligence—ability to understand logical reasoning and problem solving (math, science, patterns, sequences)

- Bodily-Kinesthetic Intelligence—ability to use the physical body skillfully and to take in knowledge through bodily sensation (coordination, working with hands)

- Visual-Spatial Intelligence—ability to understand spatial relationships and to perceive and create images (visual art, graphic design, charts and maps)

- Interpersonal Intelligence—ability to relate to others, noticing their moods, motivations, and feelings (social activity, cooperative learning, teamwork)

- Intrapersonal Intelligence—ability to understand one's own behavior and feelings (independence, time spent alone)

- Musical Intelligence—ability to comprehend and create meaningful sound (music, sensitivity to sound)

- Naturalistic Intelligence—ability to understand features of the environment (interest in nature, environmental balance, ecosystem, stress relief brought by natural environments)

TERMS

Kinesthetic
Coming from physical sensation caused by body movements and tensions.

Please complete the following assessment of your multiple intelligences, called Pathways to Learning, developed by Joyce Bishop.[5] It will help you determine which of your intelligences are most fully developed. Don't be concerned if some of your scores are low. That is true of most people, including your instructors and your authors!

Learning styles and multiple intelligences are guides to help you understand yourself. Instead of labeling yourself narrowly using one category or another, learn as much as you can about your preferences and how you can maximize your learning. Most people are a blend of styles and preferences, with one or two being dominant. In addition, you may change preferences depending on the situation. For example, a student might find it easy to take notes in outline style when the instructor lectures in an organized way. However, if another instructor jumps from topic to topic, the student might choose to use the Cornell system or a think link (Chapter 7 goes into detail about note-taking styles).

The final assessment (beginning on page 66) focuses on how you relate to others through its evaluation of personality types.

PATHWAYS TO LEARNING

Directions: Rate each statement as follows: rarely 1; sometimes 2; usually 3; always 4.

Write the number of your response (1–4) in the box next to the statement and total each set of the six questions.

Developed by Joyce Bishop, Ph.D., and based upon Howard Gardner, *Frames of Mind: The Theory of Multiple Intelligences.*

---

1. I enjoy physical activities.
2. I am uncomfortable sitting still.
3. I prefer to learn through doing.
4. When sitting I move my legs or hands.
5. I enjoy working with my hands.
6. I like to pace when I'm thinking or studying.
   TOTAL for Bodily/Kinesthetic

7. I use maps easily.
8. I draw pictures/diagrams when explaining ideas.
9. I can assemble items easily from diagrams.
10. I enjoy drawing or photography.
11. I do not like to read long paragraphs.
12. I prefer a drawn map over written directions.
    TOTAL for Visual/Spatial

13. I enjoy telling stories.
14. I like to write.
15. I like to read.
16. I express myself clearly.
17. I am good at negotiating.
18. I like to discuss topics that interest me.
    TOTAL for Verbal/Linguistic

19. I liked math in high school.
20. I like science.
21. I problem-solve well.
22. I question how things work.
23. I enjoy planning or designing something new.
24. I am able to fix things.
    TOTAL for Logical/Mathematical

25. I listen to music.
26. I move my fingers or feet when I hear music.
27. I have good rhythm.
28. I like to sing along with music.
29. People have said I have musical talent.
30. I like to express my ideas through music.
    TOTAL for Musical

31. I like doing a project with other people.
32. People come to me to help settle conflicts.
33. I like to spend time with friends.
34. I am good at understanding people.
35. I am good at making people feel comfortable.
36. I enjoy helping others.
    TOTAL for Interpersonal

37. I need quiet time to think.
38. I think about issues before I want to talk.
39. I am interested in self-improvement.
40. I understand my thoughts and feelings.
41. I know what I want out of life.
42. I prefer to work on projects alone.
    TOTAL for Intrapersonal

43. I enjoy nature whenever possible.
44. I think about having a career involving nature.
45. I enjoy studying plants, animals, or oceans.
46. I avoid being indoors except when I sleep.
47. As a child I played with bugs and leaves.
48. When I feel stressed, I want to be out in nature.
    TOTAL for Naturalistic

Write each of your eight intelligences in the column where it fits below. For each, choose the column that corresponds with your total in that intelligence.

SCORES OF 20–24 HIGHLY DEVELOPED		SCORES OF 14–19 MODERATELY DEVELOPED		SCORES BELOW 14 UNDERDEVELOPED	
Scores	Intelligences	Scores	Intelligences	Scores	Intelligences

Keys to Success, 2/e, by Carter et al., ©1998. Reprinted by permission of Prentice-Hall, Inc., Upper Saddle River, NJ.

Personality Spectrum

A system that simplifies learning styles into four personality types has been developed by Joyce Bishop (1997). Her work is based on the Myers-Briggs and Keirsey and Bates theories discussed earlier in the chapter. The Personality Spectrum will give you a personality perspective on your learning styles. Please complete the assessment on page 67. When you have tallied your scores, plot them on Figure 3-1 to create a visual representation of your spectrum.

Your Personality Spectrum assessment can help you maximize your functioning at school and at work. Each personality type has its own abilities that improve work and school performance, suitable learning techniques, and interpersonal relationships. Table 3-2 explains what suits each type.

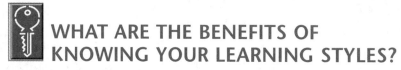

WHAT ARE THE BENEFITS OF KNOWING YOUR LEARNING STYLES?

Determining your learning styles profile takes work and self-exploration. For it to be worth your while, you need to understand what knowing your profile can do for you. The following sections will discuss benefits specific to study skills as well as more general benefits.

PERSONALITY SPECTRUM

Step 1. Rank all four responses to each question from **most** like you (4) to **least** like you (1). Place a 1, 2, 3, or 4 in each box next to the responses, and use each number only once per question.

1. I like instructors who
   ☐ a. tell me exactly what is expected of me.
   ☐ b. make learning active and exciting.
   ☐ c. maintain a safe and supportive classroom.
   ☐ d. challenge me to think at higher levels.

2. I learn best when the material is
   ☐ a. well organized.
   ☐ b. something I can do hands-on.
   ☐ c. about understanding and improving the human condition.
   ☐ d. intellectually challenging.

3. A high priority in my life is to
   ☐ a. keep my commitments.
   ☐ b. experience as much of life as possible.
   ☐ c. make a difference in other's lives.
   ☐ d. understand how things work.

4. Other people think of me as
   ☐ a. dependable and loyal.
   ☐ b. dynamic and creative.
   ☐ c. caring and honest.
   ☐ d. intelligent and inventive.

5. When I experience stress, I most likely
   ☐ a. do something to help me feel more in control.
   ☐ b. do something physical and daring.
   ☐ c. talk with a friend.
   ☐ d. go off by myself and think about my situation.

6. The greatest flaw someone can have is to be
   ☐ a. irresponsible.
   ☐ b. unwilling to try new things.
   ☐ c. selfish and unkind to others.
   ☐ d. an illogical thinker.

7. My vacations could best be described as
   ☐ a. traditional.
   ☐ b. adventuresome.
   ☐ c. pleasing to others.
   ☐ d. a new learning experience.

8. One word that best describes me is
   ☐ a. sensible.
   ☐ b. spontaneous.
   ☐ c. giving.
   ☐ d. analytical.

Step 2. Add up the total points for each column.

Total for (A)	Total for (B)	Total for (C)	Total for (D)
☐	☐	☐	☐
Organizer	Adventurer	Giver	Thinker

Step 3. Plot these numbers on the brain diagram on page 69.

From *Keys to Success: How to Achieve Your Goals,* 2/e, by Carter et al., © 1998. Reprinted by permission of Prentice-Hall, Inc., Upper Saddle River, NJ.

TABLE 3-2	PERSONALITY	STRENGTHS AT WORK AND SCHOOL	INTERPERSONAL RELATIONSHIPS
	Organizer	■ Can efficiently manage heavy work loads ■ Good organizational skills ■ Natural leadership qualities	■ Loyal ■ Dependable ■ Traditional
	Adventurer	■ Adaptable to most changes ■ Creative and skillful ■ Dynamic and fast-paced	■ Free ■ Exciting ■ Intense
	Giver	■ Always willing to help others ■ Honest and sincere ■ Good people skills	■ Giving ■ Romantic ■ Warm
	Thinker	■ Good analytical skills ■ Can develop complex designs ■ Is thorough and exact	■ Quiet ■ Good problem solver ■ Inventive

Personality spectrum at school and work.

Study Benefits

Most students aim to maximize learning while minimizing frustration and time spent studying. If you know your particular learning style, you can use techniques that complement it. Such techniques take advantage of your highly developed areas while helping you through your less-developed ones. For example, say you perform better in smaller, discussion-based classes. When you have the opportunity, you might choose a course section that is smaller or that is taught by an instructor who prefers group discussion. You might also apply specific strategies to improve your retention in a lecture situation.

This section describes the techniques that tend to complement the strengths and shortcomings of each style. Students in Professor Soloman's program made many of these suggestions according to what worked for their own learning styles. Concepts from different assessments that benefit from similar strategies are grouped together. In Figure 3-2, you can see which styles tend to be dominant among students.

Remember that you may have characteristics from many different styles, even though some are dominant. Therefore, you may see suggestions for styles other than your dominant ones that may apply to you. What's important is that you use what works. Note the boxes next to the names of each style or type. In order to spot your best suggestions quickly, mark your most dominant styles or types by making check marks in the appropriate boxes.

Are You Active or Reflective?

Active learners □ include **Bodily-Kinesthetic** □ and **Interpersonal** □ **learners as well as Adventurers.** □ They like to apply the information to the real world, experience it in their own actions, or discuss or explain to others what they have learned.

| FIGURE 3-1 | Personality spectrum—Thinking preferences and learning styles. |

Place a dot on the appropriate number line for each of your four scores and connect the dots. A new shape will be formed inside each square. Color each shape in a different color.

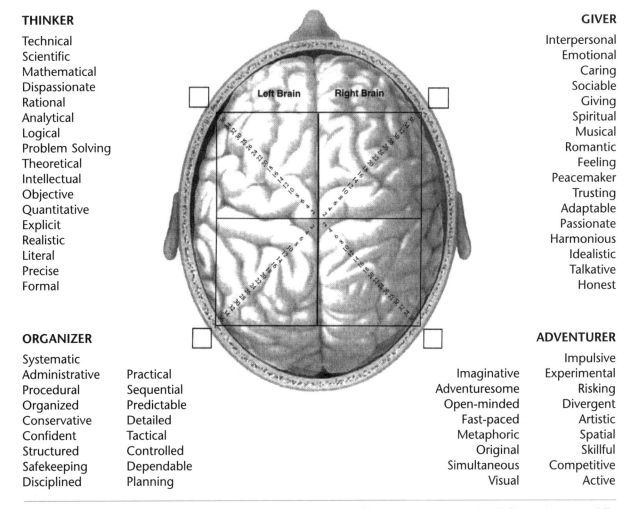

THINKER

Technical
Scientific
Mathematical
Dispassionate
Rational
Analytical
Logical
Problem Solving
Theoretical
Intellectual
Objective
Quantitative
Explicit
Realistic
Literal
Precise
Formal

GIVER

Interpersonal
Emotional
Caring
Sociable
Giving
Spiritual
Musical
Romantic
Feeling
Peacemaker
Trusting
Adaptable
Passionate
Harmonious
Idealistic
Talkative
Honest

ORGANIZER

Systematic
Administrative   Practical
Procedural   Sequential
Organized   Predictable
Conservative   Detailed
Confident   Tactical
Structured   Controlled
Safekeeping   Dependable
Disciplined   Planning

ADVENTURER

Impulsive
Imaginative   Experimental
Adventuresome   Risking
Open-minded   Divergent
Fast-paced   Artistic
Metaphoric   Spatial
Original   Skillful
Simultaneous   Competitive
Visual   Active

Source: Understanding Psychology, 3/e, by Morris, © 1996. Adapted by permission of Prentice-Hall, Inc., Upper Saddle River, NJ.

Student-suggested strategies for active learners:

- Study in a group in which members take turns explaining topics to each other and then discussing them.
- Think of practical uses for the course material.
- Pace and recite while you learn.
- Act out material or design games.
- Use flashcards with other people.
- Teach the material to someone else.

FIGURE 3-2

Percentages of students with particular learning styles.

VISUAL		VERBAL
80%		20%

ACTIVE		REFLECTIVE
80%		20%

FACTUAL		THEORETICAL
70%		30%

LINEAR		HOLISTIC
85%		15%

Source: Barbara Soloman, North Carolina State University.

Reflective learners □ **include Intrapersonal** □ **and Logical/Mathematical** □ **learners as well as Thinkers.** □ They retain and understand information better after they have taken time to think about it.

Student-suggested strategies for reflective learners:

- Study in a quiet setting.
- When you are reading, stop periodically to think about what you have read.
- Don't just memorize material; think about why it is important and what it relates to, considering the causes and effects involved.
- Write short summaries of what the material means to you.

Are You Factual or Theoretical?

Factual learners □ **and Organizers** □ **prefer concrete and specific facts, data, and detailed experimentation.** They like to solve problems with standard methods and are patient with details. They don't respond well to surprises and unique complications that upset normal procedure. They are good at memorizing facts.

Student-suggested strategies for factual learners:

- Ask the instructor how ideas and concepts apply in practice.
- Ask for specific examples of the ideas and concepts.
- Brainstorm specific examples with classmates or by yourself.
- Think about how theories make specific connections with the real world.

Theoretical learners □ **are often also logical/mathematical and prefer innovation and theories.** They are good at grasping new concepts and big-picture ideas. They dislike repetition and fact-based learning. They are comfortable with symbols and abstractions, often connecting them with prior knowledge and experience. Most classes are aimed at theoretical learners.

Student-suggested strategies for theoretical learners:

- If a class deals primarily with factual information, try to think of concepts, interpretations, or theories that link the facts together.
- Because you become impatient with details, you may be prone to careless mistakes on tests. Read directions and entire questions before answering, and be sure to check your work.
- Look for systems and patterns that arrange facts in a way that makes sense to you.
- Spend time analyzing the material.

Are You Visual/Spatial or Verbal/Linguistic?

Visual/Spatial learners ☐ **remember best what they see: diagrams, flowcharts, time lines, films, and demonstrations.** They tend to forget spoken words and ideas. Classes generally don't include that much visual information. Note that although words written on paper or shown with an overhead projector are something you see, visual learners learn most easily from visual cues that don't involve words.

Student-suggested strategies for visual/spatial learners:

- Add diagrams to your notes whenever possible. Dates can be drawn on a time line; math functions can be graphed; percentages can be drawn in a pie chart.
- Organize your notes so that you can clearly see main points and supporting facts and how things are connected. You will learn more about different styles of note-taking in Chapter 7.
- Connect related facts in your notes by drawing arrows.
- Color-code your notes using different colored highlighters so that everything relating to a particular topic is the same color.

Verbal/Linguistic learners ☐ **(often also interpersonal) remember much of what they hear and more of what they hear and then say.** They benefit from discussion, prefer verbal explanation to visual demonstration, and learn effectively by explaining things to others. Because written words are processed as verbal information, verbal learners learn well through reading. The majority of classes, since they present material through the written word, lecture, or discussion, are geared to verbal learners.

Student-suggested strategies for verbal learners:

- Talk about what you learn. Work in study groups so that you have an opportunity to explain and discuss what you are learning.
- Read the textbook and highlight no more than 10 percent.
- Rewrite your notes.
- Outline chapters.
- Recite information or write scripts and debates.

Are You Linear or Holistic?

Linear learners ☐ **find it easiest to learn material presented in a logical, ordered progression.** They solve problems in a step-by-step manner. They can work with sections of material without yet fully understanding the whole picture. They tend to be stronger when looking at the parts of a whole rather than understanding the whole and then dividing it up into parts. They learn best when taking in material in a progression from easiest to more complex to most difficult. Many courses are taught in a linear fashion.

Student-suggested strategies for linear learners:

- If you have an instructor who jumps around from topic to topic, spend time outside of class with the instructor or a classmate who can help you fill the gaps in your notes.
- If class notes are random, rewrite the material according to whatever logic helps you understand it best.
- Outline the material.

Holistic learners ☐ **learn in fits and starts.** They may feel lost for days or weeks, unable to solve even the simplest problems or show the most basic understanding, until they suddenly "get it." They may feel discouraged when struggling with material that many other students seem to learn easily. Once they understand, though, they tend to see the big picture to an extent that others may not often achieve. They are often highly creative.

Student-suggested strategies for the holistic learner:

- Recognize that you are not slow or stupid. Don't lose faith in yourself. You will get it!
- Before reading a chapter, preview it by reading all the subheadings, summaries, and any margin glossary terms. The chapter may also start with an outline and overview of the entire chapter.
- Instead of spending a short time on every subject every night, try setting aside evenings for specific subjects and immerse yourself in just one subject at a time.
- Try taking difficult subjects in summer school when you are handling fewer courses.
- Try to relate subjects to other things you already know. Keep asking yourself how you could apply the material.

Study Techniques for Additional Multiple Intelligences

People who score high in the Musical/Rhythmic ☐ **intelligence have strong memories for rhymes and can be energized by music.** They often have a song running through their minds and find themselves tapping a foot or their fingers when they hear music.

Student-suggested strategies for musical/rhythmic people:

- Create rhymes out of vocabulary words.
- Beat out rhythms when studying.

- Play instrumental music while studying if it does not distract you, but first determine what type of music improves your concentration the most.
- Take study breaks and listen to music.
- Write a rap song about your topic.

Naturalistic learners ☐ feel energized when they are connected to nature. Their career choices and hobbies reflect their love of nature. Student-suggested strategies for naturalistic people:

- Study outside whenever practical but only if it is not distracting.
- Explore subject areas that reflect your love for nature. Learning is much easier when you have a passion for it.
- Relate abstract information to something concrete in nature.
- Take breaks with something you love from nature—a walk, watching your fish, or a nature video. Use nature as a reward for getting other work done.

Study Techniques for Different Personality Types

The different personality types of the Personality Spectrum combine the learning styles and multiple intelligences you have explored. Table 3-3 shows learning techniques that benefit each type.

TABLE 3-3 Types and learning techniques.

PERSONALITY TYPES	RELATED LEARNING STYLES	LEARNING TECHNIQUES TO USE
Organizer	Factual, Linear	■ Organize material before studying. ■ Whenever possible, select instructors who have well-planned courses. ■ Keep a daily planner and to-do list.
Adventurer	Active, Bodily-Kinesthetic	■ Keep study sessions moving quickly. ■ Make learning fun and exciting. ■ Study with other Adventurers but also with Organizers.
Giver	Interpersonal	■ Form study groups. ■ Help someone else learn. ■ Pick classes that relate to your interest in people.
Thinker	Reflective, Intrapersonal, Logical-Mathematical, Theoretical	■ Study alone. ■ Allow time to think about material. ■ Pick classes and instructors who are intellectually challenging.

General Benefits

Although schools have traditionally favored verbal-linguistic students, there is no general advantage to one style over another. The only advantage is in discovering your profile through accurate and honest analysis. Following are three general benefits of knowing your learning styles:

1. You will have a better chance of avoiding problematic situations. If you don't explore what works best for you, you risk forcing yourself into career or personal situations that stifle your creativity, development, and happiness. Knowing how you learn and how you relate to the world can help you make smarter choices.

2. You will be more successful on the job. Your learning style is essentially your working style. If you know how you learn, you will be able to look for an environment that suits you best and you'll be able to work effectively on work teams. This will prepare you for successful employment in a nursing career in the twenty-first century.

3. You will be better able to target areas that need improvement. The more you know about your learning styles, the more you will be able to pinpoint the areas that are more difficult for you. That has two advantages. One, you can begin to work on difficult areas, step by step. Two, when a task comes up requiring a skill that is tough for you, you can either take special care with it or suggest someone else whose style may be better suited to it.

Your learning style profile is one important part of self-knowledge. Next you will explore other important factors that help to define you.

 ## HOW DO YOU EXPLORE WHO YOU ARE?

You are an absolutely unique individual. Although you may share individual characteristics with others, your combination of traits is one-of-a-kind. It will take a lifetime to learn everything there is to know about yourself, because you are constantly changing. However, you can start by exploring these facets of yourself: self-perception, interests, habits, abilities, and limitations.

Self-Perception

TERMS

Self-perception
How one views
oneself, one's
opinion of
oneself.

Having an accurate image of yourself is difficult. Unfortunately, many people do not have an accurate self-image. Feeling inadequate from time to time is normal, but a constantly negative self-perception can have destructive effects. Look at people you know who think that they are less intelligent, capable, or attractive than they really are. Observe how that shuts down their confidence and motivation. You do the same when you perceive yourself in a poor light.

For example, say you think you can't pass a certain course. Since you feel you don't have a chance, you don't put as much effort into the work for that course. Sure enough, at the end of the semester, you don't pass. The worst part is that you may see your failure as proof of your incapability, instead of realizing that you didn't allow yourself to try. This chain of events can occur in many situations. When it happens in the workplace, people lose jobs. When it happens in personal life, people lose relationships.

Refine your self-image so that it reflects more of your true self. These strategies might help.

- **Believe in yourself.** If you don't believe in yourself, others may have a harder time believing in you. Work to eliminate negative self-talk, for example, "I have a math block." Have faith in your abilities. When you set your goals, stick to them. Know that your mind and will are very powerful.
- **Talk to other people whom you trust.** People who know you well often have a more realistic perception of you than you do of yourself. Ask them what they think about your abilities and strengths.
- **Take personal time.** Stress makes having perspective on your life more difficult. Take time out to clear your mind and think realistically about who you are, who you want to be, and what is most important in your life.
- **Look at all of the evidence.** Mistakes can loom large in your mind. Consider what you do well and what you have accomplished as carefully as you consider your stumbles.

Building a positive self-perception is a lifelong challenge. If you maintain a bright but realistic vision of yourself, it will take you far along the road toward achieving your goals.

Interests

Taking some time now to explore your interests will help you later when you select a major and a career. You may be aware of many of your general interests already. For example, you can ask yourself:

- What areas of study do I like?
- What activities make me happy?
- What careers seem interesting to me?
- What kind of daily schedule do I like to keep (early riser, night owl)?
- What type of home and work environment do I prefer?

Interests play an important role in your life and in the workplace. Many people, however, do not take their interests seriously when choosing a career. Some make salary or stability their first priority. Some feel they have to take the first job that comes along. Some may not realize they can do better. Not considering what you are interested in may lead to an area of study or a job that leaves you unhappy, uninterested, or unfulfilled.

S—*Say* you want a registered nurse caring for you at the bedside.

A—*Ask* what other personnel will be caring for you and how, so you'll know what to expect.

F—*Firmly* insist that an RN assess your condition at least once per shift and provide you with medications.

E—*Express* any serious concerns immediately to the Director of Nursing or Director of Patient Care Services.

AMERICAN NURSES ASSOCIATION (ANA)

DAWN E. BEDELL

Sophomore, Truman College, Chicago, Illinois

I first heard about learning styles in a vocational class that I took my freshman year in college. The instructor explained that each student has their own unique way to learn. I liked the idea that learning could be a fun adventure, instead of just something you do to get a good grade.

Since then, I've noticed a few things about how I learn. For example, I usually need a little background noise to stay focused when I'm studying, so I turn on the television. And, unlike some students, I prefer straight lecture. If a teacher uses visual aids, like an overhead projector, I can't concentrate on taking notes. I also don't find graphs or charts helpful, even when they're in textbooks.

Something else that really affects my learning is the teacher's attitude. Last year I had a science teacher who seemed impatient. He acted annoyed when student's asked questions, and he made me feel incapable of learning. Instead, I like teachers who joke around and who show that they care about you. For instance, I had a figure drawing class that I thought was going to be too hard for me. The teacher saw that I was struggling, and he took the time to encourage me. I got an A in that class, and I discovered that I have a natural ability to draw.

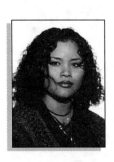

Another interest I have is writing. I like to write poetry, and I've been keeping a journal ever since high school. My mother is a Chippewa Indian, and I'm proud of that heritage. I especially like to write about the American Indian's freedom of expression through dance. I also enjoy reading literature.

I've always done well in lab work, too. This semester I'm taking a microbiology course, and I love working with the microscopes. I wish you could see my lab book; I've made some really cool sketches of the human brain and heart. Now, I'm planning to major in forensic medicine. I knew I really liked science, and with my interest in art, the field of forensics seems to click for me. When I tell people that someday I want to do autopsies or work in a mortuary, they look at me like I'm crazy. But their reaction just confirms how we each have different interests and abilities.

Although I've noted a few things here about how I learn, it just seems like a mixed bag of likes and dislikes. I don't see any clear patterns. What more can I do to understand and develop my learning potential?

M. KAY CRESCI, PH.D., R.N., C.C.R.N.

Instructor, The Johns Hopkins University School of Nursing, Baltimore, Maryland

As health care professionals in the information age, we must become lifelong learners. Therefore, recognizing how you learn best and your personal 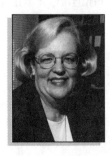 learning preferences can help you maximize your learning strengths. This is referred to as your learning style, or the way you take in and process information (R. Felder, 1996).[6] To identify your learning style, you need to think about how you learn and your preferred learning modalities: physical, environmental, cognitive, affective, and socioeconomic. Using this information allows you to not only develop successful learning strategies but also assists you in showing teachers and mentors how to best guide you.

There are a number of instruments available for determining your learning style. The Center for Teaching and Learning at Indiana University has a website listing a number of these inventories and their authors (http://web.indstate.edu/ctl/styles/invent.html) and where available direct links to on-line instruments. The inventories are categorized according to major learning style approaches: instructional preferences, social interaction models, information processing, and personality levels. You may also find on-line learning style inventories through a search engine such as altavista (http://www.altavista.com). In the search box, type "learning style" within quotation marks. Many of these authors give you immediate feedback on your learning style and appropriate learning strategies to use based on that style. Felder (1993) stresses that to function effectively in any professional capacity requires that you develop your skills in most learning style modes.[7]

In the literature, models of learning styles tend to identify four dimensions of learning: perceiving, organizing, processing, and understanding. Do you perceive information through your senses (visual or verbal) or intuitively through your thoughts and ideas? Do you organize information using facts and observations (inductive) or through deducing outcomes from given principles? Do you process information actively through engagement with others or reflectively through introspection? Finally, do you understand information through a logical sequence of steps or though seeing the global picture (Felder, 1993)? Answering these questions can help you find clues to your learning puzzle.

Another approach to exploring learning styles is the Theory of Multiple Intelligences by Howard Gardner (1991).[8] He has identified eight potential ways we may process information: verbal/linguistic, logical/mathematical, visual/spatial, bodily/kinesthetic, musical, interpersonal, intrapersonal, and naturalistic. When using this theory, it's important to recognize that intelligence and learning style are not one and the same. Intelligence is the capacity or ability to learn a designated area of knowledge, where as learning style exhibits a tendency toward learning in a specific direction (Winters, E.).[9]

Choosing to consider your interests and happiness takes courage but brings benefits. Think about your life. You spend hours of time both attending classes and studying outside of class. You will spend at least eight hours a day, five or more days a week, up to fifty or more weeks a year as a working contributor to the world. Although your studies and work won't always make you deliriously happy, it is possible to spend your school and work time in a manner that suits you.

For instance, you may be a nursing major because everyone told you that you'd never get a job, or make money, as a writer—what you really wanted to study in college. Rather than choosing one or the other, combining them may be a possibility. You can continue as a nursing major and take plenty of writing and literature courses as electives. Plan on continuing your study of literature as a lifelong pursuit *and* working as a nurse. Your various interests are not mutually exclusive; they can actually enhance each other. Creativity helps you in nursing, while nursing can help in your other pursuits. Echo Heron, RN, has written several best sellers about her experiences in critical care. Nursing is *the* place to learn about human nature and to participate in plenty of fascinating stories.

Here are two positive effects of focusing on your interests.

1. You will have more energy. Think about how you feel when you are looking forward to seeing a special person, participating in a favorite sports activity, or enjoying some entertainment. When you're doing something you like, time seems to pass very quickly. You will be able to get much more done in a subject or career area that you enjoy.

2. You will perform better. When you were in high school, you probably got your best grades in your favorite classes and excelled in your favorite activities. That doesn't change as you get older. The more you like something, the harder you work at it—and the harder you work, the more you will improve.

Habits

A preference for a particular action that you do a certain way, and often on a regular basis or at certain times, is a habit. You might have a habit of showering in the morning, eating raisins, channel surfing with the TV remote control, hitting the snooze button on your clock, talking for hours on the phone, or studying late at night. Your habits reveal a lot about you. Some habits you consider to be good habits, and some may be bad habits.

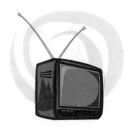

Bad habits earn that title because they can prevent you from reaching important goals. Some bad habits, such as, chronic lateness or smoking, cause obvious problems. Other habits, such as, renting movies three times a week, may not seem bad until you realize that you needed to spend those hours studying. People maintain bad habits because they offer immediate, enjoyable rewards, even if later effects are negative. For example, going out to eat frequently may drain your budget, but at first it seems easier than shopping for food, cooking, and washing dishes.

Good habits are those that have positive effects on your life. You often have to wait longer and work harder to see a reward for good habits, which makes them harder to maintain. If you cut out fattening foods, you wouldn't lose weight in two days. If you reduced your nights out to gain study time, your grades wouldn't improve in a week. When you strive to maintain good habits, trust that the rewards are somewhere down the road.

Take time to evaluate your habits. Look at the positive and negative effects of each, and decide which are helpful and which are harmful to you. Changing a habit can be a long process. Here are steps you can take to change a habit, to successfully make a behavior change.

1. Be honest about your habits. Admitting negative or destructive habits can be hard to do. You can't change a habit until you admit that it is a habit.
2. Recognize the habit as troublesome. Sometimes the trouble may not seem to come directly from the habit. For example, spending every weekend working on the house may seem important, but you may be overdoing it and ignoring friends and family members.
3. Decide to change. You might realize what your bad habits are but do not yet care about their effects on your life. Until you are convinced that you will receive something positive and useful from changing, your efforts will not get you far.
4. Start today. Don't put it off until after this week, after the family reunion, or after the semester. Each day lost is a day you haven't had the chance to benefit from a new lifestyle.
5. Change one habit at a time. Changing or breaking habits is difficult. Trying to spend more time with your family, reduce TV time, increase studying, and save more money all at once can bring on a fit of deprivation, sending you scurrying back to all your old habits. Easy does it.

6. Reward yourself appropriately for positive steps taken. If you earn a good grade, avoid slacking off on your studies the following week. Choose a reward that will not encourage you to stray from your target.

7. Keep it up. To have the best chance at changing a habit, be consistent for at least three weeks. Your brain needs time to become accustomed to the new habit. If you go back to the old habit during that time, you may feel like you're starting all over again.

8. Don't get too discouraged. Rarely does someone make the decision to change and do so without a setback or two. Being too hard on yourself might cause frustration that tempts you to give up and go back to the habit.

Abilities

Everyone's abilities include both strengths and limitations. And both can change. Examining both strengths and limitations is part of establishing the kind of clear vision of yourself that will help you to live up to your potential.

Strengths

As you think about your preferences, your particular strengths will come to mind, because you often like best the things you can do well. Some strengths seem to be natural—things you learned to do without ever having to work too hard. Others you struggled to develop and continue to work hard to maintain. Asking yourself these questions may help you define more clearly what your abilities are:

- What have I always been able to do well?
- What have others often praised about me?
- What do I like most about myself, and why?
- What is my learning style profile?
- What are my accomplishments—at home, at school, at work?

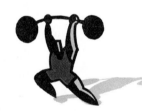

As with your preferences, knowing your abilities will help you find a job that makes the most of them. When your job requires you to do work you like, you are more likely to perform to the best of your ability. Keep that in mind as you explore nursing career areas. Assessments and inventories that will help you further assess your abilities may be available at your school's career center or library. Once you know yourself, you will be more able to set appropriate goals.

Limitations

Being human means that nobody is perfect, and no one is good at everything. Everyone has limitations. However, that doesn't mean they are easy to take. Limitations can make you feel frustrated, stressed, or angry. You may feel as though no one else has the limitations you have, or that no one else has as many.

"Strive for excellence with the understanding that learning is a life long process. Don't be afraid to question or admit you don't know something. The only stupid questions are those that go unasked."

MARY ANNE DUMAS, RN, PHD, CFNP

There are three ways to deal with your limitations. The first two—ignoring them or dwelling on them—are the most common. Neither is wise. The third way is to face them and to work to improve them while keeping the strongest focus on your abilities.

Ignoring your limitations can cause you to be unable to accomplish your goals. For example, say you are an active, global learner with a well-developed interpersonal intelligence. You have limitations in logical-mathematical intelligence and in linear thought. Ignoring that fact, you decide that you want to be a nurse and sign up for math courses. You certainly won't fail automatically. However, if you ignore your limitations related to those courses and don't seek extra help, you may have more than a few stumbles.

Dwelling on your limitations can make you forget you have any strengths at all. This results in negative self-talk and a poor self-perception. Continuing the example, if you were to dwell on your limitations in math, you might very likely stop trying altogether.

Facing limitations and working to improve them is the logical response. A healthy understanding of your limitations can help you avoid troublesome situations. In the example, you could face your limitations in math and explore other career areas that use your more well-developed abilities and intelligences. If you decided to stick with nursing, you could study an area of the field that focuses on management and interpersonal relationships.

Sabiduría

In Spanish, the term *sabiduría* represents the two sides of learning—both knowledge and wisdom. Knowledge—building what you know about how the world works—is the first part. Wisdom—deriving meaning and significance from knowledge, and deciding how to use that knowledge—is the second. As you continually learn and experience new things, the *sabiduría* you build will help you make knowledgeable and wise choices about how to lead your life.

Think of this concept as you discover more about how you learn and receive knowledge in all aspects of your life—in school, work, and personal situations. As you learn how your unique mind works and how to use it, you can more confidently assert yourself. As you expand your ability to use your mind in different ways, you can create lifelong advantages for yourself.

Applications   Chapter 3

KEY INTO YOUR LIFE
Opportunities to Apply What You Learn

 3.1 *How Do You Learn Best?*

Start by writing your scores next to each term.
Circle your highest preferences (largest numbers) for each assessment.

LEARNING STYLES INVENTORY	PATHWAYS TO LEARNING	PERSONALITY SPECTRUM
_____ Active	_____ Bodily-Kinesthetic	_____ Organizer
_____ Reflective	_____ Visual-Spatial	_____ Adventurer
_____ Factual	_____ Verbal-Linguistic	_____ Giver
_____ Theoretical	_____ Logical-Mathematical	_____ Thinker
_____ Visual	_____ Musical	
_____ Verbal	_____ Interpersonal	
_____ Linear	_____ Intrapersonal	
_____ Holistic	_____ Naturalist	

What positive experiences have you had at work and school that you can link
to the strengths you circled?

_____

_____

_____

_____

_____

_____

What negative experiences have you had that may be related to your least-developed learning styles or intelligences?

_____

_____

_____

_____

_____

 ## *Making School More Enjoyable*

List two required classes that you are not necessarily looking forward to taking. Discuss what parts of your learning style profile may relate to your lack of enthusiasm. Name learning styles–related study techniques that may help you get the most out of the class and enjoy it more.

CLASS	REASON FOR LACK OF ENTHUSIASM	LEARNING OR STUDY TECHNIQUES
1.		
2.		

 ## *Your Habits*

You have the power to change your habits. List three habits that you want to change. Discuss the effects of each and how those effects keep you from reaching your goals.

HABIT	EFFECTS THAT PREVENT YOU FROM REACHING GOALS
1.	
2.	
3.	

Out of these three, put a star by the habit you want to change first. Write down a step you can take today toward overcoming that habit.

_____

_____

_____

What helpful habit do you want to develop in its place? For example, if your problem habit were a failure to express yourself when you are angry, a replacement habit might be to talk calmly about situations that upset you as soon as they arise. If you have a habit of cramming for tests at the last minute, you could replace it with a regular study schedule that allows you to cover your material bit by bit over a longer period of time.

_____

_____

_____

One way to help yourself abandon your old habit is to think about how your new habit will improve your life. List two benefits of your new habit.

1. _____

2. _____

Give yourself one month to complete your habit shift. Set a specific deadline. Keep track of your progress by indicating on a chart or calendar how well you did each day. If you avoided the old habit, write an X below the day. If you used the new one, write an N. Therefore, a day when you only avoided the old habit will have an X; a day when you did both will have both letters; and a day when you did neither will be left blank. You can use the chart below or mark your own calendar. Try pairing up with another student and arranging to check up on each other's progress.

1	2	3	4	5	6	7	8	9	10	11	12	13	14	15	16
17	18	19	20	21	22	23	24	25	26	27	28	29	30	31	

Don't forget to reward yourself for your hard work. Write here what your reward will be when you feel you are on the road to a new and beneficial habit.

_____

_____

_____

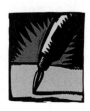

KEY TO SELF-EXPRESSION
Discovery Through Journal Writing

To record your thoughts, use a separate journal or the lined pages at the end of the chapter.

Your Learning Style Profile. Discuss the insights you have gained, through exploring your learning style profile, about your strengths and struggles at school and work. What new strengths have come to your attention? What struggles have you become aware of that you couldn't explain before? Talk about how your insights may have changed the way you see yourself as a nursing major.

Journal

Journal

Name _____   Date _____

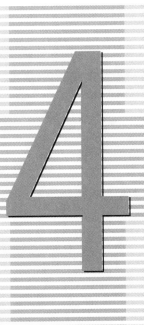

4

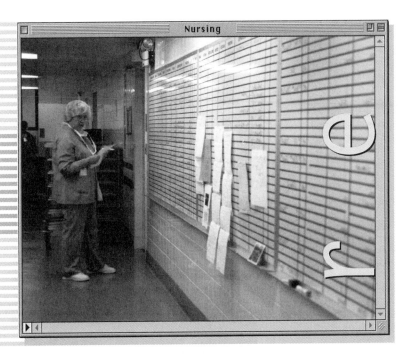

Goal Setting and Time Management

Mapping Your Course

People dream of what they want out of life, but not everyone knows how to turn dreams into reality. Often dreams seem far off in time, too difficult, or even completely unreachable. You can build paths to your dreams, however, by identifying the goals you need to achieve, one by one, to arrive at your destination. When you set goals, prioritize, and manage your time effectively, you increase your ability to take those steps to achieve your long-term goals.

This chapter explains how taking specific steps toward your goals can help you turn your dreams into reality. You will explore how your values relate to your goals, how to create a framework for your life's goals, how to set long-term and short-term goals, and how to set priorities. The section on time management will discuss how to translate those goals into daily, weekly, monthly, and yearly steps. Finally, you will explore the effects of procrastination.

In this chapter, you will explore answers to the following questions:

- What defines your values?
- How do you set and achieve goals?
- What are your priorities?
- How can you manage your time?
- Why is procrastination a problem?

WHAT DEFINES YOUR VALUES?

TERMS

Values
Principles or qualities that one considers important, right, or good.

Your personal values are the beliefs that guide your choices. Examples of values include family togetherness, a good education, caring for others, working to protect the environment, and worthwhile employment. The sum total of all your values is your *value system*. You demonstrate your particular value system in the priorities you set, how you communicate with others, your family life, your educational and career choices, even the material things with which you surround yourself, and your lifestyle.

Choosing and Evaluating Values

"Organization is the power of the day. Without it, nothing great is accomplished."
SOPHIA PALMER, 1897

Examining the sources of your values can help you define those values, trace their origin, and question the reasons why you have adopted them. Value sources, however, aren't as important as the process of considering each value carefully to see if it makes sense to you. Some of your current values may have come from television or other media but still ring true. Some may come from what others have taught you. Some you may have constructed from your own personal experience and opinion. You make the final decision about what to value, regardless of the source.

Each individual value system is unique, even if many values come from other sources. Your value system is yours alone. Your responsibility is to make sure that your values are your own choice, not the choice of others. Make value choices for yourself based on what feels right for you, for your life, and for those who are touched by your life.

You can be more sure of making choices that are right for you if you try to always question and evaluate your values. Before you adopt a value, ask yourself: Does it feel right? What effects might it have on my life? Am I choosing it to please someone else, or is it truly my choice? Values are a design for life, and you are the one who has to live the life you design.

Because life changes and new experiences may bring a change in values, try to continue to evaluate values as time goes by. Periodically evaluate the effects that having each value has on your life, and see if a shift in values might suit your changing circumstances. For example, losing your sight may cause you to value your hearing intensely. The difficulty of a divorce may have a positive result: a new value of independence and individuality. After growing up in a homogeneous community, a student who meets other students from unfamiliar backgrounds may learn a new value of living in a diverse community. Your values will grow and develop as you do if you continue to think them through.

How Values Relate to Goals

Understanding your values will help you set your nursing career and personal goals, because the most ideal goals help you achieve what you value. Values of financial independence or simple living may generate goals, such as working while going to school and keeping credit card debt low, that reflect the value. If you value helping others, try to make time for volunteer work.

Goals enable you to put values into practice. When you set and pursue goals that are based on values, you demonstrate and reinforce values through taking action. The strength of those values, in turn, reinforces your goals. You will experience a much stronger drive to achieve if you build goals around what is most important to you.

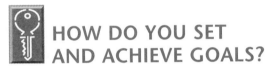

HOW DO YOU SET AND ACHIEVE GOALS?

TERMS

Goal
An end toward which effort is directed; an aim or intention.

A goal can be something as concrete as taking biochemistry next semester or as abstract as working to control your temper. When you set goals and work to achieve them, you engage your intelligence, abilities, time, and energy in order to move ahead. From major life decisions to the tiniest day-to-day activities, setting goals will help you define how you want to live and what you want to achieve.

Paul Timm, a best-selling author and teacher who is an expert in self-management, feels that focus is a key ingredient in setting and achieving goals. "Focus adds power to our actions. If somebody threw a bucket of water on you, you'd get wet, and probably get mad. But if water was shot at you through a high-pressure nozzle, you might get injured. The only difference is focus."[1] Each part of this section will explain ways to focus your energy through goal setting. You can set and achieve goals by defining a personal mission statement, placing your goals in long-term and short-term time frames, evaluating goals in terms of your values, and linking your goals to your values.

Identifying Your "Personal Mission Statement"

Some people go through their lives without ever really thinking about what they can do or what they want to achieve. If you choose not to set goals or explore what you want out of life, you may look back on your past with a sense of emptiness. You may not know what you've done or why you did it.

By periodically taking a few steps back and thinking about where you've been and where you want to be, you'll live more consciously.

One helpful way to determine your general direction is to write a *personal mission statement*. Dr. Stephen Covey, author of the best-seller *The Seven Habits of Highly Effective People*, defines a mission statement as a philosophy that outlines what you want to be (character), what you want to do (contributions and achievements), and the principles by which you live. Dr. Covey compares the personal mission statement to the Constitution of the United States, a statement of principles that gives this country guidance and standards in the face of constant change.[2]

Your personal mission isn't written in stone. It should change as you move from one phase of life to the next—from single person to spouse, from parent to single parent to caregiver of an older parent. Stay flexible and reevaluate your personal mission from time to time.

Here is an example of author Janet Katz's personal mission statement:

> My mission is to uphold the nursing profession's value of advocating for those in need by promoting the health and well-being of people of all ages, backgrounds, and economic levels through local and international community health efforts. I intend to celebrate life through service to others and caring for myself and my family.

Here is a mission statement from Immunex Corporation, a biotechnology company based in Seattle, Washington:

> Immunex is a biopharmaceutical company dedicated to developing immune system science to protect human health. The company's products offer hope to patients with cancer, inflammatory and infectious diseases.

Another example is from The Nature Conservancy, a nonprofit organization responsible for the protection of more than 10 million acres in the United States and Canada and partnerships in Latin America, the Caribbean, the Pacific, and Asia:

> The mission of The Nature Conservancy is to preserve plants, animals, and natural communities that represent the diversity of life on Earth by protecting the lands and waters they need to survive.

You will have an opportunity to write your own personal mission statement at the end of this chapter. Writing a mission statement is much more than an in-school exercise. It is truly for you. Thinking through your personal mission can help you begin to take charge of your life. It helps to put you in control instead of allowing circumstances and events to control you. If you frame your mission statement carefully so that it truly reflects your goals, it can be your guide in everything you do.

Placing Goals in Time

Everyone has the same 24 hours in a day, but it often doesn't feel like enough. Have you ever had a busy day flash by so quickly that it seems you accomplished nothing? Have you ever felt that way about a longer period of time, like a month or even a year? Your commitments can overwhelm you unless you decide how to use time to plan your steps toward goal achievement.

If developing a personal mission statement establishes the big picture, placing your goals within particular time frames allows you to bring individual areas of that picture into the foreground. Planning your progress step-by-step will help you maintain your efforts over the extended time period often needed to accomplish a goal. Goals fall into two categories: long-term and short-term.

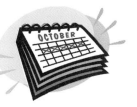

Setting Long-Term Goals

Establish first the goals that have the largest scope; that is, the *long-term goals* that you aim to attain over a lengthy period of time, up to a few years or more. As a student, you know what long-term goals are all about. You have set yourself a goal to attend school and earn a degree. Becoming educated is an admirable goal that takes a good number of years to attain.

Some long-term goals are lifelong, such as a goal to continually learn more about yourself and the world around you. Others have a more definite end, such as a goal to complete a course successfully. To determine your long-term goals, think about what you want out of your professional, educational, and personal life. Here is Janet Katz's long-term goal statement.

Janet's Goals: To accomplish my mission through writing books and journal articles, teaching nursing students, and developing improved methods for promoting the profession of nursing and its values. To create and maintain a lifestyle that is conducive to my own physical and mental health and that of my family.

For example, you may establish long-term goals such as these:

- I will graduate from college with the degree I most desire, having learned and understood as much as I could in a wide range of subjects.
- I will build my science inquiry into nursing research skills through work, volunteering, and internships or through relationships with course instructors, other nursing professionals, classmates, and coworkers.

Long-term goals can change later in your life. To begin long-term goal setting, start with next year. Deciding what you want to accomplish in the next year and writing it down will help you to focus clearly on productive actions. These goals are not like New Year's resolutions; they are based on what you really are willing to work toward and accomplish. Janet's goals focused on what she wanted to accomplish next year.

1. Finish current book project and begin investigating dissertation topic for Ph.D.
2. To exercise daily, eat six to seven servings of fruits and vegetables per day, and read books for my own enjoyment. Make time to reflect on my life and the life around me.

In the same way that Janet's goals are tailored to her personality and interests, your goals should reflect who you are. Personal missions and goals are as unique as each individual. Continuing the example above, you might adopt these goals for the coming year:

- I will earn passing grades in all my classes.
- I will volunteer and assist my biology professor in her current research project.

Setting Short-Term Goals

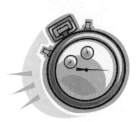

When you divide your long-term goals into smaller, manageable goals that you hope to accomplish within a relatively short time, you are setting *short-term goals*. Short-term goals narrow your focus, helping you to maintain your progress toward your long-term goals. They are the steps that take you where you want to go. Say you have set the two long-term goals you just read in the previous section. To stay on track toward those goals, you may want to accomplish these short-term goals in the next six months:

- I will pass Chemistry I, so that I can move on to Chemistry II.
- I will read three journal articles pertinent to my biology professor's research project.

These same goals can be broken down into even smaller parts, such as in one month:

- I will complete the last week's lab write-up and do the reading for the next week's lab by Sunday night of each week.
- I will read a research article from the *Journal of Nursing Research* and prepare a brief report on it for next month's Nursing Student club's brown bag seminar.

In addition to monthly goals, you may have short-term goals that extend a week, a day, or even a couple of hours in a given day. Take as an example the article you planned to present for next month's Nursing Student club's brown bag seminar. Such short-term goals may include the following:

- Three weeks from now: Attend the seminar ready to present a 10-minute clear summary of a research article from the *Journal of Nursing Research*.
- Two weeks from now: Have a final draft of the presentation and ask another club member to review it.
- One week from now: Have a first draft of an outline ready, and ask the seminar instructor to read it.
- Today by the end of the day: Find an interesting research article, and submit it to the seminar instructor.
- By 3 P.M. today: Brainstorm ideas of topics, and go to the library to start searching the *Journal of Nursing Research*.

As you consider your long-term and short-term goals, notice how all of your goals are linked to one another. As Figure 4-1 shows, your long-term

FIGURE 4-1   Linking goals together.

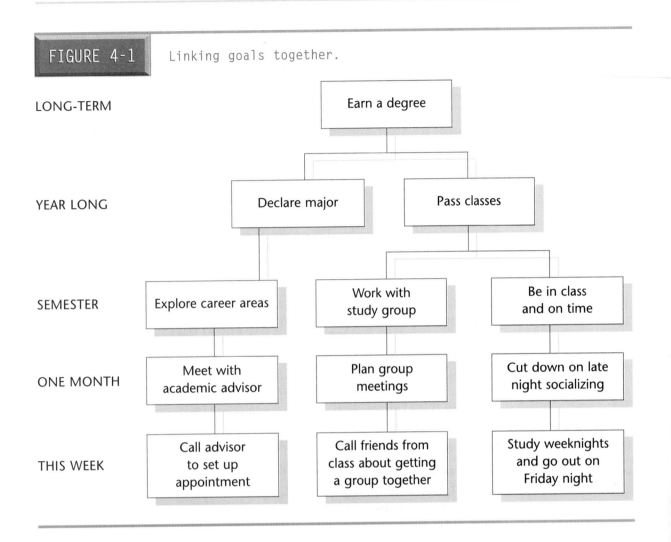

goals establish a context for the short-term goals. In turn, your short-term goals make the long-term goals seem clearer and more reachable. The whole system works to keep you on track.

Linking Goals with Values

If you are not sure how to start formulating your mission, look to your values to guide you. Define your mission and goals based on what is important to you.

If you value physical fitness, your mission statement might emphasize your commitment to staying in shape throughout your life. Your long-term goal might be to run a marathon, while your short-term goals might involve your weekly exercise and eating plans. Similarly, if you value a close family, your personal mission might emphasize how you want to maintain family ties and stability. In this case, your long-term goals might involve finding a job that allows for family time or living in a town close to your parents. Your short-term goals may focus on helping your son learn a musical instrument or having dinner with your family at least twice a week.

"The common good for which we strive can be stated in six words—better schools, better nurses, better service."

ISABEL McISAAC, 1912

Current and Personal Values Mean Appropriate Goals

When you use your values as a compass for your goals, make sure the compass is pointed in the direction of your real feelings. Watch out for the following two pitfalls that can occur.

Setting goals according to other peoples' values. Friends or family may encourage you to strive for what they think you should value, rather than what is right for you. If you follow their advice without believing in it, you may have a harder time sticking to your path. For example, someone who attends school primarily because a parent or spouse thought it was right may have less motivation and initiative than someone who made an independent decision to become a student. Look hard at what you really want, and why. Staying in tune with your own values will help you make decisions that are right for you.

Setting goals that reflect values you held in the past. What you felt yesterday may no longer apply, because life changes can alter your values. The best goals reflect what you believe today. For example, a person who has been through a near-fatal car accident may experience a dramatic increase in how he or she values time with friends and family, and a drop in how he or she values material possessions. Someone who survives a serious illness may value healthy living above all else. Keep in touch with your life's changes so your goals can reflect who you are.

Values Can Help You Identify Educational Goals

Education is a major part of your life right now. In order to define a context for your school goals, explore what you value about pursuing an education. People have many reasons for attending college. You may identify with one or more of the following possible reasons:

- I want to earn a higher salary.
- I want to build marketable skills.
- My supervisor at work says that a degree will help me move ahead in my career.
- Most of my friends were going.
- I want to be a student and learn all that I can.
- It seems like the only option for me right now.
- I am recently divorced and need to find a way to earn money.
- Everybody in my family goes to college; it's expected.
- I don't feel ready to jump into the working world yet.
- I got a scholarship.
- My friend loves her job and encouraged me to take courses in the field.
- My parent (or a spouse or partner) pushed me to go to college.
- I am pregnant and need to increase my skills so I can provide for my baby.
- I am studying for a specific career.
- I don't really know.

All of these answers are legitimate, even the last one. Being honest with yourself is crucial if you want to discover who you are and what life paths make sense for you. Whatever your reasons are for being in school, you are at the gateway to a journey of discovery.

It isn't easy to enroll in college, pay tuition, decide what to study, sign up for classes, gather the necessary materials, and actually get yourself to the school and into the classroom. Many people drop out at different places along the way, but somehow your reasons have been compelling enough for you to have arrived at this point. Thinking about why you value your education will help you stick with it.

Achieving goals becomes easier when you are realistic about what is possible. Setting priorities will help you make that distinction.

 ## WHAT ARE YOUR PRIORITIES?

When you set a priority, you identify what's important at any given moment. *Prioritizing* helps you focus on your most important goals, even when they are difficult to achieve. If you were to pursue your goals in no particular order, you might tackle the easy ones first and leave the tough ones for later. The risk is that you might never reach for goals that are important to your success. Setting priorities helps you focus your plans on accomplishing your most important goals.

To explore your priorities, think about your personal mission and look at your goals in the five life areas: personal, family, school/career, finances, and lifestyle. These five areas may not all be equally important to you right now. At this stage in your life, which two or three are most critical? Is one particular category more important than others? How would you prioritize your goals from most important to least important?

You are a unique individual, and your priorities are yours alone. What may be top priority to someone else may not mean that much to you, and vice versa. You can see this in Figure 4-2, which compares the priorities of two very different students. Each student's priorities are listed in order, with the first priority at the top and the lowest priority at the bottom.

First and foremost, your priorities should reflect your personal goals. In addition, they should reflect your relationships with others. For example, if you are a parent, your children's needs will probably be high on the priority list. You may decide to go back to school so you can get a better job, earn more money, and give them a better life. If you are in a committed relationship, you may consider the needs of your partner. You may schedule your classes so that you and your partner are home together as often as possible. Even as you consider the needs of others, though, never lose sight of your personal goals. Be true to your goals and priorities so that you can make the most of who you are.

Setting priorities moves you closer to accomplishing specific goals. It also helps you begin planning to achieve your goals within specific time frames. Being able to achieve your goals is directly linked to effective time management.

TERMS

Priority
An action or intention that takes precedence in time, attention, or position.

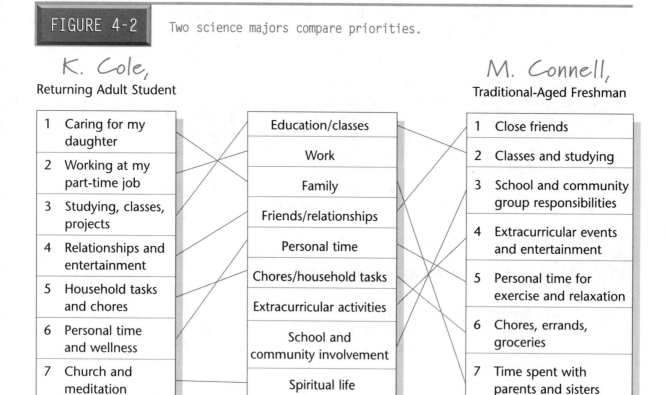

FIGURE 4-2   Two science majors compare priorities.

 ## HOW CAN YOU MANAGE YOUR TIME?

Time is one of your most valuable and precious resources. Unlike money, or opportunity, or connections, time doesn't discriminate—everyone has the same twenty-four hours in a day, every day. Your responsibility and your potential for success lie in how you use yours. You cannot manipulate or change how time passes, but you can spend it taking steps to achieve your goals. Efficient time management helps you achieve your goals in a steady, step-by-step process.

Classes, especially science classes, can be time-consuming because they often include lab time and many hours of study. As a pre-nursing or nursing major, you can promote your own success by learning to creatively and accurately manage your time.

People have a variety of different approaches to time management. Your learning style (explained in more detail in Chapter 3) can help you identify the particular way you currently use your time. For example, factual and linear learners tend to organize activities within a framework of time. Because they stay aware of how long it takes them to do something or travel somewhere, they are usually prompt. Theoretical and holistic learners tend to miss the passing of time while they are busy thinking of something else. Because they focus on the big picture, they may neglect details such as structuring their activities within available time. They frequently lose track of time and can often be late without meaning to be.

Time management, like physical fitness, is a lifelong pursuit. No one can plan a perfect schedule or build a terrific physique and then be "done." You'll work at time management throughout your life, and it can be tiring. Your ability to manage your time will vary with your mood, your stress level, how busy you are, and other factors. You're human; don't expect perfection. Just do your best. Time management involves building a schedule and making your schedule work through lists and other strategies.

Building a Schedule

Being in control of how you manage your time is a key factor in taking responsibility for yourself and your choices. When you plan your activities with an eye toward achieving your most important goals, you are taking personal responsibility for how you live. Building a schedule helps you be responsible.

Just as a road map helps you travel from place to place, a *schedule* is a time-and-activity map that helps you get from the beginning of the day (or week, or month) to the end as smoothly as possible. A written schedule helps you gain control of your life. Schedules have two major advantages: They allocate segments of time for the fulfillment of your daily, weekly, monthly, and longer-term goals, and they serve as a concrete reminder of tasks, events, due dates, responsibilities, and deadlines. Few moments are more stressful than suddenly realizing you have forgotten to pick up a prescription, take a test, or be on duty at work. Scheduling can help you avoid events like these. Learning these skills now will really help you later on in nursing school when you will be studying extremely hard.

Keep a Date Book

Gather the tools of the trade: a pen or pencil and a *date book* (sometimes called a planner). Some of you already have date books and may have used them for years. Others may have had no luck with them or have never tried. Even if you don't feel you are the type of person who would use one, give it a try. A date book is indispensable for keeping track of your time. Paul Timm says, "Most time management experts agree that rule number one in a thoughtful planning process is: Use some form of a planner where you can write things down."

There are two major types of date books. The *day-at-a-glance* version devotes a page to each day. While it gives you ample space to write the day's activities, this version makes it difficult to see what's ahead. The *week-at-a-glance* book gives you a view of the week's plans but has less room to write per day. If you write out your daily plans in detail, you might like the day-at-a-glance version. If you prefer to remind yourself of plans ahead of time, try the book that shows a week's schedule all at once. Some date books contain additional sections that allow you to note plans and goals for the year as a whole and for each month. You can also create your own sheets for yearly and monthly notations in a notepad section, if your book has one, or on plain paper that you can then insert into the book.

PATRICIA CURTIS

Junior, Georgetown University, Washington, D.C.

I plan to become a pediatric nurse with a special-ty in HIV/AIDS. During my clinicals, I've had the opportunity to take care of several HIV babies. Since I'm a student and only care for one patient during clinical rotations, I've felt gratified know-ing that I made their hospital stay a little more bearable by giving them the extra attention that they may need. Although I'm confident that I'll like the profession I've chosen, I still feel over-whelmed at times by the stress of preparing to become a nurse.

For one thing, I'm concerned about the diffi-culty I have in talking with the parents of the children. I'm more comfortable than I was at the start of clinicals, but it's still an issue. I find that parents don't seem to have a lot of faith in what I'm saying. For example, I had to tell the mother of one of my patients about a procedure on her son. She was asking me a lot of questions, and I

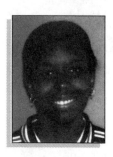

thought I did a thorough job answering her concerns. But when we finished our discus-sion, she still wanted to talk with the doctor.

I know I look pretty young for my age so that may be one reason why parents don't take me seriously, but I wonder if it will continue being this way once I graduate. Also, I find it diffi-cult when parents get upset with me about a procedure that I need to do on their child. How can I effectively communicate with them?

Another stress I face in college is time man-agement. There's always so much to do that I feel guilty relaxing or having fun. I'm doing well in my classes but sometimes I feel like it's killing me. This semester I have two courses that require a total of 12 hours of clinical work plus 200 pages of reading a week. I also work part-time as a student supervisor at the main campus library. Luckily I have an understanding boss that allows me flexible hours. With regard to extracurricular activities, I'm involved in the Student Nurses Association that includes volun-teer work at health organizations and fund-raising. Finding time for exercise seems next to impossible, but without exercise I don't have an outlet for the stress.

The nurses I work with in clinicals tell me time management continues to be a problem for them even though they are no longer in school. It's ironic that we are health care professionals and yet we have a hard time knowing how to take care of ourselves. Do you have any suggestions about how I can manage my time more efficiently so that I feel less stressed?

DR. LINA BADR

Associate Professor, University of California, Los Angeles, California

Being comfortable communicating with parents doesn't come with a degree. Confidence as a nurse comes with experience, which is why age gives wisdom. Feeling unsure is a good sign. This shows that you realize you have more to learn. I've seen nurses who are overly confident, and they often make mistakes because of it.

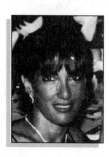

When you feel incompetent you make an effort to be more careful.

Pediatric nursing is a won-derful career choice. The HIV babies need lots of love because they can feel this at a time when they need it most.

Keep in mind that the parents of a sick child are going through a very traumatic experience, too. So it's natural for them to ask lots of questions and to seek out the doctor's advice. This is their baby you're talking about, a person more precious to them than anything else on earth. Therefore, parents need for you to explain things thoroughly to them. And expect to repeat those explanations several times because they may have difficulty concentrating, particularly if their child is seriously ill. Be patient with the parents and with yourself.

Time management is a crucial issue in this culture. It's no secret that American women are very stressed. I've traveled all over the world and have seen this to be true. We have many freedoms and opportunities here, but with these privileges come so much responsibility. I used to work full-time while I was in nursing school, and I thought I would never graduate! As a professional I must continue to use my time efficiently. One of the first things I do in the morning is make a list of the things I want to achieve that day. When I finish a task, I cross it off my list. I may only complete 50% or 60% of what I set out to do, but I still have a sense of accomplishment at the end of the day.

As a student, and especially once you begin your career, avoid comparing yourself to others. We all have competencies. Some people require only four hours of sleep a night, whereas others need a full eight hours. If you need more sleep and exercise, then you must cut back on your other activities. Maybe try alternating the activities you really want to do from one semester to another. That way you'll expose yourself to a variety of experiences, but with more sanity. And remember: You're not supposed to know as much as a nurse who has been working for twenty years. You cannot rush this kind of knowledge; you have to grow into it.

Another option to consider is an *electronic planner*. These are compact minicomputers that can hold a large amount of information. You can use them to schedule your days and weeks, make to-do lists, and create and store an address book. Electronic planners are powerful, convenient, and often fun. On the other hand, they certainly cost more than the paper version, and you can lose a lot of important data if something goes wrong with the computer inside. Evaluate your options and decide what you like best.

Set Weekly and Daily Goals

The most ideal time management starts with the smallest tasks and builds to bigger ones. Setting short-term goals that tie in to your long-term goals lends the following benefits:

- Increased meaning for your daily activities
- Shaping your path toward the achievement of your long-term goals
- A sense of order and progress

For college students as well as working people, the week is often the easiest unit of time to consider at one shot. Weekly goal setting and planning allows you to keep track of day-to-day activities while giving you the larger perspective of what is coming up during the week. Take some time before each week starts to remind yourself of your long-term goals. Keeping long-term goals in mind will help you determine related short-term goals you can accomplish during the week to come.

Figure 4-3 shows parts of a daily schedule and a weekly schedule.

Link Daily and Weekly Goals with Long-Term Goals

After you evaluate what you need to accomplish in the coming year, semester, month, week, and day in order to reach your long-term goals, use your schedule to record those steps. Write down the short-term goals that will enable you to stay on track. Here is how a student might map out two different goals over a year's time.

FIGURE 4-3

Daily and weekly
schedules.

Monday, March 20

TIME	TASKS	PRIORITY
7:00 AM	Up at 7am — finish lab writing	
8:00	Review lab protocol	☆
9:00		
10:00	Writing class	
11:00	Renew driver's license @ DMV	☆
12:00 PM		
1:00	Lunch	
2:00	Chem lab	☆
3:00		
4:00	↓	
5:00	5:30 work out	
6:00	↳6:30	
7:00	Dinner	
8:00	Read two chapters for Bio	
9:00		
10:00		
11:00		

Monday, March 20

8	BIO 212	Call: Maggie Blair	1
9		Finanical Aid Office	2
10		CPR instructor course	3
11	CHEM 203		4
12			5

EVENING 6pm yoga class

Tuesday, March 21

8	Finish reading assignment	Work @ library	1
9			2
10	ENG 112	(study for quiz)	3
11	↓		4
12		↓	5

EVENING until 7pm

Wednesday, March 22

8		Meet w/advisor	1
9	BIO 212		2
10		CPR course	3
11	CHEM 203 ☆Quiz		4
12		Pick up photos	5

EVENING 6pm Aerobics

This year:	Complete enough courses to graduate.
	Improve my physical fitness.
This semester:	Complete my applied mathematics course with a B average or higher.
	Lose 10 pounds and exercise regularly.
This month:	Set up study group schedule to coincide with quizzes.
	Begin walking and weight lifting.
This week:	Meet with study group; go over material for Friday's quiz.
	Go for a fitness walk three times; go to weight room twice.
Today:	Go over Chapter 3 in applied mathematics and do problems 1–5.
	Walk for 40 minutes.

Prioritize Goals

Prioritizing enables you to use your date book with maximum efficiency. On any given day, the necessity of completing your goals will vary. Record your goals first, and then label them according to how important they are to complete using these categories: priority 1, priority 2, and priority 3. Identify these categories using any code that makes sense to you. Some people use numbers, as above. Some use letters (A, B, C). Some write activities in different colors according to priority level. Some use symbols (*, +, –).

Priority 1 activities are the most necessary or critical to complete. They may include attending class, picking up a child from day care, putting gas in the car, and paying bills.

Priority 2 activities are part of your routine. Examples include grocery shopping, working out, participating in a school organization, or cleaning. Priority 2 tasks are important but more flexible than priority 1 activities.

Priority 3 activities are those you would like to do but can reschedule without much sacrifice. Examples might be a trip to the mall, a visit to a friend, a social phone call, a sports event, a movie, or a hair appointment. As much as you would like to accomplish them, you don't consider them urgent. Many people don't enter priority 3 tasks in their date books until they are sure they have time to get them done. You may want to list priority 3 tasks separately and refer to the list when you have some extra time.

Prioritizing your activities is essential for two reasons. First, some activities are more necessary to complete than others, and effective time management requires that you focus most of your energy on priority 1 items. Second, looking at all your priorities helps you plan when you can get things done. Often, it's not possible to get all your priority 1 activities done early in the day, especially if these activities involve scheduled classes or meetings. Prioritizing helps you set priority 1 items and then schedule priority 2 and 3 items around them as they fit.

"The right time is any time that one is still so lucky as to have. . . . Live!"

HENRY JAMES

Keep Track of Events

Your date book also enables you to schedule *events*. Rather than thinking of events as separate from goals, tie them to your long-term goals just as you would your other tasks. For example, attending a wedding in a few months contributes to your commitment to spending time with your family. Being aware of quiz dates, due dates for assignments, and meeting dates will aid your goals to achieve in school and become involved.

Note events in your date book so that you can stay aware of them ahead of time. Write them in daily, weekly, monthly, or even yearly sections, where a quick look will remind you that they are approaching. Writing them down will also help you see where they fit in the context of all your other activities. For example, if you have three big tests and a presentation all in one week, you'll want to take time in the weeks before to prepare for them all.

Following are some kinds of events worth noting in your date book:

- Due dates for papers, projects, presentations, and tests
- Important meetings, medical appointments, or due dates for bill payments
- Birthdays, anniversaries, social events, holidays, and other special occasions
- Benchmarks for steps toward a goal, such as due dates for sections of a project or a deadline for losing five pounds on your way to losing twenty

Time Management Strategies

Managing time takes thought and energy. Here are some additional strategies to try.

1. **Plan your schedule each week.** Before each week starts, note events, goals, and priorities. Look at the map of your week to decide where to fit activities like studying and priority 3 items. For example, if you have a test on Thursday, you can plan study sessions on the days up until then. If you have more free time on Tuesday and Friday than on other days, you can plan workouts or priority 3 activities at those times. Looking at the whole week will help you avoid being surprised by something you had forgotten was coming up.

2. **Make and use to-do lists.** Use a *to-do list* to record the things you want to accomplish. If you generate a daily or weekly to-do list on a separate piece of paper, you can look at all tasks and goals at once. This will help you consider time frames and priorities. You might want to prioritize your tasks and transfer them to appropriate places in your date book. Some people create daily to-do lists right on their date book pages. You can tailor a to-do list to an important event such as exam week or an especially busy day when you have a family gathering or a presentation to make. This kind of specific to-do list can help you prioritize and accomplish an unusually large task load.

3. Post monthly and yearly calendars at home. Keeping a calendar on the wall will help you stay aware of important events. You can purchase one or draw it yourself, month by month, on plain paper. Use a yearly or a monthly version (Figure 4-4 shows part of a monthly calendar) and keep it where you can refer to it often. If you live with family or friends, make the calendar a group project so that you stay aware of each other's plans. Knowing each other's schedules can also help you avoid scheduling problems such as two people who need the car at the same time or one partner's scheduling a get-together when the other has to work.

4. Schedule down time. When you're wiped out from too much activity, you don't have the energy to accomplish much with your time. A little down time will refresh you and improve your attitude. Even half an hour a day will help. Fill the time with whatever relaxes you—having a snack, reading, watching TV, playing a game or sport, walking, writing, or just doing nothing. Make down time a priority.

5. Be flexible. Since priorities determine the map of your day, week, month, or year, any priority shift can jumble your schedule. Be ready to reschedule your tasks as your priorities change. On Monday, a homework assignment due in a week might be priority 2. By Saturday, it has become priority 1. On some days a surprise priority such as a medical emergency or a family situation may pop up and force you to cancel everything else on your schedule. Other days a class may be canceled and you will have extra time on your hands. Adjust to whatever each day brings.

TERMS

Down time
Quiet time set aside for relaxation and low-key activity.

FIGURE 4-4   Monthly calendar.

OCTOBER 2000

SUNDAY	MONDAY	TUESDAY	WEDNESDAY	THURSDAY	FRIDAY	SATURDAY
1	2 WORK	3 Turn in English paper	4 Dentist 2pm	5 Chem. test	6	7
8 Frank's B-day	9 Psych test WORK	10 6:30 pm Meeting at Student Center	11 Statistics quiz WORK	12 History study group	13 WORK	14 WORK
15	16 WORK	17	18 WORK	19	20	21
22	23	24	25	26	27	28
29	30	31				

No matter how well you schedule your time, you will have moments when it's hard to stay in control. Knowing how to identify and avoid procrastination and other time traps will help you get back on track.

 ## WHY IS PROCRASTINATION A PROBLEM?

Procrastination
The act of putting off something that needs to be done.

Procrastination occurs when you postpone unpleasant or burdensome tasks. People procrastinate for different reasons. Having trouble with goal setting is one reason. People may project goals too far into the future, set unrealistic goals that are too frustrating to reach, or have no goals at all. People also procrastinate because they don't believe in their ability to complete a task or don't believe in themselves in general. As natural as these tendencies are, they can also be extremely harmful. If continued over a period of time, procrastination can develop into a habit that will dominate a person's behavior. Following are some ways to face your tendencies to procrastinate and *just do it!*

Strategies to Fight Procrastination

Weigh the benefits (to you and others) of completing the task versus the effects of procrastinating. What rewards lie ahead if you get it done? What will be the effects if you continue to put it off? Which situation has better effects? Chances are you will benefit more in the long term from facing the task head-on.

Set reasonable goals. Plan your goals carefully, allowing enough time to complete them. Unreasonable goals can be so intimidating that you do nothing at all. "Pay off the credit card bill next month" could throw you. However, "Pay off the credit card bill in six months" might inspire you to take action.

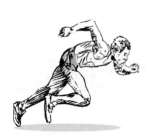

Get started. Going from doing nothing to doing something is often the hardest part of avoiding procrastination. Once you start, you may find it easier to continue.

Break the task into smaller parts. If it seems overwhelming, look at the task in terms of its parts. How can you approach it step-by-step? If you can concentrate on achieving one small goal at a time, the task may become less of a burden. To start, tell yourself, "I only have to read the first two pages, break, and continue."

Ask for help with tasks and projects at school, work, and home. You don't always have to go it alone. For example, if you have put off an intimidating assignment, ask your instructor for guidance. If you need accommodations due to a disability, don't assume that others know about it. Once you identify what's holding you up, see who can help you face the task.

Don't expect perfection. No one is perfect. Most people learn by starting at the beginning and wading through plenty of mistakes and confusion. It's better to try your best than to do nothing at all.

Procrastination is natural, but it can cause you problems if you let it get the best of you. When it does happen, take some time to think about the causes. What is it about this situation that frightens you or puts you off? Answering that question can help you address what causes lie underneath the procrastination. These causes might indicate a deeper problem that needs to be solved.

In Hebrew, the word *chai* means "life," representing all aspects of life—spiritual, emotional, family, educational, and career. Individual Hebrew characters have number values. Because the characters in the word *chai* add up to 18, the number 18 has come to be associated with good luck. The word *chai* is often worn as a good luck charm. As you plan your goals, think about your view of luck. Many people feel that a person can create his or her own luck by pursuing goals persistently and staying open to possibilities and opportunities. Canadian novelist Robertson Davies once said, "What we call luck is the inner man externalized. We make things happen to us."

Consider that your vision of life may largely determine how you live. You can prepare the way for luck by establishing a personal mission and forging ahead toward your goals. If you believe that the life you want awaits you, you will be able to recognize and make the most of luck when it comes around. *L'chaim*—to life, and good luck.

Applications   **Chapter 4**

KEY INTO YOUR LIFE
Opportunities to Apply What You Learn

 4.1 *Your Values*

Begin to explore your values by rating the following values on a scale from 1 to 4, 1 being least important to you and 4 being most important. If you have values that you don't see in the chart, list them in the blank spaces and rate them.

VALUE	RATING	VALUE	RATING
Knowing yourself		Mental health	
Physical health		Fitness and exercise	
Spending time with your family		Having an intimate relationship	
Helping others		Education	
Being well paid		Being employed	
Being liked by others		Free time/vacations	
Enjoying entertainment		Time to yourself	
Spiritual/religious life		Reading	
Keeping up with the news		Staying organized	
Being financially stable		Close friendships	
Creative/artistic pursuits		Self-improvement	
Lifelong learning		Facing your fears	

Considering your priorities, write your top five values here:

1. _____

2. _____

3. _____

4. _____

5. _____

4.2   *Why Are You Here?*

Why did you decide to enroll in school? Do any of the reasons listed in the chapter fit you? Do you have other reasons all your own? Many people have more than one answer. Write up to five here.

_____

_____

_____

_____

_____

Take a moment to think about your reasons. Which reasons are most important to you? Why? Prioritize your reasons above by writing 1 next to the most important, 2 next to the second most important, etc.

How do you feel about your reasons? You may be proud of some. On the other hand, you may not feel comfortable with others. Which do you like or dislike and why?

_____

_____

_____

_____

_____

4.3   *Short-Term Scheduling*

Take a close look at your schedule for the coming month, including events, important dates, and steps toward goals. On the calendar layout on p. 109, fill in the name of the month and appropriate numbers for the days. Then record what you hope to accomplish, including the following:

- Due dates for papers, projects, and presentations
- Test dates
- Important meetings, medical appointments, and due dates for bill payments
- Birthdays, anniversaries, and other special occasions
- Steps toward long-term goals

This kind of chart will help you see the big picture of your month. To stay on target from day to day, check these dates against the entries in your date book and make sure that they are indicated there as well.

 ## 4.4 *To-Do Lists*

Make a to-do list for what you have to do tomorrow. Include all tasks—priority 1, 2, and 3—and events.

TOMORROW'S DATE: _____

1. _____
2. _____
3. _____
4. _____
5. _____
6. _____
7. _____
8. _____
9. _____
10. _____

Use a coding system of your choice to indicate priority level of both tasks and events. Place a check mark by the items that are important enough to note in your date book. Use this list to make your schedule for tomorrow in the date book, making a separate list for priority 3 items. At the end of the day, evaluate this system. Did the to-do list help you? How did it make a difference? If you liked it, use this exercise as a guide for using to-do lists regularly.

_____

_____

_____

_____

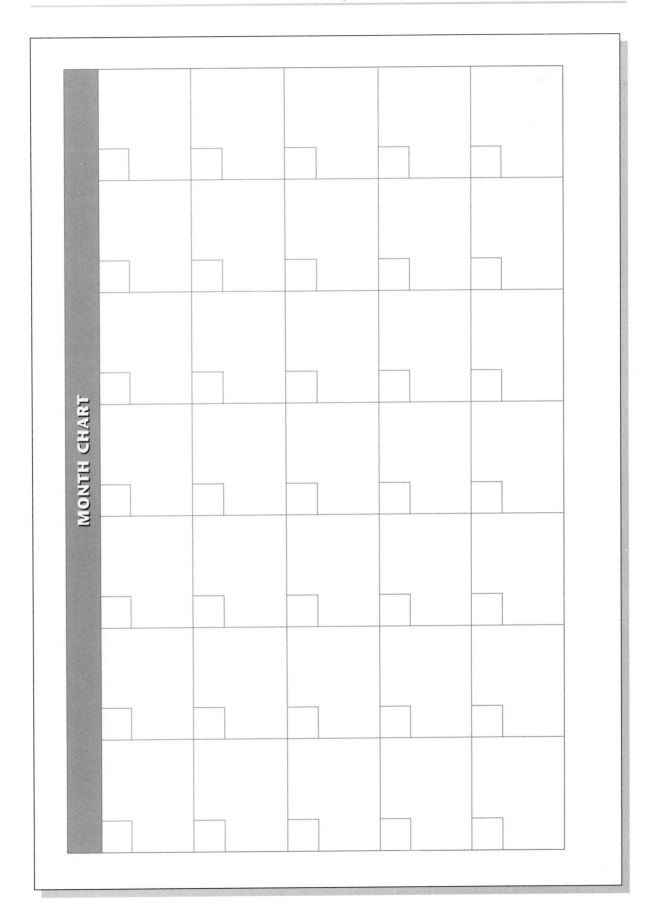

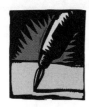

KEY TO SELF-EXPRESSION
Discovery Through Journal Writing

To record your thoughts, use a separate journal or the lined pages at the end of the chapter.

Using the personal mission statement examples in the chapter as a guide, consider what you want out of your life and create your own personal mission statement. You can write it in paragraph form, in a list of long-term goals, or in the form of a think link. Take as much time as you need in order to be as complete as possible.

Name _____ Date _____

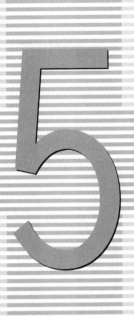

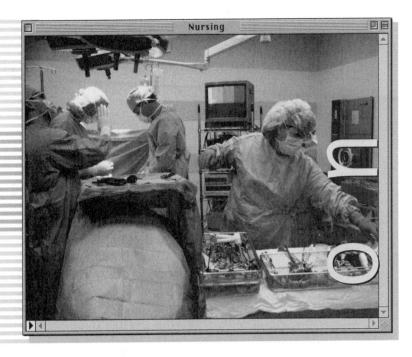

5

Scientific Inquiry

Critical and Creative Thinking in Nursing

Your mind's powers show in everything you do, from the smallest chores (comparing prices on cereals at the grocery store) to the most complex situations (figuring out how to earn money after being laid off). Your mind is able to process, store, and create with the facts and ideas it encounters. Critical and creative thinking are what enable those skills to come alive.

Understanding how your mind works is the first step toward critical thinking. When you have that understanding, you can perform the essential critical-thinking task: asking important questions about ideas and information. This chapter will show you both the mind's basic actions and the thinking processes that use those actions. You will explore what it means to be an open-minded critical and creative thinker able to ask and understand questions that promote your success as a nursing major, in your career, and in life.

In this chapter, you will explore answers to the following questions:

- What is critical thinking?
- How is critical thinking critical in nursing?
- How does your mind work?
- How does critical thinking help you succeed in nursing?
- Why shift your perspective?
- Why plan strategically?
- How can you develop creativity?

 ## WHAT IS CRITICAL THINKING?

Critical thinking is thinking that goes beyond the basic recall of information. If the word *critical* sounds negative to you, consider that the dictionary defines its meaning as "indispensable" and "important." Critical thinking is important thinking that involves asking questions. This is called essential questioning. Using critical thinking, you question established ideas, create new ideas, turn information into tools to solve problems and make decisions, and take the long-term view as well as the day-to-day view.

A critical thinker asks as many kinds of questions as possible. The following are examples of possible questions about a given piece of information: *Where did it come from? What could explain it? In what ways is it true or false, and what examples could prove or disprove it? How do I feel about it, and why? How is this information similar to or different from what I already know? Is it good or bad? What causes led to it, and what effects does it have?* Critical thinkers also try to transform information into something they can use. They ask themselves whether the information can help them solve a problem, make a decision, create something new, or anticipate the future. Such questions help the critical thinker learn, grow, and create.

Not thinking critically means not asking questions about information or ideas. A person who does not think critically tends to accept or reject information or ideas without examining them. Table 5-1 compares how a critical thinker and a noncritical thinker might respond to particular situations.

Asking questions (the focus of the table), considering as many responses as you can, choosing responses that are as complete and accurate as possible, and having insight into your own biases are some primary ingredients that make up the skill of critical thinking. You must be willing to make mistakes and ask questions.

TABLE 5-1   Not thinking critically vs. thinking critically.

YOUR ROLE	SITUATION	NON-QUESTIONING RESPONSE	QUESTIONING RESPONSE
STUDENT	Instructor is lecturing on the causes of congestive heart failure.	You assume that everything your instructor tells you is true.	You consider what the instructor says; you write down questions about issues you want to clarify; you initiate discussion with the professor or other classmates.
PARENT	Teacher discovers your child lying about something at school.	You're mad at your child and believe the teacher, or you think the teacher is lying.	You ask both teacher and child about what happened, and you compare their answers, evaluating who you think is telling the truth; you discuss the concepts of lying/honesty with your child.
SPOUSE/ PARTNER	Your partner feels that he or she no longer has quality time with you.	You think he or she is wrong and defend yourself.	You ask how long he or she has felt this way; you ask your partner and yourself why this is happening; you explore how you can improve the situation.
EMPLOYEE	You are angry at your supervisor.	You ignore or avoid your supervisor.	You are willing to discuss the situation.
NEIGHBOR	People different from you move in next door.	You ignore or avoid them; you think their way of living is weird.	You introduce yourself; you offer to help if they need it; you respectfully explore what's different about them.
CITIZEN	You encounter a homeless person.	You avoid the person and the issue.	You examine whether the community has a responsibility to the homeless, and if you find that it does, you explore how to fulfill that responsibility.
CONSUMER	You want to buy a car.	You decide on a brand-new car and don't think through how you will handle the payments.	You consider the different effects of buying a new car vs. buying a used car; you examine your money situation to see what kind of payment you can handle each month.

Critical Thinking Is a Skill

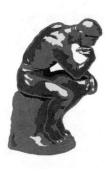

Anyone can develop the ability to think critically. Critical thinking is a skill that can be taught to students at all different levels of ability. One of the most crucial components of this skill is learning information. For instance, part of the skill of critical thinking is comparing new information with what you already know. Your prior knowledge provides a framework within which to ask questions about and evaluate a new piece of information. Without a solid base of knowledge, critical thinking is harder to achieve. For example, thinking critically about the statement "Shakespeare's character King Richard III is like an early version of Adolf Hitler" is impossible without basic knowledge of World War II and Shakespeare's play *Richard III*.

The skill of critical thinking focuses on generating questions about statements and information. To examine potential critical-thinking responses in more depth, explore the different questions that a critical thinker may have about one particular statement.

A Critical-Thinking Response to a Statement

Consider the following statement of opinion: *"My obstacles are keeping me from succeeding in school. Other people make it through school because they don't have to deal with the obstacles that I have."*

Non-questioning thinkers may accept an opinion such as this as an absolute truth, believing that their obstacles will hinder their success. As a result, on the road to achieving their goals, they may lose motivation to overcome those obstacles. In contrast, critical thinkers would take the opportunity to examine the opinion through a series of questions. Here are some examples of questions one student might ask.

"What exactly are my obstacles? Examples of my obstacles are a heavy work schedule, single parenting, being in debt, and returning to school after 10 years out."

"Who has problems that are different from mine? I do have one friend who is going through problems worse than mine, and she's getting by. I also know another guy who doesn't have too much to deal with that I can tell, and he's struggling just like I am."

"Who has problems that are similar to mine? Well, if I consider my obstacles specifically, I might be saying that single parents and returning adult students will all have trouble in school. That is not necessarily true. People in all kinds of situations may still become successful."

"Why do I think this? Maybe I am scared of returning to school and adjusting to a new environment. Maybe I am afraid to challenge myself, which I haven't done in a long time. Whatever the cause, the effect is that I feel bad about myself and don't work to the best of my abilities, and that can hurt both me and my family who depends on me."

"What is an example of someone who has had success despite having to overcome obstacles? What about Oseola McCarty, the cleaning woman who saved money all her life and raised $150,000 to create a scholar-

ship at the University of Southern Mississippi? She didn't have what anyone would call advantages, such as a high-paying job or a college education."

"What conclusion can I draw from my questions? From thinking about my friend and about Oseola McCarty, I would say that people can successfully overcome their obstacles by working hard, focusing on their abilities, and concentrating on their goals."

"How do I evaluate the effects of my statement? I think it's harmful. When we say that obstacles equal difficulty, we can damage our desire to try to overcome those obstacles. When we say that successful people don't have obstacles, we might overlook that some very successful people have to deal with hidden disadvantages such as learning disabilities or abusive families."

The Value of Critical Thinking

Critical thinking has many important advantages. Following are some of the positive effects, or benefits, of putting energy into critical thinking.

You will increase your ability to perform thinking processes that help you reach your goals in nursing. Critical thinking is a learned skill, just like shooting a basketball or using a new software program on the computer. As with any other skill, the more you use it, the better you become. The more you ask questions, the better thinker you become. The better you think, the more effective you will be when learning in school, managing your personal life, and performing and being valued in your career.

You can produce knowledge, rather than just reproduce it. The interaction of new information with what you already know creates new knowledge. The usefulness of such knowledge can be judged by how you apply it to new situations. For instance, it won't mean much for a nursing major to list the major drug categories on an exam unless he or she can make judgments about drug interactions when on the job.

You can be a valuable employee. You certainly won't be a failure in the workplace if you follow directions. However, as a nurse you must think critically and ask strategic questions about how to make improvements, large or small. Questions could range from "Is there a better way to deliver phone messages?" to "How can we find new grant money to keep our research project going?" Showing initiative and thinking critically will be more likely to earn you greater responsibility and promotions.

You can increase your creativity. You cannot be a successful critical thinker without being able to come up with new and different questions to ask, possibilities to explore, and ideas to try. Creativity is essential in producing what is new. Being creative generally improves your outlook, your sense of humor, and your perspective as you cope with problems. Later in this chapter, you will look at ways to awaken and increase your natural creativity.

"Caring requires a commitment... and a willingness to do the unlovely. Neither education nor experience quite prepares you for doing the unlovely...Caring demands listening and observing with your whole person...To care means to be trustworthy... Caring is costly. It takes a great amount of physical, emotional, and spiritual energy."

ROBERTA LYDER PAIGE, MA, RN AND JANE FINKBINER LOONEY, MS, RN 1

HOW IS CRITICAL THINKING CRITICAL IN NURSING?

Critical thinking in science and in nursing is a process of inquiry that tries to gain a better understanding of the world—from stars and meteors to the human brain and behavior to entire ecosystems. Inquiry is based on a standard set of rules known as the scientific method. The scientific method is important because it provides a regulated process for conducting research:

- Essential questioning: asking questions
- Possible answers: forming hypotheses
- Testing hypotheses: looking for answers

The scientific method is a process that other nurse researchers can then follow and repeat to reproduce and validate your results. Repetition of research studies gives the results more strength by increasing the amount of supporting evidence. For instance, you'd like to know that a medication you give a client to fight a bacterial infection had been researched using a standard method, tested repeatedly, and had strong evidence supporting its effectiveness. Furthermore, you would want to be confident that it worked on the specific bacteria your client had and that it didn't have any dangerous side effects.

The main ingredient of the scientific method is the ability to think, which sounds pretty easy, perhaps like breathing. But, you can learn to improve your thinking as you progress through college course work. Even thinking about your own thinking, called reflection, can help you. Reflection helps you understand your own biases, or your particular way of looking at phenomena, so that you can find out how your previous views might be getting in the way when what you need is a fresh perspective.

Observation is a critical skill in inquiry, and you can learn to become an astute observer through practicing the journal exercises in Chapters 1 and 2. Another thinking skill you can learn is making connections between what you already know and what you are learning. This skill will help you put information together to make new discoveries or to come up with new solutions to old problems.

Inquiry in nursing relies on asking critical questions. Questions help direct your inquiry; they help you decide where to go for information, what tests to perform, or what experiments to design. The more you improve your thinking through practice and experience, the better you will be at coming up with questions about the world, or your area of practice, and finding methods for answering those questions.

In the next section, you will read about the seven basic actions your mind performs when asking important questions. These actions are the basic blocks you will use to build the critical-thinking processes you will explore later in the chapter.

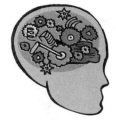

HOW DOES YOUR MIND WORK?

Critical thinking depends on a thorough understanding of the workings of the mind. Your mind has some basic moves, or actions, that it uses to understand relationships among ideas and concepts. Sometimes it uses one action by itself, but most often it uses two or more in combination.

Brain research has advanced rapidly in the past decade. The discovery of new technologies, or new uses for old technologies, has led to discoveries about memory, moods, and the learning process. For instance, researchers have used brain-scanning technology to show how parts of the brain respond to depression. This in turn has helped other researchers develop medications that work on a cellular level in brain tissue to effectively treat depression.

Brain-scanning techniques are also used to study a person's brain while they are learning. For instance, while learning to play the piano, brain scans found that the brain recruited other areas of the cerebral cortex to help in the learning process. Once the learning was complete and the function became automatic, like learning to ride a bicycle, those borrowed areas went back to their normal functions. This helps to explain how the mind works to learn new information.

Mind Actions: The Thinktrix

You can identify your mind's actions using a system called the Thinktrix, originally conceived by educators Frank Lyman, Arlene Mindus, and Charlene Lopez[1] and developed by numerous other instructors. They studied how students think and named seven mind actions that are the basic building blocks of thought. These actions are not new to you, although some of their names may be. They represent the ways in which you think all the time.

Through exploring these actions, you can go beyond just thinking and learn *how* you think. This will help you take charge of your own thinking. The more you know about how your mind works, the more control you will have over thinking processes such as problem solving, decision making, creating, and strategic planning.

Following are explanations of each of the mind actions. Each explanation names the action, defines it, and explains it with examples. As you read, follow the instructions and write your own examples in the blank spaces provided. Each action is also represented by a picture, or *icon*, that helps you visualize and remember it.

Recall: *Facts, sequence, and description.* This is the simplest action. When you **recall** you describe facts, objects, or events, or put them into sequence. *Examples:*

- Naming the steps of a geometry proof, in order
- Remembering the valence electron arrangement for calcium, chloride, and nitrogen

Your example: Recall some important events this month. _____

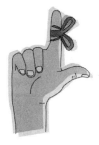

_____

_____

_____

The icon: A string tied around a finger is a familiar image of recall or remembering.

Similarity: *Analogy, likeness, comparison.* This action examines what is **similar** about one or more things. You might compare situations, ideas, people, stories, events, or objects. *Examples:*

■ Comparing notes with another student to see what facts and ideas you both have considered important.

■ Analyzing the arguments you've had with your roommate or partner this month and seeing how they all seem to be about the same problem.

Your example: Tell what is similar about the numbers 2, 4, 8, 12, and 16. ____

_____

_____

_____

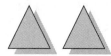

The icon: Two alike objects, in this case triangles, indicate similarity.

Difference: *Distinction, contrast, comparison.* This action examines what is **different** about one or more situations, ideas, people, stories, events, or objects, contrasting them with one another. *Examples:*

■ Seeing how three mammals differ in anatomy (horse, human, leopard)

■ Contrasting a weekday where you work half the day and go to school half the day with a weekday when you attend class and then have the rest of the day to study

Your example: Explain what about one course makes it easier to learn the material than in another course. _____

_____

_____

_____

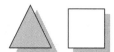

The icon: Two differing objects, in this case a triangle and a square, indicate difference.

Cause and effect: *Reasons, consequences, prediction.* Using this action, you look at what has **caused** a situation, or event, and what **effects,** or consequences, come from it. In other words, you examine both what led up to something and what will follow because of it. *Examples:*

■ You see how staying up late at night causes you to oversleep, which has the effect of your being late to class. This causes you to miss some of the material, which has the further effect of your having problems on the test.

■ When you pay your phone and utility bills on time you create effects such as a better credit rating, uninterrupted service, and a better relationship with your service providers.

Your example: Name probable causes for the days' becoming shorter in winter.

_____

_____

_____

The icon: The water droplets making ripples indicate causes and their resulting effects.

Example to principle: *Inductive reasoning, generalization, classification, conceptualization.* From one or more **examples** (facts or events), you develop a general **principle** or principles. Grouping facts or events into patterns may allow you to make a general statement about several of them at once. Classifying a fact or event helps you build knowledge. This mind action moves from the specific to the general. *Examples:*

- Molecules such as hydrochloric acid, sulfuric acid, and acetic acid all easily lose a proton (examples). Therefore, all molecules with a certain structure are an acid (principle).
- You see a movie (example), and you decide it is mostly about pride (principle).

Your example: You drop a pencil and it falls down; you see an apple fall from a tree.

Name the principle: _____

_____

_____

_____

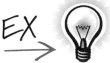

The icon: The arrow and "Ex" pointing to a light bulb on their right indicate how an example or examples lead to the principle, or idea (the light bulb, lit up).

Principle to example: *Deductive reasoning, categorization, substantiation, proof.* In a reverse of the previous action, you take a **principle** or principles and think of **examples** (events or facts) that support or prove that idea. This mind action moves from the general to the specific. *Examples:*

- When you write a paper, you start with a thesis statement, which communicates the central idea: "Men are favored over women in the modern workplace." Then you gather examples to back up that idea: Men make more money on average than women in the same jobs; there are more men in upper management positions than there are women; women can be denied advancement when they make their families a priority.
- You talk to your instructor about changing your major, giving examples that support your idea: You have worked in the field you want to change to, you have fulfilled some of the requirements for that major already, and you are unhappy with your current course of study.

Your example: Air pressure changes with altitude changes (principle). Name an example you might experience that supports the principle. _____

_____

_____

_____

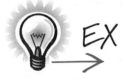

The icon: In a reverse of the previous icon, this one starts with the light bulb and has an arrow pointing to "Ex." This indicates that you start with the principle, or idea, the light bulb, and then branch into the supporting example or examples.

Evaluation: *Analysis, value, judgment, rating.* Here you **judge** whether something is useful or not useful, important or unimportant, good or bad, or right or wrong by identifying and weighing its positive and negative effects (pros and cons). Be sure to consider the specific situation at hand (a cold drink might be good on the beach in August, but not so good in the snowdrifts in January). With the facts you have gathered, you determine the value of something in terms of both predicted effects and your own needs. Cause and effect analysis always accompanies evaluation. *Examples:*

■ You decide to try taking classes later in the day for a semester. You schedule classes in the afternoons and spend your nights on the job. You find that instead of getting up early to use the morning time, you tend to sleep in and then get up not too long before you have to be at school. From those harmful effects, you evaluate that it doesn't work for you. You decide to schedule earlier classes next time.

■ Someone offers you a chance to cheat on a test. You evaluate the potential effects if you are caught. You also evaluate the long-term effects on you of not actually learning the material. You decide that it isn't worth your while to participate in the plan to cheat.

Your example: Evaluate your mode of transportation to school. _____

_____

_____

_____

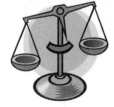

The icon: A set of scales out of balance indicates how you weigh positive and negative effects to arrive at an evaluation.

You may want to use a *mnemonic device*—a memory tool, explained in more detail in Chapter 8—to remember the seven mind actions. You can make a sentence of words that each start with a mind action's first letter. Here's an example: "Really Smart Dogs Cook Enchiladas Producing Energy" (the first letter of each word stands for one of the mind actions).

How Mind Actions Build Thinking Processes

The seven mind actions are the fundamental building blocks that your mind uses every day. Note that you will rarely use them one at a time in a step-by-step process, as they are presented here. You will usually combine them, overlap them, and repeat them more than once, using different actions for different situations. For example, when you want to say something nice at the end of a date, you might consider past comments that had an effect *similar* to what you want now. When a test question asks you to explain what prejudice is, you might name similar *examples* that confirm a principle, or theory, on prejudice.

When you combine mind actions in working toward a specific goal, you are performing a thinking process. The next few sections will explore some of the most important critical-thinking processes: solving problems, making decisions, shifting your perspective, and planning strategically. Each thinking process helps you succeed by directing your critical thinking toward the achievement of your goals. Figure 5-4, appearing later in the chapter, shows all of the mind actions and thinking processes together and reminds you that the mind actions form the core of the thinking processes.

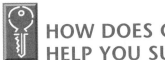

HOW DOES CRITICAL THINKING HELP YOU SUCCEED IN NURSING?

Problem solving and decision making are probably the two most crucial and common thinking processes used in nursing. Each one requires various mind actions. They overlap somewhat, because every problem that needs solving requires you to make a decision. Each process will be considered separately here. You will notice similarities in the steps involved in each.

Although both of these processes have multiple steps, you will not always have to work your way through each step. As you become more comfortable with solving problems and making decisions, your mind will automatically click through the steps you need whenever you encounter a problem or decision. Also, you will become more adept at evaluating which problems and decisions need serious consideration and which can be taken care of more quickly and simply. In becoming an expert nurse, learning these skills will take many years of experience and reflection—so, start now!

Problem Solving and Inquiry

Problem solving starts with asking questions. Asking questions is the fundamental step in inquiry. Problems to solve can range from very small, such as how to learn not to lose your car keys, to very large, such as how to care for a sick relative, manage a custody plan after a divorce, or protect the ozone layer. A problem, however, is not always necessarily a problem, that is, something that has to be fixed. In nursing, a problem is something to investigate and gain understanding about. For instance, the problem I want to learn more about is how people respond to aerobic exercise that is alternated with short bursts of anaerobic exercise.

Solving a problem can occur quickly or over many years of investigation. How quickly a solution is reached may depend on two things: (1) The urgency of the problem; and (2) the complexity of the problem.

Solving the problem of the AIDS virus is extremely urgent; it is a problem that affects people of all ages throughout the world. It is also a complex problem. Another complex problem, but one that may be judged as less urgent, is finding out how to slow down the aging process. An urgent problem requiring a quick solution is an emergency. For instance, if you have the signs and symptoms of a heart attack while playing soccer, you have an urgent, but fairly simple problem (although it may be complex in the long run). The solution doesn't require much critical thinking or take much time to come up with. Someone calls 911, and you go to the emergency department of the nearest hospital. More complex problems require more complex thinking, or critical thinking.

Use the following steps to solve problems:

1. Observe

State the problem clearly. To do this, figure out what you already know about the problem by noting what objective, or observable, evidence you have. If you are failing physics quizzes, you may think the problem is that you don't understand the material. Not understanding the material is not the problem; it is a possible *cause* of the observable problem: your failing grades.

2. Assess and Analyze

After the problem is defined, "I am failing my physics quizzes," it is time to assess what else you need to know in order to develop a solution. This is when you formulate questions. In this case you might ask yourself: "What are possible causes of my poor grades—lack of sleep or too much TV watching?" And to determine the urgency of the problem: "What is the consequence of failing these quizzes?" "Will I fail the course?" "Will my plan to go into nursing be ruined?" "Will I ever be happy again?"

3. Brainstorm

TERMS

Brainstorming
The spontaneous, rapid generation of ideas or solutions, undertaken by a group or an individual, often as part of a problem-solving process.

Brainstorming helps loosen up your thinking and creativity. Brainstorming is done without judging your answers, or ideas; thus, you remove a major barrier to creativity: fear that your answer will be wrong. That is the beauty of brainstorming—there are no right or wrong answers. This gives you the freedom to let your mind come up with all kinds of possibilities, some useful, some useless. Again, ask yourself: "What are possible causes of my failing grades?" Now, think up every cause you can, focusing just on possible causes, *not* solutions.

4. Plan

Explore possible solutions. This stage is like the scientific process stage of coming up with testable hypotheses. For instance, you determine that lack of sleep may be the biggest cause of your misunderstanding the physics material and hence, the problem—failing the quizzes. One hypothesis: "Increasing sleep to at least eight hours will increase alertness and receptiveness to understanding the physics material. Now you can test the hypothetical solution: getting more sleep. If this doesn't work (except to make you feel better, which counts, too), you may test a second hypothesis: "A tutor will improve grades."

5. Implement

Choose and implement the solution you think is most probable in improving your grades. Record your data on a calendar so you can follow your progress.

6. Evaluate

Evaluate the results you get from testing your hypothesis. In the physics student's case, did getting more sleep or working with a tutor help her grades? Look at the pros and cons of the solution. Getting eight hours of sleep may make you feel better—a pro, but it didn't help your grades—a con. Using a tutor helped your grades—a pro, but it took up time you wanted to use for skiing or other activities—a con. You must weigh the pros against the cons. Less skiing and good grades today will help you find a job later. One you enjoy and that pays well enough for you to enjoy plenty of skiing in your off hours as a nurse in Vail, Colorado.

7. Refine

Problem solving is not linear; it is circular. There is no definite beginning or end. As you work on a problem, new information will arise. Perhaps the method or instruments you are using do not measure what you want to measure. Then you will rethink your problem and method and possibly change your instrument. Refining means rethinking. It means weighing the pros and cons of your method, or of your solutions. The physics student may decide to continue to study regularly, but after several weeks, to drop the tutoring. Although the original plan was to use the tutor for longer, the student found it possible to apply, on her own, what was learned from the tutor. Thus, more time for other activities was now possible.

Using this process will enable you to solve personal, educational, and workplace problems in a thoughtful, comprehensive way. Figure 5-1 is a think link that demonstrates a way to visualize the flow of problem solving. Figure 5-2 contains a sample of how one person used this plan to solve a problem. Figure 5-3 leaves space for writing so that it can be used in your problem-solving process. These problem-solving steps essentially make up the nursing process: assessment, diagnosis, planning, implement, and evaluate.

Decision Making

Decisions are choices. Although every problem-solving process involves making a decision (when you decide which solution to try), not all decisions involve solving problems. Making a choice, or decision, requires thinking critically through all of the possible choices and evaluating which will work best for you and for the situation. Decisions large and small come up daily,

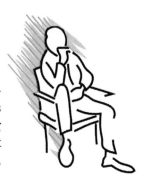

FIGURE 5-1

Problem-solving plan.

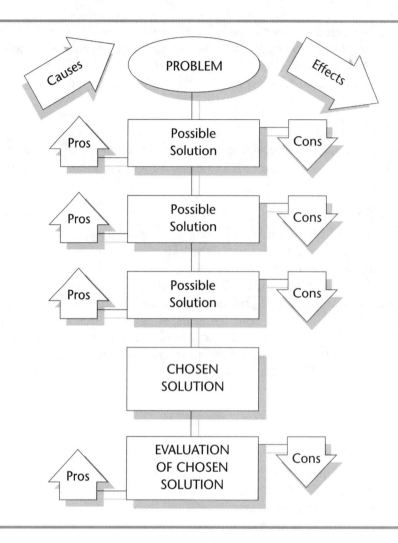

hourly, even every few minutes. Do you call your landlord when the heat isn't coming on? Do you drop a course? Should you stay in a relationship? Can you work part-time without interfering with school?

Before you begin the decision-making process, evaluate the level of the decision you are making. Do you have to decide what to have for lunch (usually a minor issue), or whether to quit a good job (often a major life change)? Some decisions are little day-to-day considerations that you can take care of quickly on your own. Others require thoughtful evaluation, time, and perhaps the input of others you trust. The following is a list of steps to take in order to think critically through a decision:

1. Decide on a goal. Why is this decision necessary? In other words, what result do you want from this decision, and what is its value? It is useful in the long run to consider your personal goals as well as your professional goals. Considering the *effects* you want can help you formulate your goal. For example, say a student currently attends a small private college. Her goal is to become a physical therapist. The school has a good program, but her financial situation has changed and has made this school too expensive for her.

FIGURE 5-2   How one student worked through a problem.

LIST CAUSES OF PROBLEM:

Must go to school to take classes

Can't have child with me in class

No one else at home to watch child

STATE PROBLEM HERE:

Need some way to provide child-care while I'm at school

LIST EFFECTS OF PROBLEM:

Missed exams and classes sometimes

Logistics take extra time, transport

Stress created for me and child

Lack of routine & comfort

Use boxes below to list possible solutions:

List potential POSITIVE effects for each solution:

Care is consistent

Reliable and familiar setting

Doesn't matter if child is sick

SOLUTION #1

Have a nanny at home

List potential NEGATIVE effects for each solution:

Expensive

Hard to find someone to trust

Person must follow my schedule

SOLUTION #2

Join child-care co-op

Meet parents like myself

Child has playmates

Inexpensive

Must trust other parents

Sick child might get others sick

SOLUTION #3

Get school to provide child care on campus

Close by to classes

Reliable care

No extra transport time

Costs school money

Need to find space and create facility

Restrictions & waiting lists

Now choose the solution you think is best—and try it.

CHOSEN SOLUTION

Join child-care co-op

List the actual POSITIVE effects for each solution:

Met some helpful people who understand me

My child likes the other three children

Low cost helps my budget

List the actual NEGATIVE effects for each solution:

When it's my turn, I have to care for four children

Sometimes our schedules clash

Can't let a sick child participate

FINAL EVALUATION: Was it a good or bad choice?

All in all, I think this is the best I could do on my budget. There are times when I have to stay home with a sick child, buy I'm mostly able to stay committed to both parenting and school.

Source: Adapted from a heuristic developed by Frank T. Lyman Jr., Ph.D., University of Maryland, 1983.

FIGURE 5-3   Use this form to work through one or more problem(s) of your own.

LIST CAUSES OF PROBLEM: STATE PROBLEM HERE: LIST EFFECTS OF PROBLEM:

_____   _____
_____   _____
_____   _____
_____   _____

Use boxes below to
list possible solutions:

List potential POSITIVE   SOLUTION #1   List potential NEGATIVE
effects for each solution: effects for each solution:

_____   _____
_____   _____
_____   _____

SOLUTION #2

_____   _____
_____   _____
_____   _____

SOLUTION #3

_____   _____
_____   _____
_____   _____

Now choose the solution
you think is best—and try it.

CHOSEN SOLUTION

List the actual POSITIVE   List the actual NEGATIVE
effects for each solution: effects for each solution:

_____   _____
_____   _____
_____   _____
_____   _____

FINAL EVALUATION: Was it a good or bad choice?

Source: Adapted from a heuristic developed by Frank T. Lyman Jr., Ph.D., University of Maryland, 1983.

2. Establish needs. *Recall* the needs of everyone (or everything) involved in the decision. The student needs a school with a full physical therapy program; she and her parents need to cut costs (her mother changed jobs and her family cannot continue to afford the current school); she values the education environment of her current school.

3. Name, investigate, and evaluate available options. Brainstorm possible choices, and then look at the facts surrounding each. *Evaluate* the pros and cons of each possibility. Weigh these and judge the best course of action. Here are some possibilities that the student in the college example might consider:

   ■ *Continue at the current college.* **Positive effects:** I wouldn't have to adjust to a new place or to new people. I could continue my course work as planned. **Negative effects:** I would have to find a way to finance most of my tuition and costs on my own, whether through loans, grants, or work. I'm not sure I could find time to work as much as I would need to, and I don't think I would qualify for as much aid as I now need.

   ■ *Transfer to the state college.* **Positive effects:** I might be able to reconnect with people there that I know from high school. Tuition and room costs would be cheaper than at my current school. I could transfer credits. **Negative effects:** I would still have to work some or find minimal financial aid. The physical therapy program is small and not very strong.

4. Decide on a plan of action and pursue it. Make a choice based on your evaluation, and act on your choice. In this case, the student might decide to move back in with her family and transfer to a public school to earn a bachelor's degree. Although she might lose some independence and contact with friends, the positive effects are money saved, opportunity to spend time on studies rather than working to earn tuition money.

5. Evaluate the result. Was it useful? Not useful? Some of both? Weigh the positive and negative effects. The student may find with her transfer decision that it can be hard living at home, although her parents are adjusting to her independence and she is trying to respect their concerns as parents. Fewer social distractions result in her getting more work done. The financial situation is much more favorable. All things considered, she evaluates that this decision was a good one.

Making important decisions can take time. Think through your decision thoroughly, considering your own ideas as well as those of others you trust, but don't hesitate to act once you have your plan. You cannot benefit from your decision until you act upon it and follow through.

 ## WHY SHIFT YOUR PERSPECTIVE?

Seeing the world from your perspective, or point of view, without trying to see things from another's point of view is inflexible, limiting, and frustrating. You probably know how hard it can be to relate to someone who cannot understand you—a coworker who's annoyed that you leave early on

Perspective
A mental point of view or outlook, based on a cluster of related assumptions, incorporating values, interests, and knowledge.

TONI M. RIEHM

Senior, Indiana University South Bend,
South Bend, Indiana

As a nontraditional student, I've been taking college courses for nine years on a part-time basis. I've worked on and off during this time, but for the most part, I've been a stay-at-home mom. In thinking about preparing for a future career, I wanted a degree that would allow me diversity in the job market and fulfillment as a person. Nursing offers much flexibility and personal rewards like no other career. The BSN program requires prerequisite classes in fields such as humanities and the sciences. Taking these courses enabled me to take about six to eight credit hours per semester while my children were small, and now that they are more independent, I can manage clinicals.

I'm very happy about my choice to become a nurse. There are many disciplines within the nursing

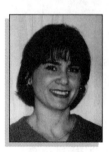

profession to choose from, and I see nursing as very purposeful because of the opportunity to assist people in achieving their optimal level of health. Sometimes you're helping patients face dramatic life changes because their current illness is forcing them to live a

new way. Other times you're helping people at the end of their lives to make that transition as gracefully as possible. In my clinical practice, I like taking a holistic approach to caring for people. Nursing teaches me to assist them with not only their immediate sickness but with how their health concerns affect their whole life.

In light of all these positives, I sometimes struggle to balance the completion of a bachelor's degree in nursing with all of my other responsibilities. This semester, in particular, has been very stressful. Last year my mother was diagnosed with lung cancer. She lived in Florida so I spent much of the summer there and then went back again this fall to be with her when she died. Juggling the needs of my family with the responsibilities of being a nursing student took a lot out of me. I continue to deal with the loss I'm experiencing, and so much of what I'm feeling has to be put on hold.

I realize many students encounter difficult situations like mine in which family priorities have to be balanced with the demands of school. I've also noticed that dedicated nursing students are high achievers who are dissatisfied if they aren't producing their best work. This is my dilemma now, too. My test scores have dropped some recently which bothers me because I know I am capable of doing better. With so many life happenings going on however, my mind is scattered on other things in addition to my classwork. There have even been times I've wanted to quit, but I know the regret I'd feel if I did that. My family has seen all the hard work I've put in so far, and my close friends and instructors have given me so much support along the way. I also think it's been a good example for my children to learn that making an effort and struggling to achieve does produce results. How can I manage all my responsibilities and still achieve my goals in pursuing my nursing degree?

SUSANNA CUNNINGHAM, B.S.N., PH.D., F.A.A.N.

Professor of Biobehavioral Nursing and Health
Systems, University of Washington, Seattle,
Washington

We have students here who are doing similar kinds of balancing acts. Managing our lives requires creative thinking of the highest order. The students who seem to do the best job at making these kinds

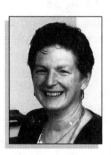

of life decisions are those who sort through their priorities. Then they slowly step through what they know they have to do. When I was in my postdoctoral program I made the decision to treat school like a job. I constrained it to certain hours and made my family the priority.

Although I have a doctoral degree, my secondary degree is in vacationing. I just returned from two weeks of scuba diving in Maui with my adult children. You need to play with your family. Trying new things leads us into different thinking processes. You don't have to get A's in order to prove you're smart. You're already a long way in achieving your goals, and you've proven that you have the skills for a successful nursing career. You'll do better later once you've given yourself time to recover. I consider it an act of courage when a student takes time to deal with personal issues rather than ignore them. The more important issue is, "What am I learning?" If you're going to class and focusing on the material in front of you, then you're learning and that's what matters.

Our brain is a miraculous organ. It has the ability to process information on various levels even when we're off doing something else. For example, I like to do crossword puzzles. If I can't figure out several words on a given day, I'll put it aside. I've noticed that when I come back to it another day with fresh spirit, the words often pop out. We as a society seem to think that doing more and running faster is a virtue, which is a strange thought. As nurses, we need to model self-care. Depending on your program's requirements, perhaps you could take only one or two classes the next quarter or even postpone school for a semester. In any case, slowing down is a smart decision.

Another strategy is to integrate what you're learning into family time. When I had statistics, I included my kids by having them draw diagrams. By teaching your kids what you're learning, you also refine your thoughts on the subject. The most creative people in science, and in other fields as well, are those who have taken ideas from different worlds and put them together in a new way. They can look at a problem from one field and put it with what they know from another field and find that it fits.

Losing our parents is a universal experience that often causes us to sit back and evaluate life more deeply. You need to honor the loss of your mother. I hope you're talking and thinking about her. Perhaps seeing a school counselor or enlisting the support of other students who are facing similar challenges can help. In so doing, you not only help yourself, you also demonstrate healthy ways to cope with loss for your children. So my main message to you is this: Be kind to yourself. Why should you be disheveled in the time you're alive? This is your life. It's not your boss', or your professor's, or your spouse's; it's yours. Make the most of it.

Thursdays for physical therapy, a parent who doesn't see why you can't take a study break to visit, a friend who can't understand why you would date someone of a different ethnicity. Seeing beyond one's own perspective can be difficult, especially when life problems and fatigue leave you feeling stressed.

On the other hand, when you shift your perspective to consider someone else's, you can open the lines of communication. Trying to understand what other people feel, need, and want makes you more responsive to them. They may feel respected by you and respond to you in turn. For example, if you want to add or drop a course and your advisor says it's impossible, not waiting to hear you out, the last thing you may feel like doing is pouring your heart out. On the other hand, if your advisor asks to hear your point of view, you may sense that you are respected. Because the advisor wants to hear from you, you feel valued; that may encourage you to respond, or even to change your mind.

Every time you shift your perspective, you can also learn something new. There are worlds of knowledge and possibilities outside your individual existence. You may learn that what you eat daily may be against someone else's religious beliefs. You may discover people who don't fit a stereotype.

Shifting your perspective is invaluable in helping you find fresh solutions. In nursing, a fresh view is extremely useful in understanding and interacting with others. It is critical that you develop this skill.

Asking questions like these will help you maintain flexibility and openness in your perspective.

- What is similar and different about this person/belief/method and me/my beliefs/my methods?
- What positive and negative effects come from this different way of being/acting/believing? Even if this perspective seems to have negative effects for me, how might it have positive effects for others and therefore have value?
- What can I learn from this different perspective? Is there anything I could adopt

for my own life—something that would help me improve who I am or what I do? Is there anything I wouldn't do myself but that I can still respect and learn from?

Shifting your perspective is at the heart of all successful communication. Each person is unique. Even within a group of people similar to yourself, there will be a great variety of perspectives. Whether you see that each world community has different customs or you understand that a friend can't go out on weekends because he spends that time with his mother, you have increased your wealth of knowledge and shown respect to others. Being able to shift perspective and communicate more effectively may mean the difference between success and failure in today's diverse working world.

 ## WHY PLAN STRATEGICALLY?

Strategy
A plan of action designed to accomplish a specific goal.

If you've ever played a game of chess or checkers, participated in a wrestling or martial arts match, planned an event, or had a drawn-out argument, you have had experience with strategy. In those situations and many others, you have to think through and anticipate the moves the other person is about to make. Often you have to think about several possible options that person could put into play, and you consider what you would counter with should any of those options occur. In competitive situations, you try to outguess the other person with your choices. The extent of your strategic skills can determine whether you will win or lose.

Strategy is the plan of action, the method, the "how" behind any goal you want to achieve. Specifically, strategic planning means having a plan for the future, whether you are looking at the next week, month, year, 10 years, or 50 years. It means exploring the future positive and negative effects of the choices you make and actions you take today. You are planning strategically right now just by being in school. You made a decision that the requirements of attending college are a legitimate price to pay for the skills, contacts, and opportunities that will help you in the future. As a student, you are challenging yourself to achieve. You are learning to set goals for the future, analyze what you want in the long term, and prepare for the job market to increase your career options. Being strategic with yourself means challenging yourself as you would challenge a competitor, urging yourself to work toward your goals with conviction and determination.

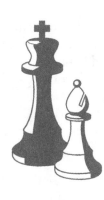

What are the benefits, or positive effects, of strategic planning?

Strategy is an essential skill in the workplace. A food company that wants to develop a successful health-food product needs to examine the anticipated trends in health consciousness. A nurse practitioner needs to think through every aspect of the client's case, anticipating how to manage a disease, medications, and other treatments. Strategic planning creates a vision into the future that allows the planner to anticipate all kinds of possibilities and, most importantly, to be prepared for them.

Strategic planning powers your short-term and long-term goal setting. Once you have set goals, you need to plan the steps that will help you achieve those goals over time. For example, a strategic thinker who wants to own a home in five years' time might drive a used car and cut out luxuries, put a small amount of money every month into a mutual fund, and keep an eye on current mortgage percentages. In class, a strategic planner will think critically about the material presented, knowing that information is most useful later on if it is clearly understood.

Strategic planning helps you keep up with technology. As technology develops more and more quickly, some jobs become obsolete and others are created. It's possible to spend years in school training for a career area that will be drying up when you are ready to enter the work force. When you plan strategically, you can take a broader range of courses or choose a nursing area that is expanding. This will make it more likely that your skills will be in demand well after you graduate.

Effective critical thinking is essential to strategic planning. Here are some tips for becoming a strategic planner:

Develop a rational plan. What approach is most likely to achieve your goal? What steps will you need to take this year, or in 5, 10, or 20 years from now?

Anticipate all possible outcomes of your actions. What are the pros and cons?

Ask the question "how?" How do you achieve your goals? How do you learn effectively and remember what you learn? How do you develop a productive idea on the job? How do you distinguish yourself at school and at work?

Use human resources. Use information from talking to people who are where you want to be, professionally or personally. What caused them to get there? Ask them what they believe are the important steps to take, degrees to have, training to experience, and knowledge to gain.

In each thinking process, seen in Figure 5-4, use your imagination and creativity to come up with ideas, examples, causes, effects, and solutions. You have a capacity to be creative, whether you are aware of it or not. Open up your mind and awaken your creativity. It will enhance your critical thinking, make you a better student, and make life more enjoyable.

 ## HOW CAN YOU DEVELOP CREATIVITY?

Everyone is creative. Although the word "creative" may seem to refer primarily to artists, writers, musicians, and others who work in fields whose creative aspects are in the forefront, creativity comes in many other forms. It is the power to create anything, whether it is a solution, idea, approach, tangible product, work of art, system, program—anything at all. To help expand your concept of creativity, the list below offers examples of day-to-day creative thinking.

- Figuring out an alternative plan when your baby sitter unexpectedly cancels on you

TERMS

Creativity
The ability to produce something new through imaginative skill.

FIGURE 5-4

The wheel of thinking.

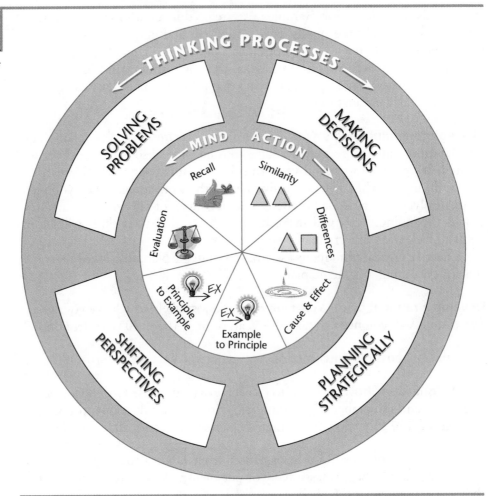

- Planning how to coordinate your work and class schedules
- Talking through a problem with an instructor, and finding a way to understand each other

Creative innovations introduced by all kinds of people continually expand and change the world. Here are some that have had an impact:

- Susan B. Anthony and other women fought for and won the right for women to vote.
- Florence Nightingale promoted hand washing for health care workers and saved thousands of lives, even though the reason it helped, it eliminates bacteria, was not known.
- Henry Ford introduced the assembly line method of automobile construction, making cars cheap enough to be available to the average citizen.
- Rosa Parks refused to give up her seat on the bus to a white person, thus setting off a chain of events that gave rise to the civil rights movement.
- Alicia Diaz, director of the Center of Hispanic Policy, Research, and Development, developed corporate partnerships and internship programs that have become models for small, efficient government.

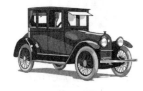

Even though these particular innovations had wide-ranging effects, the characteristics of these influential innovators can be found in all people who exercise their creative capabilities.

Characteristics of Creative People

Creative people think in fresh new ways that improve our understanding of the world. Roger van Oech, an expert on creativity, highlights this kind of flexibility.[2] "I've found that the hallmark of creative people is their mental flexibility," he says. "Like race-car drivers who shift in and out of different gears depending on where they are on the course, creative people are able to shift in and out of different types of thinking depending on the needs of the situation at hand. . . . They're doggedly persistent in striving to reach their goals."

Creativity in nursing and science leads to many discoveries. Although many scientific discoveries occur accidentally, which is called *serendipity*, it takes creativity to recognize that the accidental discovery, or result, is valuable. Serendipity is common in science, it occurs when something is discovered while in the process of trying to discover something else. Serendipity is "the gift of finding valuable or agreeable things not sought for."[3]

Examples of creativity and serendipity in science abound and include:

- Velcro by George deMestral. Velcro was accidentally discovered by deMestral when he returned home from a walk and noticed a cocklebur stuck tightly to the fabric of his clothing. On close examination, he noticed how well the bur's hooks held onto the fabric and used that same system to make Velcro.

- Penicillin by Sir Alexander Fleming. In 1928, Fleming worked in a bacteriology laboratory preparing influenza cultures in petri dishes. He noticed a clear area in the dish where a piece of mold had fallen. He isolated the mold and found it belonged to the genus *Penicillium*. Out of the thousands of species of molds, this one happened to fall in Fleming's petri dish, but more importantly, he noticed its effect and followed up by asking why the bacteria culture was cleared away by this particular substance. Fleming's intelligence is what made the discovery. He is quoted as saying, "The story of penicillin has a certain romance in it and helps to illustrate the amount of chance, or fortune, or fate, or destiny, call it what you will, in anybody's career."[4]

Discoveries are not dependent on accidents alone, creativity is needed to think of new ways to do things and to make sense of what you observe. Louis Pasteur, who made exceptional breakthroughs in microbiology and medicine, put it this way: "In the fields of observation, chance favors only the prepared mind." Yes, accidents do happen, and they can lead to major discoveries; but if you aren't ready, you won't know them when you see them. Unless the mind is thoroughly charged beforehand, the proverbial spark of genius, if it should manifest itself, probably will find nothing to ignite.[5]

Another form of creativity is in asking the right questions. The 1998 Columbus scholar Marek Elbaum, a scientist at Electro-Optical Sciences, was interested in how he could help cancer specialists detect melanoma, one of the deadliest forms of cancer. He asked the following question and produced a creative answer:

> We went to oncologists and we asked, "What is difficult for you?" And they said, "If you could help us discriminate early melanoma from benign pigmented lesions, this would be of great help." And we said with great arrogance, "Yes, we can do such things."[6]

The next question Elbaum and his colleagues asked was if the malignant lesions looked different than benign ones under different light frequencies. This turned out to be the case, and they created an imaging device that detects melanoma in less than a minute.

Creating science out of everyday observations is what the web-based Beachcombers group and the Oceanography Society are doing by studying and recording the flotsam that washes up on beaches around the world. The idea behind this documentation is to discover social and economic clues about global shipping and how pollution travels, by harnessing members of the Beachcombers' natural enthusiasm for observation of vast stretches of the world's coastlines. The website, "Beachcombers' Alert!" provides potential data collectors instructions for joining the search.

Overall, your chance of making a miracle discovery is minimal, but you can significantly add to the body of knowledge that builds toward such discoveries. Nobel laureate Paul Flory, upon receiving the Priestley Medal, the American Chemical Society's highest award, said:

> Significant inventions are not mere accidents . . . happenstance usually plays a part, to be sure, but there is much more to invention than the popular notion of a bolt out of the blue. Knowledge in depth and breadth are virtual prerequisites.[7]

Brainstorming Toward a Creative Answer

As discussed earlier in the chapter, you are brainstorming when you approach a problem by letting your mind free-associate and come up with as many possible ideas, examples, or solutions as you can, without immediately evaluating them as good or bad. Brainstorming is also referred to as divergent thinking—you start with the issue or problem and then let your mind diverge, or go in as many different directions as it wants, in search of ideas or solutions. You can use brainstorming for problem solving, decision making, preparing to write an essay, or any time you want to open your mind to new possibilities. You can continue to use this important technique in your nursing career. It works with all sorts of groups, teams, and even with clients and families.[8] Here are some rules for successful brainstorming.

Don't evaluate or criticize an idea right away. Write down your ideas so that you remember them. Evaluate later, after you have had a chance to think about them. Try to avoid criticizing other people's ideas as well. Students often become stifled when their ideas are evaluated during brainstorming.

Notice your tendency to say that things are right or wrong, black or white, and instead let things be gray—unknown.

Focus on quantity; don't worry about quality until later. Try to generate as many ideas or examples as you can. The more thoughts you generate, the better the chance that one may be useful. Brainstorming works well in groups. Group members can become inspired by, and make creative use of, one another's ideas.

Let yourself consider wild and wacky ideas. Trust yourself to fall off the edge of tradition when you explore your creativity. Sometimes the craziest ideas end up being the most productive, positive, workable solutions around.

Remember, creativity can be developed if you have the desire and patience. Be gentle with yourself in the process. Most people are harsher with themselves and their ideas than is necessary. Your creative expression will become more free with practice.

Creativity and Critical Thinking

Critical thinking and creativity work hand in hand. Critical thinking is inherently creative, because it requires you to take the information you are given and come up with original ideas or solutions to problems. For example, you can brainstorm to generate possible causes of a certain effect. If the effect you were examining was fatigue in afternoon classes, you might come up with possible causes such as lack of sleep, too much morning caffeine, a diet heavy in carbohydrates, a natural tendency toward low energy at that time, or an instructor who doesn't inspire you. Through your consideration of causes and solutions, you have been thinking both creatively and critically.

Creative thinkers and critical thinkers have similar characteristics—both consider new perspectives, ask questions, don't hesitate to question accepted assumptions and traditions, and persist in the search for answers. Only through thinking critically and creatively can you freely question, brainstorm, and evaluate in order to come up with the most fitting ideas, solutions, decisions, arguments, and plans.

You use critical-thinking mind actions throughout everything you do in school and in your daily life.

Κριveιv

The word "critical" is derived from the Greek word *krinein*, which means to separate in order to choose or select. To be a mindful, aware critical thinker, you need to be able to separate, evaluate, and select ideas, facts, and thoughts.

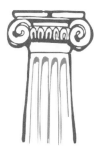

Think of this concept as you apply critical thinking to your reading, writing, and interaction with others. Be aware of the information you take in and of your thoughts, and be selective as you process them. Critical thinking gives you the power to make sense of life by deliberately selecting how to respond to the information, people, and events that you encounter.

Applications   **Chapter 5**

KEY INTO YOUR LIFE
Opportunities to Apply What You Learn

 Brainstorming on the Idea Wheel

Your creative mind can solve problems when you least expect it. Many people report having sudden ideas while exercising, driving, showering, upon waking, or even when dreaming. When the pressure is off, the mind is often more free to roam through uncharted territory and bring back treasures.

To make the most of this "mind-float," grab ideas right when they surface. If you don't, they roll back into your subconscious as if on a wheel. Since you never know how big the wheel is, you can't be sure when that particular idea will roll to the top again. That's one of the reasons why writers carry notebooks—they need to grab thoughts when they come to the top of the wheel.

On the blank supplied below, name a problem, large or small, to which you haven't yet found a satisfactory solution. Do a brainstorm without the time limit. Be on the lookout for ideas, causes, effects, solutions, or similar problems coming to the top of your wheel. The minute it happens, grab this book and write your idea(s) next to the problem. Take a look at your ideas later, and see how your creative mind may have pointed you toward some original and workable solutions. You may want to keep a book by your bed to catch ideas that pop up before, during, or after sleep.

Problem: _____

Ideas: _____

_____

_____

_____

_____

_____

_____

_____

_____

5.2 *Brainstorming in a Group*

In a group, brainstorm some answers to the following questions. Remember, in brainstorming there are no right or wrong answers. This is a time to be creative and let the ideas flow.

THEMES IN THE STUDY OF LIFE	QUESTIONS
Life is organized on many structural levels.	What are the structural levels?
Cells are the organism's basic unit of structure and function.	What purpose do cells serve in the function of organisms and their structure?
Continuity of life is based on inheritable information—DNA.	What are the structure and function of DNA in the inheritance of traits?
Study of organisms enriches the study of life.	What differences are there between an organism as a whole functioning unit and its structures?
Structure and function correlate at all levels of biological organization.	How does anatomy determine function?
Organisms are open systems that interact continuously with their environments.	How does the environment affect the function or structure of an organism?
Diversity and unity are the dual faces of life on earth.	In what ways do organisms differ and in which ways are they alike?
Evolution is the core theme of biology.	What are the hallmarks of evolution, and how does it unify, or connect, life on earth?
Science is a process of inquiry that often involves hypothetical and deductive thinking.	What is an example of deductive inquiry?

Source: Adapted from Campbell, N. A. (1997) *Biology* (4th ed.). Menlo Park: Benjamin Cummings, pages 2–24.

5.3 *Essential Questioning*

Choose one of the themes from Exercise 5.2. Considering this theme as a statement of a biological science principle, devise as many questions as you can that would help you clarify, validate, support, or dispute the principle.

_____

_____

_____
_____
_____
_____
_____
_____
_____

5.4 *Problem Solving*

Choose two of your questions from Exercise 5.3 and answer the following:

A. What further information would be helpful to work toward an answer?

Question 1: _____

_____

_____

Question 2: _____

_____

_____

B. Where could you go for this information?

Question 1: _____

_____

_____

Question 2: _____

_____

_____

C. How could you go about testing your questions?

Question 1: _____

_____

_____

Question 2: _____

_____

_____

Biases

Consider the two questions you chose in Exercise 5.4 and the theme you chose for Exercise 5.3. Make a list of what biases may have affected your choices. (Try to think of at least three.)

_____

_____

_____

_____

_____

_____

KEY TO SELF-EXPRESSION
Discovery Through Journal Writing

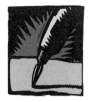

To record your thoughts, use a separate journal or the lined page at the end of the chapter.

Strategic Planning

Discuss your abilities and limitations in how you set and plan your short-term and long-term goals. Do you tend to plan ahead of time? Why or why not? What do you like and dislike about strategically planning ahead? Do you have a hard time seeing beyond the present, or do you like to predict what will happen in the future? Discuss a long-term goal in terms of what you want in one year, five years, ten years, and twenty years. How do you plan to accomplish this goal? What steps will you take? What do you want to achieve?

Journal

Name _____ Date _____

6

Reading and Studying

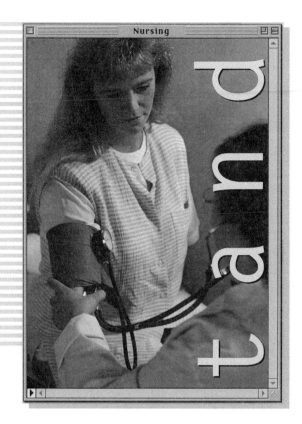

Maximizing Written Resources

S ociety revolves around the written word. As the *Condition of Education 1996* states, "In recent years, literacy has been viewed as one of the fundamental tools necessary for successful economic performance in industrialized societies. Literacy is no longer defined merely as a basic threshold of reading ability, but rather as the ability to understand and use printed information in daily activities, at home, at work, and in the community."[1]

If you read thoroughly and understand what you read and if you achieve your study goals, you can improve your capacity to learn and understand. In this chapter you will learn how you can overcome barriers to successful reading and benefit from defining a purpose every time you read. You will explore the PQ3R study technique and see how critical reading can help you maximize your understanding of any kind of nursing or science text. Finally, the chapter will provide an overview of your library's resources.

In this chapter, you will explore answers to the following questions:

- What are the challenges in science and nursing readings?
- What kind of reading will you do in nursing and the sciences?
- Why define your purpose for reading?
- How can PQ3R help you study reading materials?
- How can you read critically?
- What resources does your library offer?

 ## WHAT ARE THE CHALLENGES IN SCIENCE AND NURSING READINGS?

Whatever your skill level, you will encounter challenges that make reading more difficult, such as an excess of reading assignments, difficult texts, distractions, a lack of speed and comprehension, and insufficient vocabulary. Following are some ideas about how to meet these challenges. Note that if you have a reading disability, if English is not your primary language, or if you have limited reading skills, you may need additional support and guidance. Most colleges provide services for students through a reading center or tutoring program. Take the initiative to seek help if you need it. Many accomplished learners have benefited from help in specific areas.

Dealing with Reading Overload

Reading overload is part of almost every college experience. On a typical day, you may be faced with reading assignments that look like this:

- An entire textbook chapter on the causes of depression (psychology).
- An original research study on the stages of sleep (physiology).
- Pages 1–50 in a human biology textbook (biological science).

Reading all this and more leaves little time for anything else unless you read selectively and skillfully. You can't control your reading load. You can, however, improve your reading skills. The material in this chapter will present techniques that can help you read and study as efficiently as you possibly can, while still having time left over for other things.

Working Through Difficult Science and Nursing Texts

While many science and nursing textbooks are useful teaching tools, some can be poorly written and organized. Students using texts that aren't well written may blame themselves for the difficulty they're experiencing. Because texts are often written with the purpose of challenging the intellect, even well-written and organized texts may be dense and difficult to read. Generally, the further you advance in your education, the more complex your required reading is likely to be. For example, your physiology professor may assign a chapter on renal hemodynamics. You may feel at times as though you are reading a foreign language as you encounter new concepts, words, and terms.

Assignments can also be difficult when the required reading is from primary sources rather than from texts. *Primary sources* are original documents rather than another writer's interpretation of these documents. They include:

- Historical documents
- Scientific studies, including lab reports and accounts of experiments
- Research journal articles

The academic writing found in nursing research journal articles and scientific studies is different from other kinds of writing. Some academic writers assume that readers understand sophisticated concepts. They may not define basic terms, provide background information, or supply a wealth of examples to support their ideas. As a result, concepts may be difficult to understand.

Making your way through difficult reading material is hard work that can be accomplished through focus, motivation, commitment, and skill. The following strategies may help.

Approach your reading assignments head-on. Be careful not to prejudge them as impossible or boring before you even start to read.

Accept the fact that some texts may require some extra work and concentration. Set a goal to make your way through the material and learn, whatever it takes.

When a primary source discusses difficult concepts that it does not explain, put in some extra work to define such concepts on your own. Ask your instructor or other students for help. Consult reference materials in that particular subject area, other class materials, dictionaries, and encyclopedias. You may want to make this process more convenient by creating your own minilibrary at home. Collect reference materials that you use often, such as a dictionary, a thesaurus, a writer's style handbook, and maybe an atlas or computer manual. You may also benefit from owning reference materials in your particular areas of study. "If you find yourself going to the library to look up the same reference again and again, consider purchasing that book for your personal or office library," advises library expert Sherwood Harris.[2]

"No barrier of the senses shuts me out from the sweet, gracious discourse of my book friends. They talk to me without embarrassment or awkwardness."
HELEN KELLER

Look for order and meaning in seemingly chaotic reading materials. The information you will find in this chapter on the PQ3R reading technique and on critical reading will help you discover patterns and achieve a greater depth of understanding. Finding order within chaos is an important skill, not just in the mastery of reading, but also in life. This skill can give you power by helping you "read" (think through) work dilemmas, personal problems, and educational situations.

Managing Distractions

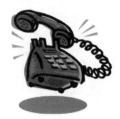

With so much happening around you, it's often hard to keep your mind on what you are reading. Distractions take many forms. Some are external: the sound of a telephone, a friend who sits next to you at lunch and wants to talk, a young child who asks for help with homework. Other distractions come from within. As you try to study, you may be thinking about your parent's health, an argument you had with a friend or partner, a paper due in art history, or a site on the Internet that you want to visit.

Identify the Distraction and Choose a Suitable Action

Pinpoint what's distracting you before you decide what kind of action to take. If the distraction is *external* and *out of your control*, such as construction outside your building or a noisy group in the library, try to move away from it. If the distraction is *external* but *within your control*, such as the television, telephone, or children, take action. For example, if the television or phone is a problem, turn off the TV or unplug the phone for an hour.

If the distraction is *internal*, there are a few strategies to try that may help you clear your mind. You may want to take a break from your studying and tend to one of the issues that you are worrying about. Physical exercise may relax you and bring back your ability to focus. For some people, studying while listening to music helps to quiet a busy mind. For others, silence may do the trick. If you need silence to read or study and cannot find a truly quiet environment, consider purchasing sound-muffling headphones or even earplugs.

Find the Best Place and Time to Read

Any reader needs focus and discipline in order to concentrate on the material. Finding a place and time that minimize outside distractions will help you achieve that focus. Here are some suggestions:

Read alone unless you are working with other readers. Family members, friends, or others who are not in study mode may interrupt your concentration. If you prefer to read alone, establish a relatively interruption-proof place and time, such as an out-of-the-way spot at the library or an after-class hour in an empty classroom. If you study at home and live with other people, you may want to place a "Quiet" sign on the door. Some students benefit from reading with one or more other students. If this helps you, plan to schedule a group reading meeting where you read sections of the assigned material and then break to discuss them.

Find a comfortable location. Many students study in the library on a hard-backed chair. Others prefer a library easy chair, a chair in their room, or even the floor. The spot you choose should be comfortable enough for hours of reading, but not so comfortable that you fall asleep. Also, make sure that you have adequate lighting and aren't too hot or too cold.

Choose a regular reading place and time. Choose a spot or two you like and return to them often. Also, choose a time when your mind is alert and focused. Some students prefer to read just before or after the class for which the reading is assigned. Eventually, you will associate preferred places and times with focused reading.

If it helps you concentrate, listen to soothing background music. The right music can drown out background noises and relax you. However, the wrong music can make it impossible to concentrate; for some people, silence is better. Experiment to learn what you prefer; if music helps, stick with the type that works best. A personal headset makes listening possible no matter where you are.

Turn off the television. For most people, reading and TV don't mix.

Building Comprehension and Speed

Most students lead busy lives, carrying heavy academic loads while perhaps working a job or even caring for a family. It's difficult to make time to study at all, let alone handle the enormous reading assignments for your different classes. Increasing your reading comprehension and speed will save you valuable time and effort.

Rapid reading won't do you any good if you can't remember the material or answer questions about it. However, reading too slowly can be equally inefficient because it often eats up valuable study time and gives your mind space to wander. Your goal is to read for maximum speed *and* comprehension. Focus on comprehension first, because greater comprehension is the primary goal and also promotes greater speed.

Methods for Increasing Reading Comprehension

Following are some specific strategies for increasing your understanding of what you read:

Continually build your knowledge through reading and studying. More than any other factor, what you already know before you read a passage will determine your ability to understand and remember important ideas. Previous knowledge, including vocabulary, facts, and ideas, gives you a context for what you read.

Establish your purpose for reading. When you establish what you want to get out of your reading, you will be able to determine what level of understanding you need to reach and, therefore, on what you need to focus.

TERMS

Context
Written or spoken knowledge that can help to illuminate the meaning of a word or passage.

WENDY CASCIATO

Senior, University of Iowa, Iowa City, Iowa

My area of interest is community health nursing. Upon graduation, I would like to pursue a career in parish or school nursing. One of the challenges I've faced as a college student is information overload. There's so much material to absorb, and sometimes my concerns aren't addressed in textbooks.

For example, I've been receiving quite a bit of advice from faculty and other nurses. They recommend that even though I know I want to be a community health nurse, I should work for a year or two at a hospital. They say floor work provides an opportunity to solidify a nurse's assessment skills. For me, this suggestion presents a real internal conflict. I'm eager to launch my career in community health, yet I also want to be fully prepared to assume the challenges of community health nursing.

This brings me to another related concern, which is the often subtle but very real insinuations I receive about community health nursing being a less respected position than that of a hospital nurse. I sense that this branch of the nursing profession isn't viewed with the same esteem as other nursing specialties. Of course, I don't believe that, but I'm not sure how to counter this stereotype. Their advice makes me wonder if my education has been enough.

As beneficial as my studies are, I realize there's more knowledge for me to tap. Today we have many written resources available at our fingertips, 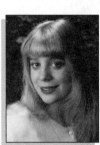 and I want to make the most of this opportunity. However, weeding through what's relevant, whether I'm on the Internet or in the library, can get overwhelming. If I could expand my understanding of how to set professional goals and what resources would best facilitate the fulfillment of these goals, I think I might have a better handle on making decisions that affect my nursing career. Can you offer suggestions for maximizing written resources?

KATHRYN H. KRAUSS, R.N., M.S.W.

Parish Nurse, Central United Methodist Church, Spokane, Washington

My nursing career spans over 40 years of experience, when I began as a hospital nurse. I've also taught parenting classes for the American Red Cross, served as a Lamaze instructor, and developed a support group for women with breast cancer, as well as many other roles in between. But I've not found any area as personally fulfilling as community health nursing.

The advice you're receiving, in my opinion, is incorrect. Although hospital work is valuable in many ways, community health nursing offers such a wide range of experiences that you'll find yourself making assessments all the time. I work as a 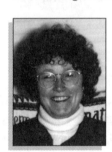 parish nurse for an inner city church. Our church serves over 25,000 meals per year to high school students, families, the poor, homeless, and mentally ill. We provide health education, do assessments and help connect folks to health care providers and agencies. We also promote health care among the residents of the low-income apartment buildings in our neighborhood. In one of the buildings, where many of the residents have mental illness, we offer art therapy classes and host an art exhibition of their work. In all of these activities, I'm constantly assessing people's needs.

Perhaps community health nursing isn't held in high esteem among the nurses you know because of the value they place on modern technology, which hospitals rely on. By contrast, community health nursing emphasizes hospitality, which isn't usually a high-tech activity. However, building relationships is a key component to effective prevention of health problems. If you can't earn the trust and respect of the people in your community, they won't allow you to educate them about their health issues.

I suggest that you not try to change anyone else's stereotype of the specialty you've chosen.

Instead, put your energy into enjoying what you do. Your intuition about the need to set professional goals is a keen observation. One goal you may want to set is to obtain certification through the ANA Credential Center. This requires rigorous and disciplined community health nursing education.

Information overload will continue to be an issue, even after you leave college. One of the most effective methods I've found for staying current is to join professional nurse organizations. I recommend the regional parish nurse organization, which publishes a monthly newsletter. The second organization worth checking out is your local parish nurse support group. The monthly meetings always contain an educational component, plus they have an e-mail bulletin board. From these resources, you can begin to develop your own library by collecting and filing inspiring articles. In the process, you will train your mind to notice interesting and pertinent information as it relates to your specialty.

Reading good literature, beyond what you were exposed to in the classroom, can also supplement your education. I have an extensive and diverse library that includes literature, philosophy, social work, nursing practice, psychology, and theology. I use these books and articles daily in many ways. For example, I crafted my personal mission statement based on the Bible, from Jesus' words: "I have come that they might have life and life in all its fullness" (John 10:10). My library also helps me serve the students under my supervision and is a useful resource when I write articles for nursing publications.

And take advantage of people resources. Enlisting the support of a spiritual director can help you define your call in life. I also suggest that you seek out a mentor who is a community health nurse. You can observe how this person handles snags in their professional life, and what habits they implement that help them succeed. Studying another person might be the best book you'll ever read.

Remove the barriers of negative self-talk. Instead of telling yourself that you cannot understand, think positively. Tell yourself: *I can learn this material. I am a good reader.* And then, if you do need help, get it.

Think critically. Ask yourself questions. Do you understand the sentence, paragraph, or chapter you just read? Are ideas and supporting examples clear to you? Could you clearly explain what you just read to someone else?

Methods for Increasing Reading Speed

The following suggestions will help increase your reading speed.

- Try to read groups of words rather than single words.
- Avoid pointing your finger to guide your reading, since this will slow your pace.
- Try swinging your eyes from side to side as you read a passage, instead of stopping at various points to read individual words.
- When reading narrow columns, focus your eyes in the middle of the column and read down the page. With practice, you'll be able to read the entire column width.
- Avoid vocalization when reading.
- Avoid thinking each word to yourself as you read it, a practice known as *subvocalization*. Subvocalization is one of the primary causes of slow reading speed.

Facing the challenges of reading is only the first step. The next important step is to look at the different kinds of reading you will encounter as a science major.

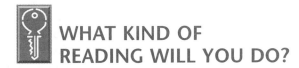

WHAT KIND OF READING WILL YOU DO?

Readings in nursing and science courses will differ from liberal arts courses in three ways.

Vocalization
The practice of
speaking the
words and/or
moving your lips
while reading.

1. Amount of new vocabulary you will need to learn. Any science you study will have new terms to describe phenomena unique to that discipline. For example, in biology words crop up like chloroplasts, isotonic, plasmolysis, and vestigial. In nursing, acronyms are the rule rather than the exception. A patient has an AMI (anterior myocardial infarction), requires q 1 ABGs (arterial blood gases monitored every hour), and is on an IABP (intra-aortic balloon pump) in preparation for a PTCA (percutaneous transluminal angioplasty) or a CABG (coronary artery bypass graft).

2. Content is generally not written in a narrative style. Therefore, following the flow of the text is more challenging. Science books, if written in typical technical writing style, can be dry and a drudgery to plow through. Fortunately, there are many technical and textbook writers who are able to present scientific information in lively and interesting ways. Hopefully, these writers will be the ones you are required to read. If not, just take extra time for your reading and ask for help interpreting the "foreign" language you are learning.

3. Content is concentrated and text is full of information, diagrams, and formulas. Science and nursing texts are concentrated, usually lacking any story, or as described above, lacking easy narrative flow. In addition, you are required to read and understand symbols, math formulas and equations, diagrams of models, and graphs, which are used to explain the material. You will be memorizing new terms and models in order to learn more complex concepts. Graphics, that is, not written text, are often used to represent ideas.

Along with your readings from textbooks, you will read from research journals and possibly other science-oriented publications like *Scientific American*, *Natural History*, or *Image: The Journal of Nursing Scholarship*. Books hold up-to-date information but not the most current, cutting edge information. From the time an author submits her manuscript for a textbook, it can take a year or more to be printed. For basic, or beginning, science courses, such as geology, physiology, or chemistry, the age of a textbook matters less than for courses dealing with information on technology or breakthrough discoveries, such as new cancer treatments.

The most up-to-date information is found in journals that publish research findings. Journals are designed to disseminate new and relevant information to the scientific community of a particular field. In nursing there is the *Journal of Advanced Nursing Science* and *Image*; in medicine, *JAMA* and the *New England Journal of Medicine*; in life sciences there is *Nature*. These are all examples of discipline-specific publications that publish research articles.

Journals serve the function of letting other researchers, or would-be researchers, see what their colleagues are doing. Repetition of studies is an important step in validating results before they are put into practice or applied to further study. Many research studies are designed to replicate research found in journals.

Another purpose of journals is to critically review the research being submitted for publication. Journals have reviewers who are asked to read and comment on an article before it is published. This review process helps ensure that published research is of high quality. However, not all research that is published is of the highest quality, and this is one very good reason why you will be learning to review research articles yourself. You have to understand the concepts of research and research methodology before you continue in a science career, because once in the field you must be able to critically review the research you read before you put it into practice.

Now, you understand better the challenges and types of reading in science. The final important step is to examine why you are reading any given piece of material.

WHY DEFINE YOUR PURPOSE FOR READING?

As with all other aspects of your education, asking important questions will enable you to make the most of your efforts. When you define your purpose, you ask yourself *why* you are reading a particular piece of material. One way to do this is by completing this sentence: "In reading this material, I intend to define/learn/answer/achieve . . ." With a clear purpose in mind, you can decide how much time and what kind of effort to expend on various reading assignments. Nearly 375 years ago, Francis Bacon, the English philosopher, recognized that

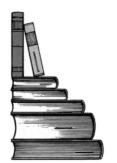

> Some books are to be tasted, others to be swallowed, and some few to be chewed and digested; that is, some books are to be read only in parts, others to be read but not curiously; and some few to be read wholly, and with diligence and attention.

Achieving your reading purpose requires adapting to different types of reading materials. Being a flexible reader—adjusting your reading strategies and pace—will help you to adapt successfully.

Purpose Determines Reading Strategy

With purpose comes direction; with direction comes a strategy for reading. Following are four reading purposes, examined briefly. You may have one or more for each piece of reading material you approach.

Purpose 1: Read to evaluate critically. Critical evaluation involves approaching the material with an open mind, examining causes and effects, evaluating ideas, and asking questions that test the strength of the writer's argument and that try to identify assumptions. Critical reading is essential for you to demonstrate an understanding of material that goes beyond basic recall of information. You will read more about critical reading later in the chapter.

Purpose 2: Read for comprehension. Much of the studying you do involves reading for the purpose of comprehending the material. The two main components of comprehension are *general principles* and *specific facts/examples*. These components depend on one another. Facts and examples help to explain or support ideas, and ideas provide a framework that helps the reader to remember facts and examples.

General Principles. General principles reading is rapid reading that seeks an overview of the material. You may skip entire sections as you focus on headings, subheadings, and summary statements in search of general principles.

Specific Facts/Examples. At times, readers may focus on locating specific pieces of information—for example, the sequence of geologic time periods. Often, a reader may search for examples that support or explain more general principles—for example, the structure of a plant cell. Because you know exactly what you are looking for, you can skim the material at a rapid rate. Reading your texts for specific information may help before taking a test.

Purpose 3: Read for practical application. A third purpose for reading is to gather usable information that you can apply toward a specific goal. When you read a computer software manual, an instruction sheet for assembling a bookshelf, or a cookbook recipe, your goal is to learn how to do something. Reading and action usually go hand in hand.

Purpose 4: Read for pleasure. Some materials you read for entertainment, such as *Rolling Stone* magazine or the latest John Grisham courtroom thriller. Entertaining reading may also go beyond materials that seem obviously designed to entertain. Whereas some people may read a Jane Austen novel for comprehension, as in a class assignment, others may read Austen's books for pleasure.

Purpose Determines Pace

George M. Usova, senior education specialist and graduate professor at the Johns Hopkins University, explains: "Good readers are flexible readers. They read at a variety of rates and adapt them to the reading *purpose* at hand, the *difficulty* of the material, and their *familiarity* with the subject area."[3] As Table 6-1 shows, good readers link the pace of reading to their reading purpose.

So far, this chapter has focused on reading. Recognizing obstacles to effective reading and defining the various purposes for reading lay the groundwork for effective *studying*—the process of mastering the concepts and skills contained in your texts.

 ## HOW CAN PQ3R HELP YOU STUDY READING MATERIALS?

When you study, you take ownership of the material you read. You learn it well enough to apply it to what you do. For example, by the time students studying to be computer hardware technicians complete their course work, they should be able to assemble various machines and analyze hardware problems that lead to malfunctions.

Studying also gives you mastery over *concepts*. For example, a dental hygiene student learns the causes of gum disease, a biology student learns what happens during photosynthesis, and a health sciences student learns about health policy analysis.

TABLE 6-1

TYPE OF MATERIAL	READING PURPOSE	PACE
Academic readings ■ Textbooks ■ Original sources ■ Articles from scholarly journals ■ Online publications for academic readers ■ Lab reports ■ Required fiction	■ Critical analysis ■ Overall mastery ■ Preparation for tests	■ Slow, especially if the material is new and unfamiliar
Manuals ■ Instructions ■ Recipes	■ Practical application	■ Slow to medium
Journalism and nonfiction for the general reader ■ Nonfiction books ■ Newspapers ■ Magazines ■ Online publications for the general public	■ Understanding of general ideas, key concepts, and specific facts for personal understanding and/or practical application	■ Medium to fast
Nonrequired ■ Fiction	■ Understanding of general ideas, key concepts, and specific facts for enjoyment	■ Variable, but tending toward the faster speeds

Linking purpose to pace.

Source: Adapted from Nicholas Reid Schaffzin, *The Princeton Review Reading Smart.* New York: Random House, 1996, p. 15.

This section will focus on a technique that will help you learn and study more effectively as you read your nursing and science textbooks.

Preview-Question-Read-Recite-Review (PQ3R)

PQ3R is a technique that will help you grasp ideas quickly, remember more, and review effectively and efficiently for tests. The symbols PQ3R stand for *preview, question, read, recite,* and *review*—all steps in the studying process. Developed more than 55 years ago by Francis Robinson, the technique is still being used today because it works.[4] It is particularly helpful for studying science texts.

Moving through the stages of PQ3R requires that you know how to skim and scan. Skimming involves rapid reading of various chapter elements, including introductions, conclusions, and summaries; the first and last lines of

TERMS

Skimming
Rapid, superficial reading of material that involves glancing through to determine central ideas and main elements.

Scanning
Reading material
in an invest-
igative way,
searching for
specific
information.

paragraphs; boldface or italicized terms; pictures, charts, and diagrams. In contrast, scanning involves the careful search for specific facts and examples. You will probably use scanning during the *review* phase of PQ3R when you need to locate and remind yourself of particular information. In a chemistry text, for example, you may scan for examples of how to apply a particular formula.

Preview

The best way to ruin a whodunit novel is to flip through the pages to find out how everything turned out. However, when reading textbooks, previewing can help you learn and is encouraged. *Previewing* refers to the process of surveying, or pre-reading, a book before you actually study it. Most textbooks include devices that give students an overview of the text as a whole as well as of the contents of individual chapters. As you look at Figure 6-1, on the following page, think about how many of these devices you already use.

Question

Your next step is to examine the chapter headings and, on your own paper, write questions linked to those headings. These questions will focus your attention and increase your interest, helping you relate new ideas to what you already know and building your comprehension. You can take questions from the textbook or from your lecture notes, or come up with them on your own when you preview, based on what ideas you think are most important.

Here is how this technique works. In the box on page 156, the column on the left contains primary- and secondary-level headings from a chapter of *Biology*, a text by Neil A. Campbell. The column on the right rephrases these headings in question form.

There is no "correct" set of questions. Given the same headings, you would create your own particular set of questions. The more useful kinds of questions are ones that engage the critical-thinking mind actions and processes found in Chapter 5.

Read

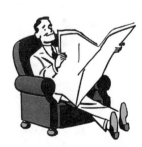

Your questions give you a starting point for *reading*, the first R in PQ3R. Read the material with the purpose of answering each question you raised. Pay special attention to the first and last lines of every paragraph, which should tell you what the paragraph is about. As you read, record key words, phrases, and concepts in your notebook. Some students divide the notebook into two columns, writing questions on the left and answers on the right. This method, known as the Cornell note-taking system, is described in more detail in Chapter 7.

If you own the textbook, marking it up—in whatever ways you prefer—is a must. The notations that you make will help you to interact with the material and make sense of it. You may want to write notes in the margins,

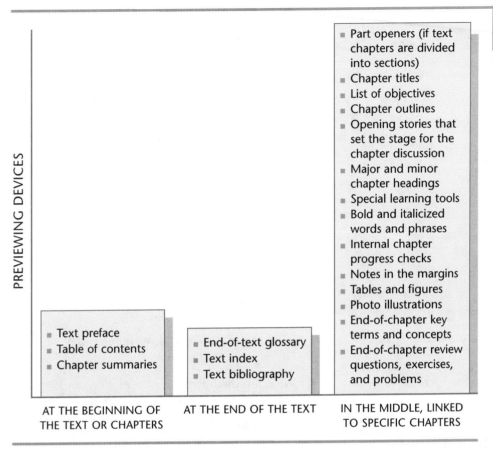

FIGURE 6-1

Text and chapter previewing devices.

circle key ideas, or highlight key sections. Some people prefer to underline, although underlining adds more ink to the lines of text and may overwhelm your eye. Although writing in a textbook makes it difficult to sell it back to the bookstore, the increased depth of understanding you can gain is worth the investment.

Highlighting may help you pinpoint material to review before an exam. Here are some additional tips on highlighting:

Get in the habit of marking the text *after* you read the material. If you do it while you are reading, you may wind up marking less important passages.

Highlight key terms and concepts. Mark the examples that explain and support important ideas. You might try highlighting ideas in one color and examples in another.

Highlight figures and tables. They are especially important if they summarize text concepts.

Avoid overmarking. A phrase or two is enough in most paragraphs. Set off long passages with brackets rather than marking every line.

Write notes in the margins with a pen or pencil. Comments like "main point" and "important definition" will help you find key sections later on.

Themes in the Study of Life	Questions
Life is organized on many structural levels.	What are the structural levels?
Cells are the organism's basic unit of structure and function.	What purpose do cells serve in the function of organisms and their structure?
Continuity of life is based on inheritable information—DNA.	What are the structure and function of DNA in the inheritance of traits?
Study of organisms enriches the study of life.	What differences are there between an organism as a whole functioning unit and its structures?
Structure and function correlate at all levels of biological organization.	How does anatomy determine function?
Organisms are open systems that interact continuously with their environments.	How does the environment affect the function or structure of an organism?
Diversity and unity are the dual faces of life on earth.	In what ways do organisms differ and in which ways are they alike?
Evolution is the core theme of biology.	What are the hallmarks of evolution, and how does it unify, or connect, life on earth?
Science is a process of inquiry that often involves hypothetical and deductive thinking.	What is an example of deductive inquiry?

Source: Adapted from Campbell, N. A. (1997). *Biology* (4th ed.). Menlo Park: Benjamin Cummings, pages 2–24.

Be careful not to mistake highlighting for learning. You will not necessarily learn what you highlight unless you review it carefully. You may benefit from writing the important information you have highlighted into your lecture notes.

One final step in the reading phase is to divide your reading into digestible segments. Many students read from one topic heading to the next, then stop. Pace your reading so that you understand as you go. If you find you are losing the thread of the ideas you are reading, you may want to try smaller segments, or you may need to take a break and come back to it later.

Recite

Once you finish reading a topic, stop and answer the questions you raised about it in the Q stage of PQ3R. You may decide to recite each answer aloud, silently speak the answers to yourself, tell the answers to another person as though you were teaching him or her, or write your ideas and answers in brief notes. Writing is often the most effective way to solidify what you have read. Use whatever techniques best suit your learning style profile (see Chapter 3).

After you finish one section, move on to the next. Then repeat the question-read-recite cycle until you complete the entire chapter. If during this process you find yourself fumbling for thoughts, it means that you do not yet "own" the ideas. Reread the section that's giving you trouble until you master its contents. Understanding each section as you go is crucial because the material in one section often forms a foundation for the next.

Review

Review soon after you finish a chapter. Here are some techniques for reviewing.

- Skim and reread your notes. Then try summarizing them from memory.
- Answer the text's end-of-chapter review, discussion, and application questions.
- Quiz yourself, using the questions you raised in the *Q* stage. If you can't answer one of your own or one of the text's questions, go back and scan the material for answers.
- Review and summarize in writing the sections and phrases you have highlighted.
- Create a chapter outline in standard outline form or think-link form.
- Reread the preface, headings, tables, and summary.
- Recite important concepts to yourself, or record important information on a cassette tape and play it on your car's tape deck or your Walkman.
- Make flashcards that have an idea or word on one side and examples, a definition, or other related information on the other. Test yourself.
- Think critically: Break ideas down into examples, consider similar or different concepts, recall important terms, evaluate ideas, and explore causes and effects.
- Make think links that show how important concepts relate to one another.

Remember that you can ask your instructor if you need help clarifying your reading material. Your instructor is an important resource. Pinpoint the material you want to discuss, schedule a meeting with her during office hours, and come prepared with a list of questions. You may also want to ask what materials to focus on when you study for tests.

If possible, you should review both alone and with study groups. Reviewing in as many different ways as possible increases the likelihood of retention. Figure 6-2 shows some techniques that will help a study group maximize its time and efforts.

Repeating the review process renews and solidifies your knowledge. That is why it is important to set up regular review sessions—for example, once a week. As you review, remember that refreshing your knowledge is easier and faster than learning it the first time.

As you can see in Table 6-2 on p. 160, using PQ3R is part of being an active reader. Active reading involves the specific activities that help you retain what you learn.

FIGURE 6-2 Study group techniques.

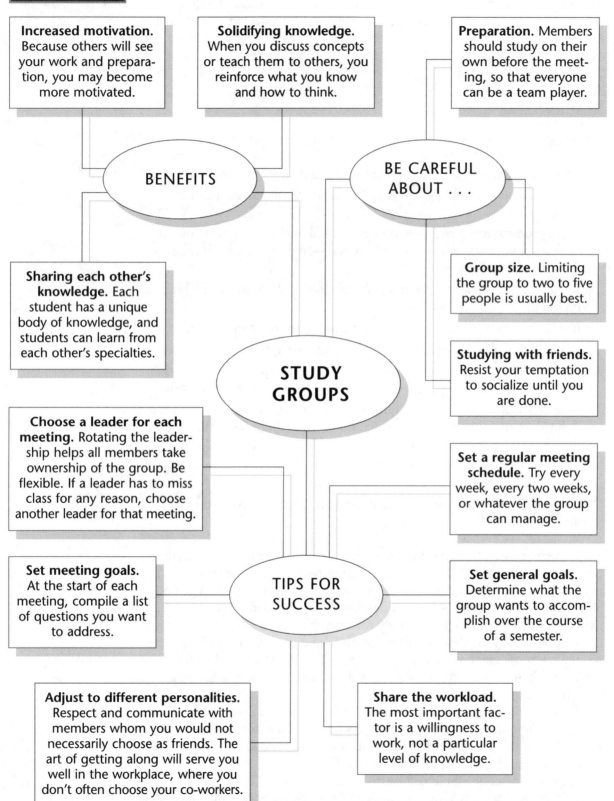

Increased motivation. Because others will see your work and preparation, you may become more motivated.

Solidifying knowledge. When you discuss concepts or teach them to others, you reinforce what you know and how to think.

Preparation. Members should study on their own before the meeting, so that everyone can be a team player.

BENEFITS

BE CAREFUL ABOUT . . .

Sharing each other's knowledge. Each student has a unique body of knowledge, and students can learn from each other's specialties.

Group size. Limiting the group to two to five people is usually best.

Studying with friends. Resist your temptation to socialize until you are done.

STUDY GROUPS

Choose a leader for each meeting. Rotating the leadership helps all members take ownership of the group. Be flexible. If a leader has to miss class for any reason, choose another leader for that meeting.

Set a regular meeting schedule. Try every week, every two weeks, or whatever the group can manage.

Set meeting goals. At the start of each meeting, compile a list of questions you want to address.

TIPS FOR SUCCESS

Set general goals. Determine what the group wants to accomplish over the course of a semester.

Adjust to different personalities. Respect and communicate with members whom you would not necessarily choose as friends. The art of getting along will serve you well in the workplace, where you don't often choose your co-workers.

Share the workload. The most important factor is a willingness to work, not a particular level of knowledge.

HOW CAN YOU READ CRITICALLY?

Your textbooks will often contain features that highlight important ideas and help you determine questions to ask while reading. As you advance in your education, however, many reading assignments will not be so clearly marked, especially if they are primary sources such as research reports in journals. You will need critical-reading skills in order to select the important ideas, identify examples that support them, and ask questions about the text without the aid of any special features or tools.

Critical reading enables you to consider reading material carefully, developing a thorough understanding of it through evaluation and analysis. A critical reader is able to discern what in a piece of reading material is true or useful, such as when using material as a source for an essay. A critical reader can also compare one piece of material to another and evaluate which makes more sense, which proves its thesis more successfully, or which is more useful for the reader's purpose.

Critical reading is reading that transcends taking in and regurgitating material. You can read critically by using PQ3R to get a basic idea of the material, asking questions based on the critical-thinking mind actions, shifting your perspective, and seeking understanding.

Use PQ3R to "Taste" Reading Material

Sylvan Barnet and Hugo Bedau, authors of *Critical Thinking, Reading, and Writing—A Brief Guide to Argument*, suggest that the active reading of PQ3R will help you form an initial idea of what a piece of reading material is all about. Through previewing, skimming for ideas and examples, highlighting and writing comments and questions in the margins, and reviewing, you can develop a basic understanding of its central ideas and contents.[5]

Summarizing, part of the review process in PQ3R, is one of the best ways to develop an understanding of a piece of reading material. To construct a summary, focus on the central ideas of the piece and the main examples that support those ideas. A summary does not contain any of your own ideas or your evaluation of the material. It simply condenses the material, making it easier for you to focus on the structure of the piece and its central ideas when you go back to read more critically. At that point, you can begin to evaluate the piece and introduce your own ideas. Using the mind actions will help you.

Summary
A concise restatement of the material, in your own words, that covers the main points.

Ask Questions Based on the Mind Actions

The essence of critical reading, as with critical thinking, is asking questions. Instead of simply accepting what you read, seek a more thorough understanding by questioning the material as you go along. Using the mind actions of the Thinktrix to formulate your questions will help you understand the material.

What parts of the material you focus on will depend on your purpose for reading. For example, if you are writing a paper on the effects of radiation on man-in-the-moon marigolds, you might spend your time focusing on how

TABLE 6-2	ACTIVE READERS TEND TO . . .	
Use PQ3R to become an active reader.	Divide material into manageable sections	Answer end-of-chapter questions and applications
	Write questions	Create chapter outlines
	Answer questions through focused note taking	Create think links that map concepts in a logical way
	Highlight key concepts	Make flash cards and study them
	Recite, verbally and in writing, the answers to questions	Recite what they learned into a tape recorder and play the tape back
	Focus on main ideas found in paragraphs, sections, and chapters	Rewrite and summarize notes and highlighted materials from memory
	Recognize summary and support devices	Explain what they read to a family member or friend
	Analyze tables, figures, and photos	Form a study group

certain causes fit your thesis. If you are comparing two pieces of writing that contain opposing arguments, you may focus on picking out their central ideas and evaluating how well the writers use examples to support these ideas.

You can question any of the following components of reading material:

- The central idea of the entire piece
- A particular idea or statement
- The examples that support an idea or statement
- The proof of a fact
- The definition of a concept

Following are some ways to critically question your reading material, based on the mind actions. Apply them to any component you want to question by substituting the component for the words "it" and "this."

  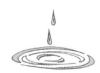

Similarity: What does this remind me of, or how is it similar to something else I know?

Difference: What different conclusions are possible? How is this different from my experience?

Cause and Effect: Why did this happen, or what caused this? What are the effects or consequences of this? What effect does the author want to have, or what is the purpose of this material? What effects support a stated cause?

Example to Principle: How would I classify this, or what is the best
principle to fit this example(s)?

How would I summarize this, or what are the
key principles?

What is the thesis or central idea?

Principle to Example: What evidence supports this, or what examples
fit this principle?

Evaluation: How would I evaluate this? Is it valid or
pertinent?

Does this example support my thesis or
central idea?

Shift Your Perspective

Your understanding of perspective will help you understand that many reading materials are written from a particular perspective. Perspective often has a strong effect on how the material is presented. For example, if a recording artist and a music censorship advocate were each to write a piece about a controversial song created by that artist, their different perspectives would result in two very different pieces of writing.

To analyze perspective, ask questions like the following:

What perspective is guiding this? What are the underlying ideas that influence this material?

Who wrote this, and what may be the author's perspective? For example, a piece on a new drug written by an employee of the drug manufacturer may differ from a doctor's evaluation of the drug.

What does the title of the material tell me about its perspective? For example, a piece entitled "New Therapies for Diabetes" may be more informational, and "What's Wrong with Insulin Injections" may intend to be persuasive.

How does the material's source affect its perspective? For example, an article on health management organizations (HMOs) published in an HMO newsletter may be more favorable and one-sided than one published in *The New York Times*.

Seek Understanding

Reading critically allows you to investigate what you read so that you can reach the highest possible level of understanding. Think of your reading process as an archaeological dig. The first step is to excavate a site and uncover the artifacts. In reading, that corresponds to your initial preview and reading of the material. As important as the excavation is, the process would be incomplete if you stopped there and just took home a bunch of items covered in dirt. The second half of the process is to investigate each item, evaluate what all of those

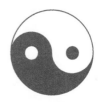

items mean, and to derive new knowledge and ideas from what you discover. Critical reading allows you to complete that crucial second half of the process.

As you work through all of the different requirements of critical reading, remember that critical reading takes *time* and *focus*. Finding a time, place, and purpose for reading, covered earlier in this chapter, is crucial to successful critical reading. Give yourself a chance to gain as much as possible from what you read.

No matter where or how you prefer to study, your school's library (or libraries) can provide many useful services to help you make the most of classes, reading, studying, and assignments.

WHAT RESOURCES DOES YOUR LIBRARY OFFER?

Your library can help you search for all kinds of information. First, learn about your library, its resources, and its layout. While some schools have only one library, other schools have a library network that includes one or more central libraries and smaller, specialized libraries that focus on specific academic areas. Take advantage of library tours, orientation, training sessions, and descriptive pamphlets. Spend time walking around the library on your own. If you still have questions, ask a reference librarian. A simple question can save hours of searching. The following sections will help you understand how your library operates.

General Reference Works

As a nursing and science student, you will spend time in the library getting to know, and use, the reference section. Getting to know the reference librarian, the library layout, and resources will save you time later on.

General reference works give you an overview and lead you to more specific information. These works cover topics in a broad, nondetailed way. General reference guides are found in the front of most libraries and are often available on CD-ROM, a compact disk that contains millions of words and images. You access this information by inserting the disk into a specially designed computer. Among the works that fall into this category are:

- encyclopedias—for example, the multivolume *Encyclopaedia Britannica*
- almanacs—*The World Almanac and Book of Facts*
- dictionaries—*Webster's New World College Dictionary*
- biographical reference works—*Webster's Biographical Dictionary*
- bibliographies—*Books in Print*

Specialized Reference Works

Look at *specialized reference works* to find more specific facts. Specialized reference works include encyclopedias and dictionaries that focus on a narrow field. The short summaries you will find there focus on critical ideas. Bibliographies

> "We are quite cosmopolitan here, and speak among us many languages. Two of my pupils seem likely to make excellent nurses; they are very devoted to the patients and the work. I find them unpunctual and noisy, but the patients are devoted to them also and we already have a reputation for nursing well."
>
> NURSE EDITH CAVELL, 1908

that accompany the articles point you to the names and works of recognized experts. Examples of specialized references include the *International Encyclopedia of Film*, the *Encyclopedia of Computer Science and Technology*, and the *Dictionary of Education*.

Library Book Catalog

Found near the front of the library, the *book catalog* lists every book the library owns. The listings usually appear in three separate categories: authors' names, book titles, and subjects. Not too long ago, most libraries stored their book catalogs on index-sized cards in hundreds of small drawers. Today, many libraries have replaced these cards with computers. Using a terminal that has access to the library's computer records, you can search by specific author, title, and subject.

The computerized catalog in your college library is probably connected to the holdings of other college and university libraries. This gives you an on-line search capacity, which means that if you don't find the book you want in your local library, you can track it down in another library and request it through an interlibrary loan. *Interlibrary loan* is a system used by many colleges to allow students to borrow materials from a library other than the one at their school. Students request materials through their own library, where the materials are eventually delivered by the outside library. When you are in a rush, keep in mind that interlibrary loans may take a substantial amount of time.

Periodical Indexes

Periodicals are magazines, journals, and newspapers that are published on a regular basis throughout the year. Examples include *Nature, Computer Science*, and *Science*. Many libraries display periodicals that are a year or two old and convert older copies to microfilm or microfiche (photocopies of materials reduced greatly in size and printed on film readable in a special reading machine—*microfilm* is a strip of film, and *microfiche* refers to individual leaves of film). Finding articles in publications involves a search of periodical indexes. The most widely used general index is the *Reader's Guide to Periodical Literature*, which is available on CD-ROM and in book form. The *Reader's Guide* indexes articles in more than 100 general-interest magazines and journals.

Electronic Research

You will also find complete source material through a variety of electronic sources, including the Internet, on-line services, and CD-ROM. Here is a sampling of the kind of information you will find: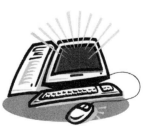

- complete articles from thousands of journals and magazines
- complete articles from newspapers around the world
- government data on topics as varied as agriculture, transportation, and labor
- business documents, including corporate annual reports

Your library is connected to the *Internet*, a worldwide computer network that links government, university, research, and business computers along the Information Superhighway. Tapping into the *World Wide Web*—a tool for searching the huge libraries of information stored on the Internet—gives you access to billions of written words and graphic images. The Internet is so vast that you may need other publications to help you explore it. Seek out tools to aid you on your journeys along the Information Superhighway. If your college has its own Internet home page, start by spending some time browsing through it.

Although most libraries do not charge a fee to access the Internet, they may charge when you connect to commercial on-line services, including Nexis, CompuServe, and Prodigy. Ask your librarian about all fees and restrictions. Libraries also have electronic databases on CD-ROM. A database is a collection of data—or, in the case of most libraries, a list of related resources that all focus on one specific subject area—arranged so that you can search through it and retrieve specific items easily. For example, the DIA-LOG Information System includes hundreds of small databases in specialized areas. CD-ROM databases are generally smaller than on-line databases and are updated less frequently. However, there is never a user's fee. Useful indexes for nursing include Cinahl (on CD-ROM) and PubMed (a free on-line journal search), www.ncbi.nlmnih.gov/PubMed.

читать

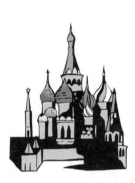

This word may look completely unfamiliar to you, but anyone who can read the Russian language and alphabet will know that it means "read." People who read languages that use different kinds of characters, such as Russian, Japanese, or Greek, learn to process those characters as easily as you process the letters of your native alphabet. Your mind learns to process individually each letter or character you see. This ability enables you to move to the next level of understanding—making sense of those letters or characters when they are grouped to form words, phrases, and sentences.

Think of this concept when you read. Remember that your mind is an incredible tool, processing unmeasurable amounts of information so that you can understand the concepts on the page. Give it the best opportunity to succeed by reading as often as you can and by focusing on all of the elements that help you read to the best of your ability.

Applications   Chapter 6

KEY INTO YOUR LIFE
Opportunities to Apply What You Learn

 6.1 *Studying a Text Page*

The following excerpt is from Evaluation and Exercise Prescription, Fardy and Yanowitz, *Cardiac Rehabilitation, Adult Fitness, and Exercise Testing,* 3rd ed.[6] Read the material using the study techniques in this chapter, and complete the questions that follow.

EXERCISE PRESCRIPTION

THE EXERCISE PRESCRIPTION represents the carefully regulated dosage of physical activity of a long-term training program. The dosage consists of a coalescence of intensity, duration, and frequency of effort that is undertaken in an exercise mode to achieve specific program objectives. The prescription should be developed in a manner similar to that of prescribing medication, that is, administered in specified amounts based on individual needs. When designed for cardiac rehabilitation and adult fitness, the exercise modes are usually selected for the purpose of enhancing cardiovascular function and lessening the risk of coronary heart disease. Other training objectives such as strength and flexibility have very different prescriptions and are addressed briefly in this chapter, although the reader is referred elsewhere for more in-depth information. The purposes of this chapter are to present the rationale for an exercise prescription that promotes cardiovascular function; to present the physiologic basis and design of the prescription, the factors that affect the prescription; and to apply the prescription formula to an exercise training program.

Physiologic Basis of the Exercise Prescription

The physiologic basis of the exercise prescription is the overload principle and the relationship between training stimuli (dosage) and adaptation (response).

Overload Principle

Overload by definition means that the training stimulus must surpass normal daily physical exertion to be beneficial. The training stimulus, however, should not provoke undue fatigue, musculoskeletal strain, or mental or emotional burnout. Optimal benefit necessitates regular updating of the overload threshold.

Dose Response

Adaptation is related to the amount of physical exertion, although the relationship is not consistently linear. Dose-response curves depicted in Figure A-1 represent a relationship illustrating that adaptation does not occur until some minimal effort is expended, that is, overload. The curves do not represent physiologic measures, but rather represent a conceptual comparison of effort versus gain under different circumstances. Training adaptation is modest or non-existent for most persons until effort approximates 50 to 60% of maximum intensity. Thereafter, gains are rapid until they plateau at the top of the curves, between 85 and 90% of maximal effort, indicating that exercise is too intense or that there is insufficient time for recovery, or both. The dose-response curves shift to the right as physical condition improves. The rate of adaptation varies among individuals, although improvements are generally similar at different ages and for males and females.

FIGURE A-1   *Improvement anticipated from effort expended.*

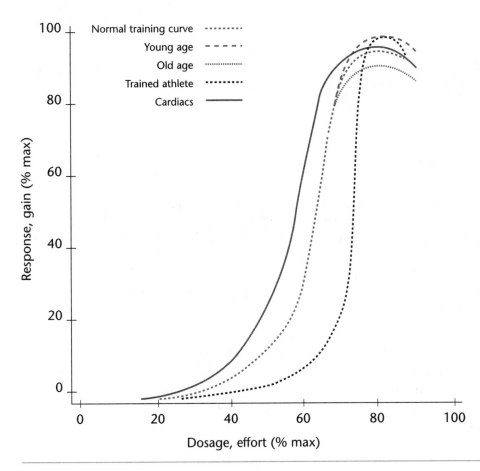

Improvement anticipated from effort expended: A conceptual diagram illustrating training curves in various populations. Note that the trained athlete is required to exercise at a greater intensity to make gains similar to those of normal persons of cardiac patients. Also note that age at onset of training affects the maximal physiologic gain. (Redrawn from Fardy PS. "Train for aerobic power." In: Burke E.J., ed., *Toward an Understanding of Human Performance.* Ithaca, NY: Movement Publications, 1977.)

Components of the Prescription

The prescription dosage consists of intensity, duration, frequency, and mode of exercise.

Intensity

The single most important factor of the exercise prescription is intensity of effort, usually expressed as a percentage of functional aerobic capacity or maximal heart rate (MHR). There is a strong and consistent correlation between oxygen uptake and heart rate as a percentage of maximum (Fig. A-2), regardless of the level of physical condition, gender, or muscle groups being compared.

Several approaches may be used to prescribe training intensity. In any case maximal exercise testing is recommended for best results. The ACSM Guidelines provide clear recommendations for testing. Heart rate prescriptions based on submaximal testing or age-estimated maximal heart rates have the potential for considerable error and, as a result, may be too strenuous and pose the risk of injury or too easy and, hence, ineffective.

The target heart rate (THR) is ordinarily established between 70 and 90% MHR, approximately 60 to 80% VO_{2max}. Those who are poorly conditioned as well as patients with cardiopulmonary disease can benefit from training at heart rates less than 70% MHR, while competitive athletes may require greater than 90% MHR for training adaptation.

Source: P.S. Fardy and F.G. Yanowitz, *Cardiac Rehabilitation, Adult Fitness, and Exercise Testing,* 3rd ed. © Williams & Wilkins, Baltimore, MD, 1995, pp. 246–247. Used with permission.

1. Identify the headings of the excerpt and the relationship among them. Which headings are primary-level headings; which are secondary; which are tertiary (third-level heads)? Which heading serves as an umbrella for the rest?

   _____

   _____

2. What do the headings tell you about the content of the excerpt?

   _____

   _____

3. Identify the terms with abbreviations after them. What does this tell you about these words? How is the graph in Figure A.1 useful?

   _____

   _____

   _____

4. After reading the chapter headings, write three study questions. List the questions below:

   _____

   _____

   _____

5. Using a marker pen, highlight key phrases and sentences. Write short marginal notes to help you review the material at a later point.

6. After reading this page, list three key concepts that you will need to study:

   a. _____

   b. _____

   c. _____

 ## 6.2 *Focusing on Your Purpose for Reading*

Read the material on the following page on kinetic and potential energy and the first law of thermodynamics taken from *Life On Earth* by Teresa Audesirk and Gerald Audesirk.[7] When you have finished, answer the questions following the selection.

Among the fundamental characteristics of all living organisms is the ability to guide chemical reactions within their bodies along certain pathways. The chemical reactions serve many functions, depending on the nature of the organism: to synthesize the molecules that make up the organism's body, to reproduce, to move, even to think. Chemical reactions either require or release energy, which can be defined simply as *the capacity to do work*, including synthesizing molecules, moving things around, and generating heat and light. In this chapter we discuss the physical laws that govern energy flow in the universe, how energy flow in turn governs chemical reactions, and how the chemical reactions within living cells are controlled by the molecules of the cell itself. Chapters 7 and 8 focus on photosynthesis, the chief "port of entry" for energy into the biosphere, and glycolysis and cellular respiration, the most important sequences of chemical reactions that release energy.

ENERGY AND THE ABILITY TO DO WORK

As you learned in Chapter 2, there are two types of energy: **kinetic energy** and **potential energy.** Both types of energy may exist in many different forms. Kinetic energy, or *energy of movement*, includes light (movement of photons), heat (movement of molecules), electricity (movement of electrically charged particles), and movement of large objects. Potential energy, or *stored energy*, includes chemical energy stored in the bonds that hold atoms together in molecules, electrical energy stored in a battery, and positional energy stored in a diver poised to spring (Fig. 4-1). Under the right conditions, kinetic energy can be transformed into potential energy, and vice versa. For example, the diver converted kinetic energy of movement into potential energy of position when she climbed the ladder up to the platform; when she jumps off, the potential energy will be converted back into kinetic energy.

To understand how energy flow governs interactions among pieces of matter, we need to know two things: (1) the quantity of available energy and (2) the usefulness of the energy. These are the subjects of the laws of thermodynamics, which we will now examine.

The Laws of Thermodynamics Describe the Basic Properties of Energy

All interactions among pieces of matter are governed by the two **laws of thermodynamics,** physical principles that define the basic properties and behavior of energy. The laws of thermodynamics deal with "isolated systems," which are any parts of the universe that cannot exchange either matter or energy with any other parts. Probably no part of the universe is completely isolated from all possible exchange with every other part, but the concept of an isolated system is useful in thinking about energy flow.

The First Law of Thermodynamics States That Energy Can Be Neither Created nor Destroyed

The **first law of thermodynamics** states that within any isolated system, energy can be neither created nor destroyed, although it can be changed in form (for example, from chemical energy to heat energy). In other words, within an isolated system *the total quantity of energy remains constant*. The first law is therefore often called the law of conservation of energy. To use a familiar example, let's see how the first law applies to driving your car (Fig. 4-2). We can consider that your car (with a full tank of gas), the road, and the surrounding air roughly constitute an isolated system. When you drive your car, you convert the potential chemical energy of gasoline into kinetic energy of movement and heat energy. The total amount of energy that was in the gasoline before it was burned is the same as the total amount of this kinetic energy and heat.

An important rule of energy conversions is this: Energy always flows "downhill," from places with a high concentration of energy to places with a low concentration of energy. This is the principle behind engines. As we described in Chapter 2, temperature is a measure of how fast molecules move. The burning gasoline in your car's engine consists of molecules moving at extremely high speeds: a high concentration of energy. The cooler air outside the engine consists of molecules moving at much lower speeds: a low concentration of energy. The molecules in the engine hit the piston harder than the air molecules outside the engine do, so the piston moves upward, driving the gears that move the car. Work is done. When the engine is turned off, it cools down as heat is transferred from the warm engine to its cooler surroundings. The molecules on both sides of the piston move at the same speed, so the piston stays still. No work is done.

T. Audesirk and G. Audesirk, *Life on Earth*. (Upper Saddle River, NJ: Prentice-Hall, 1997). Reprinted by permission of Prentice-Hall, Inc.

1. *Reading for critical evaluation.* Evaluate the material by answering these questions:

Were the ideas clearly supported by examples? If you feel one or more were not supported, give an example.

_____

_____

_____

_____

Did the author make any assumptions that weren't examined? If so, name one or more.

_____

_____

_____

_____

Do you disagree with any part of the material? If so, which part, and why?

_____

_____

_____

_____

_____

Do you have any suggestions for how the material could have been presented more effectively?

_____

_____

_____

_____

_____

2. *Reading for practical application.* Imagine you have to give a presentation on this material the next time the class meets. On a separate sheet of paper, create an outline or think link that maps out the key elements you would discuss.

3. *Reading for comprehension.* Answer the following questions to determine the level of your comprehension.

Name the two types of energy.

_____

_____

Which one "stores" energy?

_____

_____

Can kinetic energy be turned into potential energy?

_____

_____

What is the term that describes the basic properties and behaviors of energy?

_____

Mark the following statements as true (T) or false (F).

_____ Within any isolated system, energy can be neither created nor destroyed.

_____ Energy always flows downhill, from high-concentration levels to low.

_____ All interactions among pieces of matter are governed by two laws of thermodynamics.

_____ Some parts of the universe are isolated from other parts.

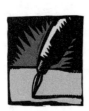

KEY TO SELF-EXPRESSION
Discovery Through Journal Writing

To record your thoughts, use a separate journal or the lined pages at the end of the chapter.

Reading Challenges

What is your most difficult challenge when reading assigned materials? A challenge might be a particular kind of reading material, a reading situation, or the achievement of a certain goal when reading. Considering the tools that this chapter presents, make a plan that addresses this challenge. What techniques might be able to help you most? How and when will you try them out? What positive effects do you anticipate they may have on you?

Name _____   Date _____

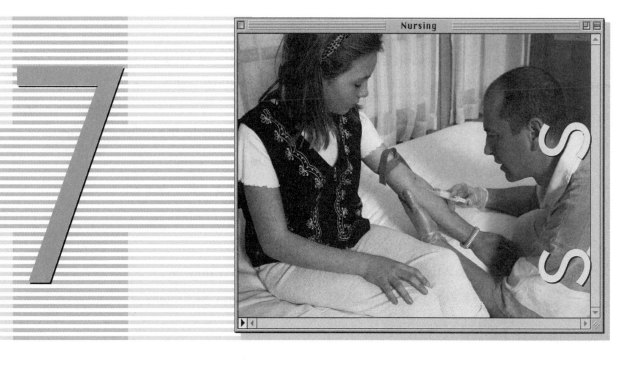

Note-Taking
and Writing

Harnessing the Power
of Words and Ideas

Words, joined to form ideas, are tools that have enormous power. Whether you write an essay, a memo to a supervisor, or a letter over e-mail, words allow you to take your ideas out of the realm of thought and give them a form that other people can read and consider. You can harness their power for your own. Set a goal for yourself: Strive continually to improve your knowledge of how to use words to construct understandable ideas.

This chapter will teach you the note-taking skills you need to record information successfully. It will show you how to express your written ideas completely and how good writing is linked to clear thinking. In class or at work, taking notes and writing well will help you stand out from the crowd.

In this chapter, you will explore answers to the following questions:

- How does taking notes help you?
- Which note-taking system should you use?
- How can you write faster when taking notes?
- Why does good writing matter in nursing?
- What are the elements of effective writing?
- What is the writing process in nursing and science?

 ## HOW DOES TAKING NOTES HELP YOU?

Notes help you learn when you are in class, doing research, or studying. Because it is virtually impossible to take notes on everything you hear or read, the act of note-taking encourages you to decide what is worth remembering. The positive effects of note-taking include:

- Your notes provide material that helps you study information and prepare for tests.
- When you take notes, you become an active, involved listener and learner.
- Note-taking helps increase your observation skills.
- Notes help you think critically and organize ideas.
- The information you learn in class or lab may not appear in any text; you will have no way to study it without writing it down.
- If it is difficult for you to process information while in class, having notes to read and make sense of later can help you learn.
- Note-taking is a skill for life that you will use on the job and in your personal life.

Recording Information in Class

Your notes have two purposes: First, they should reflect what you heard in class, and second, they should be a resource for studying, writing, or comparing with your text material.

Preparing to Take Class Notes

Taking good class notes depends on good preparation, including the following:

- If your instructor assigns reading on a lecture topic, you may choose to complete the reading before class so that the lecture becomes more of a review than an introduction.

- Use separate pieces of $8^1/_2$-by-11-inch paper for each class. If you use a three-ring binder, punch holes in papers your instructor hands out and insert them immediately following your notes for that day.

- Take a comfortable seat where you can easily see and hear, and be ready to write as soon as the instructor begins speaking.

- Choose a note-taking system that helps you handle the instructor's speaking style. While one instructor may deliver organized lectures at a normal speaking rate, another may jump from topic to topic or talk very quickly.

- Set up a support system with a student in each class. That way, when you are absent, you can get the notes you missed.

What to Do During Class

Because no one has the time to write down everything he hears, the following strategies will help you choose and record what you feel is important, in a format that you can read and understand later.

- Date each page. When you take several pages of notes during a lecture, add an identifying letter or number to the date on each page: 11/27 A, 11/27 B, . . . or 11/27—1 of 3, 11/27—2 of 3.

- Add the specific topic of the lecture at the top of the page. For example:

  11/27 A—Thermal Behavior of Gases

- If your instructor jumps from topic to topic during a single class, try starting a new page for each new topic.

- Ask yourself critical-thinking questions as you listen: Do I need this information? Is the information important or is it just a digression? Is the information fact or opinion? If it is opinion, is it worth remembering?

- Record whatever an instructor emphasizes (see Figure 7-1 for details).

- Continue to take notes during class discussions and question-and-answer periods. What your fellow students ask about may help you as well.

- Leave one or more blank spaces between points. This white space will help you review your notes, because information will appear in self-contained sections.

- Draw pictures and diagrams that help illustrate ideas.

- Indicate material that is especially important with a star, with underlining, with a highlighter pen, or by writing words in capital letters.

- If you cannot understand what the instructor is saying, leave a space and place a question mark in the margin. Then ask the instructor to explain it again after class or discuss it with a classmate. Fill in the blank when the idea is clear.

- Take notes until the instructor stops speaking. Students who stop writing a few minutes before the class is over can miss critical information.

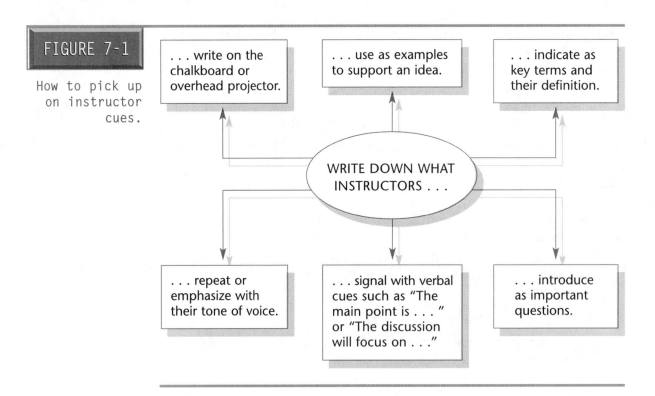

FIGURE 7-1

How to pick up
on instructor
cues.

. . . write on the chalkboard or overhead projector.

. . . use as examples to support an idea.

. . . indicate as key terms and their definition.

WRITE DOWN WHAT INSTRUCTORS . . .

. . . repeat or emphasize with their tone of voice.

. . . signal with verbal cues such as "The main point is . . . " or "The discussion will focus on . . ."

. . . introduce as important questions.

"Omit needless words. . . . This requires not that the writer make all his sentences short, or that he avoid all detail and treat his subjects only in outline, but that every word tell."

WILLIAM STRUNK, JR.

■ Make your notes as legible, organized, and complete as possible. Your notes are only useful if you can read and understand them.

Make Notes a Valuable After-Class Reference

Class notes are a valuable study tool when you review them regularly. To help you do this, try to recopy notes after class. This will help clarify points and assist your memory.

Try to begin your review within a day of the lecture. Read over the notes to learn the information, clarify abbreviations, fill in missing information, and underline or highlight key points. Try to review each week's notes at the end of that week. Think critically about the material, in writing, study group discussions, or quiet reflective thought. You might also try summarizing your notes, either as you review them or from memory.

You can take notes in many ways. Different note-taking systems suit different people and situations. Explore each system and choose what works for you.

WHICH NOTE-TAKING SYSTEM SHOULD YOU USE?

You will benefit most from the system that feels most comfortable to you. As you consider each system, remember the learning styles profile you compiled in Chapter 3. The most common note-taking systems include outlines, the Cornell system, and think links.

FIGURE 7-2

Sample formal
outline.

Impulse and Momentum

I. Key Ideas
   A. Impulse and Momentum: Forces that act between colliding objects
      1. Impulse: impulse force = average value of force times time interval
      2. Momentum: vector quantity = body's mass times velocity
   B. Conservation of Momentum: "Law of conservation of momentum"—Acceleration and change in total momentum of system determined by net external force on system.
II. Key Equations
   A. Momentum of a particle $p = mv$
   B. Impulse and Momentum
      1. Impulse $= F_{av} \Delta t = m\Delta v = \Delta(mv) = \Delta p$
      2. Conservation of momentum $= p = p_1 + p_2 =$ constant

Adapted from: Granvil C. Kyker, Jr. (1987). *Study Guide: Paul A Tipler College Physics.* New York: Worth, 81–82.

Taking Notes in Outline Form

When a reading assignment or lecture seems well organized, you may choose to take notes in outline form. *Outlining* shows the relationships among ideas and their supporting examples through the use of line-by-line phrases set off by varying indentations.

Formal outlines indicate ideas and examples using Roman numerals, capital and lowercase letters, and numbers. When you are pressed for time, such as during class, you can use an informal system of consistent indenting and dashes instead. Formal outlines also require at least two headings on the same level—that is, if you have a II A you must also have a II B. Figure 7-2 shows an outline on impulse and momentum.

Guided Notes

From time to time, an instructor may give you a guide, usually in the form of an outline, to help you take notes in the class. This outline may be on a page that you receive at the beginning of the class, on the board, or on an overhead projector.

Although *guided notes* help you follow the lecture and organize your thoughts during class, they do not replace your own notes. Because they are more of a basic outline of topics than a comprehensive coverage of information, they require that you fill in what they do not cover in detail. If you tune out in class because you think that the guided notes are all you need, you will most likely miss important information.

When you receive guided notes on paper, write directly on the paper if there is room. If not, use a separate sheet and write on it the outline categories that the guided notes suggest. If the guided notes are on the board or an overhead projector, copy them down, leaving plenty of space in between for your own notes.

Using the Cornell Note-Taking System

The *Cornell note-taking system*, also known as the T-note system, was developed more than 45 years ago by Walter Pauk at Cornell University.[1] The system is successful because it is simple—and because it works. It consists of three sections on ordinary note paper:

- *Section 1*, the largest section, is on the right. Record your notes here in informal outline form.

- *Section 2*, to the left of your notes, is the *cue column*. Leave it blank while you read or listen, then fill it in later as you review. You might fill it with comments that highlight main ideas, clarify meaning, suggest examples, or link ideas and examples. You can even draw diagrams.

- *Section 3*, at the bottom of the page, is the *summary area*, where you summarize the notes on the page. When you review, use this section to reinforce concepts and provide an overview.

When you use the Cornell system, create the note-taking structure before class begins. Picture an upside-down letter T and use Figure 7-3 as your guide. Make the cue column about 2 1/2 inches wide and the summary area 2 inches tall. Figure 7-3 shows how a student used the Cornell system to take notes in an introductory human development course.

Creating a Think Link

A *think link*, also known as a mind map, is a visual form of note-taking. When you draw a think link, you diagram ideas using shapes and lines that link ideas and supporting details and examples. The visual design makes the connections easy to see, and the use of shapes and pictures extends the material beyond just words. Many learners respond well to the power of visualization. You can use think links to brainstorm ideas for paper topics as well.

One way to create a think link is to start by circling your topic in the middle of a sheet of unlined paper. Next, draw a line from the circled topic and write the name of the first major idea at the end of that line. Circle the idea also. Then jot down specific facts related to the idea, linking them to the

TERMS

Visualization
The interpretation
of verbal ideas
through the use of
mental visual
images.

Why do some workers have a better attitude toward their work than others?

Some managers view workers as lazy; others view them as motivated and productive.

Maslow's Hierarchy

self-actualization needs (challenging job)

esteem needs (job title)

social needs (friends at work)

security needs (health plan)

physiological needs (pay)

October 3, 2000, p. 1

Understanding Employee Motivation

Purpose of motivational theories

—To explain role of human relations in motivating employee performance

—Theories translate into how managers actually treat workers

2 specific theories

—Human resources model, developed by Douglas McGregor, shows that managers have radically different beliefs about motivation.

—Theory X holds that people are naturally irresponsible and uncooperative

—Theory Y holds that people are naturally responsible and self-motivated

Maslow's Hierarchy of Needs says that people have needs in 5 different areas, which they attempt to satisfy in their work

—Physiological need: need for survival, including food and shelter

—Security need: need for stability and protection

—Social need: need for friendship and companionship

—Esteem need: need for status and recognition

—Self-actualization need: need for self-fulfillment

Needs at lower levels must be met before a person tries to satisfy needs at higher levels.

—Developed by psychologist Abraham Maslow

Two motivational theories try to explain worker motivation. The human resources model includes Theory X and Theory Y. Maslow's Hierarchy of Needs suggests that people have needs in 5 different areas: physiological, security, social, esteem, and self-actualization.

idea with lines. Continue the process, connecting thoughts to one another using circles, lines, and words.

A think link may be difficult to construct in class, especially if your instructor talks quickly. In this case, use another note-taking system during class. Then make a think link as you review. Figure 7-4 shows a think link on a sociology concept called *social stratification.*

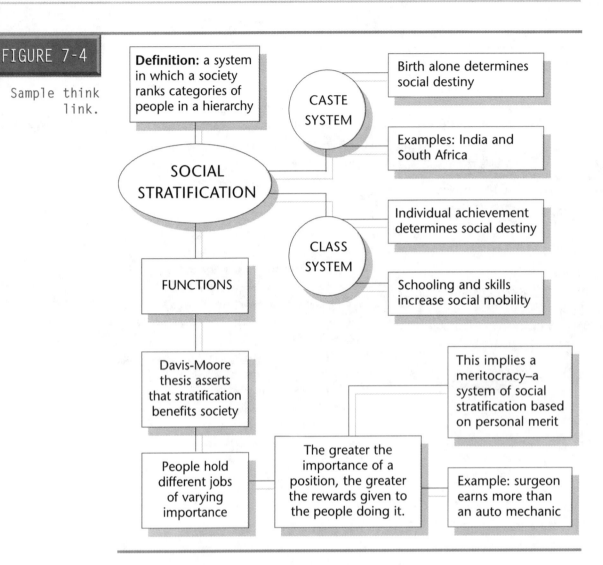

FIGURE 7-4

Sample think link.

Once you choose a note-taking system, your success will depend on how well you use it. Personal shorthand will help you make the most of whatever system you choose.

HOW CAN YOU WRITE FASTER WHEN TAKING NOTES?

When taking notes, many students feel they can't keep up with the instructor. Using some personal shorthand (not standard secretarial shorthand) can help to push the pen faster. *Shorthand* is writing that shortens words or replaces them with symbols. Because you are the only intended reader, you can use symbols and abbreviate words in ways that only you understand.

The only danger with shorthand is that you might forget what your writing means. To avoid this problem, review your shorthand notes while your abbreviations and symbols are fresh in your mind. If there is any confusion, spell out words as you review.

Here are some suggestions that will help you master this important skill:

1. Use the following standard abbreviations in place of complete words:

w/	with	cf	compare, in comparison to
w/o	without	ff	following
→	means; resulting in	Q	question
←	as a result of	p.	page
↑	increasing	*	most importantly
↓	decreasing	<	less than
∴	therefore	>	more than
∵	because	=	equals
≈	approximately	%	percent
+ or &	and	△	change
−	minus; negative	2	to; two; too
NO. or #	number	vs	versus; against
i.e.	that is,	eg	for example
etc.	and so forth	c/o	care of
ng	no good	lb	pound

2. Shorten words by removing vowels from the middle of words:

   prps   =   purpose
   Crvtte =   Corvette (as on a vanity license plate for a car)

3. Substitute word beginnings for entire words:

   assoc   =   associate; association
   info   =   information

4. Form plurals by adding s:

   prblms =   problems
   prntrs =   printers

5. Make up your own symbols and use them consistently:

   b/4   =   before
   2thake =   toothache

6. Learn to rely on key phrases instead of complete sentences: "German—nouns capitalized" instead of "In the German language, all nouns are capitalized."

While note-taking focuses on taking in ideas, writing focuses on expressing them. Next you will explore the roles that writing can play in your life.

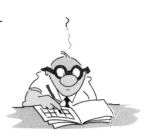

 ## WHY DOES GOOD WRITING MATTER IN NURSING?

Good writing reflects clear thinking. Therefore, a clear thought process is the best preparation for a well-written document, and a well-written document shows the reader a clear thought process. Good writing skills also depend on reading. The more you expose yourself to the work of other writers, the more you will develop your ability to express yourself well. Not only will you learn more words and ideas, but you will also learn about all the different ways a writer can put words together in order to express ideas. In addition, reading generates new ideas inside your mind, ideas you can use in your writing.

In school, almost any course you take will require you to write essays or papers in order to communicate your knowledge and thought process. In order to express yourself successfully in those essays and papers, you need good writing skills. Knowing how to write and express yourself is essential in the workplace as well.

Instructors, supervisors, and other people who see your writing judge your thinking ability based on what you write and how you write it. Over the next few years, you may write papers, essays, answers to essay test questions, job application letters, resumes, business proposals and reports, memos to co-workers, and letters to customers and suppliers. Good writing skills will help you achieve the goals you set out to accomplish with each writing task.

Your writing represents you. In science, good writing presents unique challenges because of the technical nature of scientific language. In nursing, good writing includes the qualities of science writing plus the challenge of clarity for legal purposes.

WHAT ARE THE ELEMENTS OF EFFECTIVE WRITING?

Every writing situation is different, depending on three elements. Your goal is to understand each element before you begin to write:

- *Your purpose:* What do you want to accomplish with this particular piece of writing?
- *Your topic:* What is the subject about which you will write?
- *Your audience:* Who will read your writing?

Figure 7-5 shows how these elements are interdependent. As a triangle needs three points to be complete, a piece of writing needs these three elements.

FIGURE 7-5

The three elements of writing.

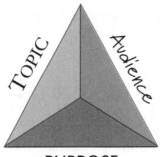

Writing Purpose

Writing without having set your purpose first is like driving without deciding where you want to arrive. You'll get somewhere, but chances are it won't be where you needed to go. Therefore, when you write, always define what you want to accomplish before you start.

There are many different purposes for writing. However, the two purposes you will most commonly use in classwork and on the job are to inform and to persuade.

The purpose of *informative writing* is to present and explain ideas. A research paper on how hospitals use donated blood to save lives informs readers without trying to mold opinion. The writer presents facts in an unbiased way, without introducing a particular point of view. Most newspaper articles, except on the opinion and editorial pages, are examples of informative writing.

Persuasive writing has the purpose of convincing readers that your point of view is correct. Often, persuasive writing seeks to change the mind of the reader. For example, as a member of the student health committee, you write a newspaper column attempting to persuade readers to give blood. Examples of persuasive writing include newspaper editorials, business proposals, and books and magazine articles with a point of view.

Additional possible writing purposes include *entertaining* the reader and *narrating* (describing an image or event to the reader). Although most of your writing in school will inform or persuade, you may occasionally need to entertain or narrate as well. Sometimes purposes will even overlap—you might write an informative essay that entertains at the same time.

Knowing Your Audience

In almost every case, a writer creates written material so that it can be read by others. The two partners in this process are the writer and the audience. Knowing who your audience is will help you communicate successfully.

TERMS

Audience
The reader or readers of any written piece of material.

Key Questions About Your Audience

In school, your primary audience will be your instructors. Instructors use your papers to evaluate the depth of your knowledge. For many assignments, instructors will want you to assume that they are typical readers rather than informed instructors. Writing for typical readers usually means that you should be as complete as possible in your explanations.

At times you may write papers that are intended to address informed instructors or a specific reading audience other than your instructors. In such cases, you may ask yourself some or all of the following questions, depending on which are relevant to your topic.

- What are my readers' ages, cultural backgrounds, interests, and experiences?
- What are their roles? Are they instructors, students, employers, customers?

- How much do they know about my topic? Are they experts in the field or beginners?
- Are they interested, or do I have to convince them to read what I write?
- Can I expect my audience to have an open or closed mind?

After you answer the questions about your audience, take what you have discovered into consideration as you write.

Your Commitment to Your Audience

Your goal is to organize your ideas so that readers can follow them. Suppose, for example, you are writing an informative research paper for a non-expert audience on using on-line services to get a job. One way to accomplish your goal is to first explain what these services are and the kinds of help they offer, then describe each service in detail, and finally conclude with how these services will change job hunting in the twenty-first century.

Effective and successful writing involves following the steps of the *writing process.*

 # WHAT IS THE WRITING PROCESS IN NURSING AND SCIENCE?

The writing process provides an opportunity for you to state and refine your thoughts until you have expressed yourself as clearly as possible. Critical thinking plays an important role every step of the way. The four main parts of the process are planning, drafting, revising, and editing. Included in this section are the writing steps unique to research writing.

Planning

Planning gives you a chance to think about what to write and how to write it. Planning involves brainstorming for ideas, defining and narrowing your topic by using prewriting strategies, conducting research if necessary, writing a thesis statement, and writing a working outline. Although the steps in preparing to write are listed in sequence, in real life the steps overlap one another as you plan your document.

Open Your Mind Through Brainstorming

Whether your instructor assigns a partially defined topic (geneticist Barbara McClintock) or a general category within which you make your own choice (women in science), you should brainstorm to develop ideas about what you want to write. Brainstorming is a creative technique that involves generating ideas about a subject without making judgments. You may want to look at the section on creativity in Chapter 5 for more details.

First, let your mind wander! Write down anything on the assigned subject that comes to mind, in no particular order. Then, organize that list into an

FIGURE 7-6

Education and employment.

A life-changing event . . .
   —Family
   —Childhood
  →Military
    —travel
   →Boot
      —physical conditioning
       • swim tests
       • intensive training
       • ENDLESS pushups
      —Chief who was our commander
      —mental discipline
       • military lifestyle
       • perfecting our appearance
      —self-confidence
       • walk like you're in control
       • don't blindly accept anything

outline or think link that helps you see the possibilities more clearly. To make the outline or think link, separate list items into general ideas or categories and sub-ideas or examples. Then associate the sub-ideas or examples with the ideas they support or fit. Figure 7-6 shows a portion of an outline a student, Michael B. Jackson, constructed from his brainstorming list. The assignment is a five-paragraph essay on a life-changing event. Here, only the subject that Michael eventually chose is shown broken down into different ideas.

Narrow Your Topic Through Prewriting Strategies

When your brainstorming has generated some possibilities, you can narrow your topic. Focus on the sub-ideas and examples from your initial brainstorming session. Because they are relatively specific, they will be more likely to point you toward possible topics.

Choose one or more sub-ideas or examples that you like and explore them using prewriting strategies such as brainstorming, freewriting, and asking journalists' questions.[2] Prewriting strategies will help you decide which of your possible topics you would most like to pursue.

TERMS

Prewriting strategies Techniques for generating ideas about a topic and finding out how much you already know before you start your research and writing.

Brainstorming. The same process you used to generate ideas will also help you narrow your topic further. Generate thoughts about the possibility you have chosen and write them down. Then, organize them into categories, noticing any patterns that appear. See if any of the sub-ideas or examples seem as if they might make good topics.

Freewriting. Another stream-of-consciousness technique that encourages you to put down ideas on paper as they occur to you is called *freewriting*. When you freewrite, you write whatever comes to mind without censoring your ideas or worrying about grammar, spelling, punctuation, or organization. Freewriting helps you think creatively and gives you an opportunity to begin weaving in information that you know. Freewrite on the sub-ideas or examples you have created to see if you want to pursue any of them. Here is a sample of freewriting:

> Boot camp for the Coast Guard really changed my life. First of all, I really got in shape. We had to get up every morning at 5 a.m., eat breakfast, and go right into training. We had to do endless military-style push-ups–but we later found out that these have a purpose, to prepare us to hit the deck in the event of enemy fire. We had a lot of aquatic tests, once we were awakened at 3 a.m. to do one in full uniform! Boot camp also helped me to feel confident about myself and be disciplined. Chief Marzloff was the main person who made that happen. He was tough but there was always a reason. He got angry when I used to nod my head whenever he would speak to me, he said that made it seem like I was blindly accepting whatever he said, which was a weakness. From him I have learned to keep an eye on my body's movements when I communicate. I learned a lot more from him too.

Asking journalists' questions. When journalists start working on a story, they ask themselves: Who? What? Where? When? Why? and How? You can use these *journalists' questions* to focus your thinking. Ask these questions about any sub-idea or example to discover what you may want to discuss. For example:

Who?   Who was at boot camp? Who influenced me the most?

What?   What about boot camp changed my life? What did we do?

When?   When in my life did I go to boot camp, and for how long? When did we fulfill our duties?

Where?   Where was boot camp located? Where did we spend our day-to-day time?

Why?   Why did I decide to go there? Why was it such an important experience?

How?   How did we train in the camp? How were we treated? How did we achieve success?

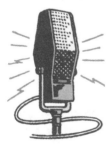

As you prewrite, don't forget to focus on the paper length, due date of your assignment, and any other requirements (such as topic area or purpose).

These requirements influence your choice of a final topic. For example, if you had a month to write an informative 20-page paper on learning disabilities, you might choose to discuss the symptoms, diagnosis, effects, and treatment of attention deficit hyperactivity disorder (ADHD). If you were given a week to write a five-page persuasive essay, you might write about how elementary students with ADHD need special training.

Prewriting will help you develop a topic broad enough to give you something with which to work but narrow enough to be manageable. Prewriting also helps you see what you know and what you don't know. If your assignment requires more than you already know, you may need to do research.

Conduct Research

Much of the writing you do in college, such as when you must write a short essay for freshman composition or for an exam, will rely on what you already know about a subject. In these cases, prewriting strategies may generate all the ideas and information you need. In other writing situations, outside sources are necessary. Try doing your research in stages. In the first stage, look for a basic overview that can help you write a thesis statement. In the second stage, go into more depth in your research, tracking down information that will help you fill in the gaps and complete your thoughts.

Write a Thesis Statement

Your work up until this point has prepared you to write a *thesis statement*, the central message you want to communicate. The thesis statement states your subject and point of view, reflects your writing purpose and audience, and acts as the organizing principle of your paper. It tells your readers what they should expect to read. Here is an example from Michael's paper:

Topic	Coast Guard boot camp
Purpose	To inform and narrate
Audience	Instructor with unknown knowledge about the topic
Thesis statement	Chief Marzloff, our Basic Training Company Commander at the U. S. Coast Guard Basic Training Facility, shaped my life through physical conditioning, developing my self-confidence, and instilling strong mental discipline.

A thesis statement is just as important in a short document, such as a letter, as it is in a long paper. For example, when you write a job application letter, a clear thesis statement will help you tell the recruiter why you deserve the job.

Write a Working Outline

The final step in the preparation process involves writing a working outline. Use this outline as a loose guide instead of a finalized structure. As you draft your paper, your ideas and structure may change many times. Only through allowing changes and refinements to happen can you get closer and closer to what you really want to say. Some students prefer a more formal outline structure, while others like to use a think link. Choose whatever form suits you best.

Create a Checklist

Use the checklist in Table 7-1 to make sure your preparation is complete. Under "Date Due," create your own writing schedule, giving each task an intended completion date. Work backwards from the date the assignment is due and estimate how long it will take to complete each step. Refer to Chapter 4 for time management skills that will help you schedule your writing process.

As you develop your schedule, keep in mind that you'll probably move back and forth between tasks. You might find yourself doing two and even three things on the same day. Stick to the schedule as best you can, while balancing the other demands of your busy life, and check off your accomplishments on the list as you complete them.

Drafting

Some people aim for perfection when they write a first draft. They want to get everything right—from word choice to tone to sentence structure to paragraph organization to spelling, punctuation, and grammar. Resist this tendency because it may lead you to shut the door on ideas before you even know they are there.

A *first draft* involves putting ideas down on paper for the first time—but not the last! You may write many different versions of the assignment until you like what you see. Each version moves you closer to communicating exactly what you want to say in the way you want to say it. The process is like starting with a muddy pond and gradually clearing the mud away until your last version is a clear body of water, showing the rocks and the fish underneath the surface. Think of your first draft as a way of establishing the pond before you start clearing it up.

TABLE 7-1	DATE DUE	TASK	IS IT COMPLETE?
Preparation checklist.		Brainstorm	
		Define and narrow	
		Use prewriting strategies	
		Conduct research if necessary	
		Write thesis statement	
		Write working outline	
		Complete research	

The elements of writing a first draft are freewriting, crafting an introduction, organizing the ideas in the body of the paper, formulating a conclusion, and citing sources.

Freewriting Your Draft

If the introduction, body, and conclusion are the three parts of the sandwich, freewriting is the process of searching the refrigerator for the ingredients and laying them all out on the table. Take everything that you have developed in the planning stages and freewrite a very rough draft. Don't censor yourself. For now, don't consciously think about your introduction, conclusion, or structure within the paper body. Focus on getting your ideas out of the realm of thought and onto the paper, in whatever form they prefer to be at the moment.

When you have the beginnings of a paper in your hands, you can start to shape it into something with a more definite form. First, work on how you want to begin your paper.

Writing an Introduction

The introduction tells your readers what the rest of the paper will contain. Including the thesis statement is essential. Here, for example, is a draft of an introduction for Michael's paper about the Coast Guard. The thesis statement is underlined at the end of the paragraph:

> Chief Marzloff took on the task of shaping the lives and careers of the youngest, newest members of the U. S. Coast Guard. During my eight weeks in training, he was my father, my instructor, my leader, and my worst enemy. He took his job very seriously and demanded that we do the same. <u>The Chief was instrumental in conditioning our bodies, developing our self-confidence, and instilling mental discipline within us.</u>

When you write an introduction, you might try to draw the reader in with an anecdote—a story that is directly related to the thesis. You can try other hooks, including a relevant quotation, dramatic statistics, and questions that encourage critical thinking. Whatever strategy you choose, be sure it is linked to your thesis statement. In addition, try to state your purpose without referring to its identity as a purpose. For example, in your introductory paragraph, state "Computer technology is infiltrating every aspect of health care," instead of, "In this paper, my purpose is to prove that computer technology is infiltrating every aspect of health care."

After you have an introduction that seems to set up the purpose of your paper, work on making sure the body fulfills that purpose.

TERMS

Hooks
Elements—including facts, quotes, statistics, questions, stories, or statements—that catch the reader's attention and encourage her to want to continue to read.

Creating the Body of a Paper

The body of the paper contains your central ideas and supporting evidence. *Evidence*—proof that informs or persuades—consists of the facts, statistics, examples, and expert opinions that you know or have gathered during research.

Look at the array of ideas and evidences within your draft in its current state. Think about how you might group certain items of evidence with the

LILIAN A. KANDA

Lewis University, Romeoville, Illinois

I have a two year associates degree in nursing, and I'm now enrolled in a bachelor's program. Writing was not emphasized much in the two-year nursing program. Students only had to take a minimum basic college English course, but this doesn't provide what you need in the real world. I work at a hospital, and I'm realizing that I need to improve my writing skills. With charting it's important to be accurate. I've tried following older nurses as my role models, but I've found that I still must adapt to my own way of charting. In the hospital, mistakes do happen. When I have to make an incident report stating what happened I wish my writing skills were better. The four-year degree involves more about writing and research, and it's giving me a chance to polish my writing skills.

One of my required courses is called "Concepts of Professional Nursing." My first paper for that class was about collaboration, in which I 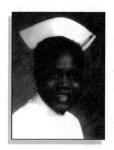 described teamwork among my coworkers. I was ready to quit the class, but the teacher was patient and I completed the course. The hardest part was doing the citations. One of the rules, of course, is that you can't use someone else's words, and I found it hard to paraphrase. If I can write about something that I'm very familiar with, the writing comes easier for me. For example, I wrote a paper about my growing up in Ghana, West Africa. That was one of my favorite writing assignments.

In some ways I think computers spoil nurses in regard to writing. Technology makes nursing easier, but it doesn't encourage nurses to write more. In school we are taught to write in narrative form, but with charting you usually have to abbreviate, so grammar is often disregarded. We do some narrative charting, but at the hospital I used to work for, we used only computer checklists for charting. Sometimes when we have new in-service programs for the computer it's so scary to me because I'm not used to anything that advanced. In spite of my apprehensions, I see the value of

writing on many levels. For example, following a charting system helps me focus on the patient and anticipate problems that I might have overlooked had I not taken the time to write out my observations. Information that might not have initially seemed important may be vital to another health care professional, especially if the patient's condition changes. The reflective aspect of writing helps me look at the patient holistically.

Last semester I had a patient with a skin integrity problem, and I noticed how writing down my interpretation of the issues facing this patient helped me coordinate an effective plan. This brings me to the heart of my concern. During clinicals, I only take care of one patient at a time. What about when I must juggle five or more patients all at once? I know the nursing profession is demanding. But without writing to stimulate my thinking, I'm concerned that I won't be able to provide the kind of care that I envision. It feels like I'm cheating myself and the patient. How can I balance time restrictions, along with a myriad of other nursing responsibilities, and still provide quality patient care?

RAY SALVA, JR.

Registered Nurse, Gottlieb Memorial Hospital, Melrose Park, Illinois

Providing quality patient care can feel like a tug-of-war game. As a nurse, you will be pulled in many directions all at once, but with experience you can 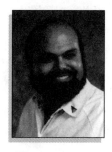 manage your patient load so that each person receives the best care possible.

One of the keys to providing quality care is organizational skills. Knowing which patients need the most care can help you set priorities during your particular shift. The severity of each patient's physical condition determines, at least in part, how much care you can and should give to them. Some patients require a lot more individual attention because of the seriousness of their condition. Remembering the basic ABCs: airway, breathing, and circulation, has helped me make this determination.

It might also help to be aware that day shifts are busier than evening shifts. Most hospital procedures, such as X-rays, are scheduled during the day and that's also when doctors and families make their visits. Since you've found it gratifying to focus on one patient at a time, you may prefer to specialize in ICU or CCU, because these patients frequently require one-on-one nursing care.

Another key of quality patient care is knowing what resources are available at your hospital. For example, knowing who to contact if a patient is having respiratory distress, or needs psychiatric care, can make a difference. When you begin your first nursing position, you should receive a policy and procedures manual which list these resources. For the sake of your patients, read through this so that you are aware of the options for them.

As you probably know, not every hospital uses SOAP notes and most hospitals are now computerized. You may find that you don't have time to do much writing and charting until near the end of your shift, after the necessary and urgent tasks are completed. At my hospital, every patient has their own computer check list and other prompts that nurses are expected to fill out. At the bottom there is a narrative section where I can be creative and make note of something important concerning the patient.

Since writing is a crucial learning tool for you, perhaps you could write about nursing in your free time. You could keep a journal and after the close of certain shifts, you could write down your observations and insights, and use these notes as a reminder of what worked for you that day and what didn't work.

Keep in mind that written care plans are only one part of the puzzle in providing quality care. Your training, your instinct, and even your individual personality all comprise the other pieces that help you become an excellent nurse. When I started my nursing career seven years ago I was a nervous wreck because I wanted to be the "perfect" nurse. Over time a more relaxed style began to emerge, and I brought "me" into the job. Once that happened I found nursing to be the kind of rewarding profession I always knew it could be.

particular ideas they support. Then, when you see the groups that form, try to find a structure that helps you to organize them into a clear pattern. Here are some strategies to consider.

Arrange ideas by time. Describe events in order or in reverse order.

Arrange ideas according to importance. You can choose to start with the idea that carries the most weight and move to ideas with less value or influence. You can also move from the least important to the most important idea.

Arrange ideas by problem and solution. Start with a specific problem; then discuss one or more solutions.

Writing the Conclusion

Your conclusion is a statement or paragraph that provides closure for your paper. Aim to summarize the information in the body of your paper, as well as to critically evaluate what is important about that information. Try one of the following devices:

- A summary of main points (if material is longer than three pages)
- A story, a statistic, a quote, a question that makes the reader think
- A call to action
- A look to the future

As you work on your conclusion, try not to introduce new facts or restate what you feel you have proved ("I have successfully proven that violent cartoons are related to increased violence in children"). Let your ideas as they are presented in the body of the paper speak for themselves. Readers should feel that they have reached a natural point of completion.

Crediting Authors and Sources

When you write a paper using any materials other than your own thoughts and recollections, the ideas you gathered in your research become part of your own writing. This does

Plagiarism
The act of using
someone else's
exact words, fig-
ures, unique
approach, or
specific reasoning
without giving
appropriate
credit.

not mean that you can claim these ideas as your own or fail to attribute them to someone. You need to credit authors for their ideas and words in order to avoid plagiarism.

To prevent plagiarism, learn the difference between a quotation and a paraphrase. A *quotation* refers to a source's exact words, which are set off from the rest of the text by quotation marks. A *paraphrase* is a restatement of the quotation in your own words, using your own sentence structure. Restatement means to completely rewrite the idea, not just to remove or replace a few words. A paraphrase may not be acceptable if it is too close to the original.

Even an acceptable paraphrase requires a citation of the source of the ideas within it. Take care to credit any source that you quote, paraphrase, or use as evidence. To credit sources, write a footnote or endnote that describes the source. Use the format preferred by your instructor. Writing manuals such as the *APA Publication Manual* contain acceptable formats.

Revising

When you *revise*, you critically evaluate the word choice, paragraph structure, and style of your first draft to see how it works. Any draft, no matter how good, can always be improved. Be thorough as you add, delete, replace, and reorganize words, sentences, and paragraphs. You may want to print out your draft and then spend time making notes and corrections on that hard copy before you make changes on a typewritten or computer-printed version. Figure 7-7 on the next page shows a paragraph from Michael's first draft, with revision comments added.

In addition to revising on your own, some of your classes may include peer review (having students read each other's work and offer suggestions). A peer reviewer can tell you what comes across well and what may be confusing. Having a different perspective on your writing is extremely valuable. Even if you don't have an organized peer-review system, you may want to ask a classmate to review your work as a favor to you.

The elements of revision include being a critical writer by checking for clarity and conciseness.

Being a Critical Writer

Critical thinking is as important in writing as it is in reading. Thinking critically when writing will help you move your papers beyond restating what you have researched and learned. Of course, your knowledge is an important part of your writing. What will make your writing even more important and unique, however, is how you use critical thinking to construct your own new ideas and knowledge from what you have learned.

The key to critical writing is asking the question, "So what?" For example, if you were writing a paper on nutrition, you might discuss a variety of good eating habits. Asking "So what?" could lead you into a discussion of *why* these habits are helpful, or what positive effects they have. If you were writing a paper on Aristotle's view of cosmology, you might list the main ideas you noticed he had on the subject. Then, asking "So what?" could lead

FIGURE 7-7

Paragraph from
first draft.

> Of the changes that ~~happened to us~~, the physical
> *military recruits undergo*
>
> transformation is the ~~biggest. When we arrived at the~~
> *most evident*   *Too much ↗*
>
> ~~training facility, it was January, cold and cloudy. At the~~
> *Maybe— upon my January arrival at the*
>
> ~~time,~~ I was a little thin, but I had been working out and
> *training facility*
>
> thought that I could physically do anything. Oh boy, was
>
> I wrong! The Chief said to us right away: "Get down,
> *← his trademark phrase*   *were*
>
> maggots!" Upon this command, we ~all to drop to the
> *endless*
>
> ground and do ~military-style push-ups. Water survival
>
> tactics were also part of the training ~~that we had to~~
> *unnecessary*
>
> ~~complete.~~ Occasionally, my dreams of home were
>
> interrupted at 3 a.m. when we had a surprise aquatic
> *resented*
>
> test. Although we ~~didn't feel too happy about~~ this
>   *mention how chief was involved*
>
> sub-human treatment at the time, we learned to
>
> appreciate how the conditioning was turning our bodies
>   *say more about this (swimming in uniform incident?)*
>
> into fine-tuned machines.

you to evaluate why Aristotle's ideas are important to our understanding of cosmology today.

As you revise, ask yourself questions that can help you think through ideas and examples, come up with your own original insights about the material, and be as complete and clear as possible. Use the mind actions to guide you. Here are some examples of questions you may ask:

Are these examples clearly connected to an idea or principle?

Are there any similar concepts or facts I know of that can add to how I support this?

What else can I recall that can help to support this idea?

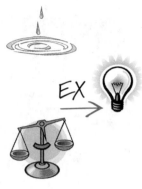

In evaluating any event or situation, have I clearly indicated the causes and effects?

What new principle or idea comes to mind when I think about these examples or facts?

How do I evaluate any effect/fact/situation? Is it good or bad, useful or not?

What different arguments might a reader think of that I should address here?

Finally, critical thinking can help you evaluate the content and form of your paper. As you start your revision, ask yourself the following questions.

- Will my audience understand my thesis and how I've supported it?
- Does the introduction prepare the reader and capture attention?
- Is the body of the paper organized effectively?
- Is each idea fully developed, explained, and supported by examples?
- Are my ideas connected to one another through logical transitions?
- Do I have a clear, concise, simple writing style?
- Does the paper fulfill the requirements of the assignment?
- Does the conclusion provide a natural ending to the paper?

Check for Clarity and Conciseness

Aim to say what you want to say in the clearest, most efficient way possible. A few well-chosen words will do your ideas more justice than a flurry of language. Try to eliminate extra words and phrases. Rewrite wordy phrases in a more concise, conversational way. For example, you can write "if" instead of "in the event that" or "now" instead of "this point in time." "Capriciously, I sauntered forth to the entryway and pummeled the door that loomed so majestically before me" might become "I skipped to the door and knocked loudly."

Editing

In contrast to the critical thinking of revising, *editing* involves correcting technical mistakes in spelling, grammar, punctuation, as well as checking style consistency for elements such as abbreviations and capitalizations. Editing comes last, after you are satisfied with your ideas, organization, and style of writing. If you use a computer, you might want to use the grammar-check and spellcheck functions to find mistakes. A spell-checker helps, but you still need to check your work on your own. While a spell-checker won't pick up the mistake in the following sentence, someone who is reading for sense will:

They are not hear on Tuesdays.

Look also for *sexist language*, which characterizes people based on their gender. Sexist language often involves the male pronoun *he* or *his*. For example "An executive often spends hours each day going through his electronic mail" implies that executives are always men. A simple change will eliminate the sexist language: "Executives often spend hours each day going through their electronic mail," or "An executive often spends hours each day going through his or her electronic mail." Another option is to alternate use of pronouns, using "him" in one section or example and "her" in another. Try to be sensitive to words that leave out or slight women. *Mail carrier* is preferable to *mailman; student* to *coed.*

Proofreading is the last stage of editing, occurring when you have a final version of your paper. Proofreading means reading every word and sentence in the final version to make sure they are accurate. Look for technical mistakes, run-on sentences, and sentence fragments. Look for incorrect word usage and references that aren't clear.

Teamwork can be a big help as you edit and proofread, because another pair of eyes may see errors that you didn't notice on your own. If possible, have someone look over your work. Ask for feedback on what is clear and what is confusing. Then ask the reader to edit and proofread for errors.

A Final Checklist

You are now ready to complete your revising and editing checklist. All the tasks listed in Table 7-2 should be complete when you submit your final paper.

Your final paper reflects all the hard work you put in during the writing process. Figure 7-8 shows the final version of Michael's paper.

"See revision as 'envisioning again.' If there are areas in your work where there is a blur or vagueness, you can simply see the picture again and add the details that will bring your work closer to your mind's picture."

NATALIE GOLDBERG

DATE DUE	TASK	IS IT COMPLETE?
	Check the body of the paper for clear thinking and adequate support of ideas	
	Finalize introduction and conclusion	
	Check word spelling and usage	
	Check grammar	
	Check paragraph structure	
	Make sure language is familiar and concise	
	Check punctuation	
	Check capitalization	
	Check transitions	
	Eliminate sexist language	

TABLE 7-2

Revising and editing checklist.

FIGURE 7-8

The final version of the paper.

March 19, 2000
Michael B. Jackson

BOYS TO MEN

His stature was one of confidence, often misinterpreted by others as cockiness. His small frame was lean and agile, yet stiff and upright, as though every move were a calculated formula. For the longest eight weeks of my life, he was my father, my instructor, my leader, and my worst enemy. His name is Chief Marzloff, and he had the task of shaping the lives and careers of the youngest, newest members of the U. S. Coast Guard. As our Basic Training Company Commander, he took his job very seriously and demanded that we do the same. Within a limited time span, he conditioned our bodies, developed our self-confidence, and instilled within us a strong mental discipline.

Of the changes that recruits in military basic training undergo, the physical transformation is the most immediately evident. Upon my January arrival at the training facility, I was a little thin, but I had been working out and thought that I could physically do anything. Oh boy, was I wrong! The Chief wasted no time in introducing me to one of his trademark phrases: "Get down, maggots!" Upon this command, we were all to drop to the ground and produce endless counts of military-style push-ups. Later, we found out that exercise prepared us for hitting the deck in the event of enemy fire. Water survival tactics were also part of the training. Occasionally, my dreams of home were interrupted at about 3 a.m. when our company was selected for a surprise aquatic test. I recall one such test that required us to swim laps around the perimeter of a pool while in full uniform. I felt like a salmon swimming upstream, fueled only by natural instinct. Although we resented this sub-human treatment at the time, we learned to appreciate how the strict guidance of the Chief was turning our bodies into fine-tuned machines.

Beyond physical ability, Chief Marzloff also played an integral role in the development of our self-confidence. He would often declare in his raspy voice, "Look me in the eyes when you speak to me! Show me that you believe what you're saying!" He taught us that anything less was an expression of disrespect. Furthermore, he appeared to attack a personal habit of my own. It seemed that whenever he would speak to me individually, I would nervously nod my head in response. I was trying to demonstrate that I understood, but to him, I was blindly accepting anything that he said. He would roar, "That is a sign of weakness!" Needless to say, I am now conscious of all bodily motions when communicating with others. The Chief also reinforced self-confidence through his own example. He walked with his square chin up and chest out, like the proud parent of a newborn baby. He always gave the appearance that he had something to do, and that

(continued)

FIGURE 7-8

Continued.

he was in complete control. Collectively, all of the methods that the Chief used were successful in developing our self-confidence.

Perhaps the Chief's greatest contribution was the mental discipline that he instilled in his recruits. He taught us that physical ability and self-confidence were nothing without the mental discipline required to obtain any worthwhile goal. For us, this discipline began with adapting to the military lifestyle. Our day began promptly at 0500 hours, early enough to awaken the oversleeping roosters. By 0515 hours, we had to have showered, shaved, and perfectly donned our uniforms. At that point, we were marched to the galley for chow, where we learned to take only what is necessary, rather than indulging. Before each meal, the Chief would warn, "Get what you want, but you will eat all that you get!" After making good on his threat a few times, we all got the point. Throughout our stay, the Chief repeatedly stressed the significance of self-discipline. He would calmly utter, "Give a little now, get a lot later." I guess that meant different things to all of us. For me, it was a simple phrase that would later become my personal philosophy on life. The Chief went to great lengths to ensure that everyone under his direction possessed the mental discipline required to be successful in boot camp or in any of life's challenges.

Chief Marzloff was a remarkable role model and a positive influence on many lives. I never saw him smile, but it was evident that he genuinely cared a great deal about his job and all the lives that he touched. This man single-handedly conditioned our bodies, developed our self-confidence, and instilled a strong mental discipline that remains in me to this day. I have not seen the Chief since March 28, 1992, graduation day. Over the years, however, I have incorporated many of his ideals into my life. Above all, he taught us the true meaning of the U. S. Coast Guard slogan, "Semper Peratus" (Always Ready).

The Research Format

Written research reports fit into a prescribed formula, making them easily identifiable in the journals you read. The sections are as follows:

Abstract. The beginning of an article is called the abstract. The abstract is approximately a 200-word summary of the entire research study.

Introduction. This section introduces the problem and often gives the research purpose and question, or hypothesis, to be tested in the study.

Literature review. The literature review justifies the need for the study by showing how other research on similar subjects leaves gaps in the knowledge base. Sometimes the literature review is not under its own heading but included in the introduction.

Theoretical framework. This is a section heading you will not always see, although sometimes the concepts are woven into the introduction. The theoretical framework is the foundation for the study. For instance, if I was studying health risk behaviors in college students, I might use a framework based on the Health Belief Model—a model that describes how a person's beliefs about health affect their health practices.

Sample and setting. This is the section that explains who or what is to be studied, the number studied, and where they/it were studied.

Methods. The research method is described in this section. Here you can see how the researchers went about designing the study, collecting data, and possible statistical tests they plan to use.

Results. The findings of the study are posted here, often in the form of tables or figures with statistical techniques applied.

Discussion. The summary of the entire study often includes recommendations for future research on the subject. This can be a good place to look for ideas for studies of your own.

Suà

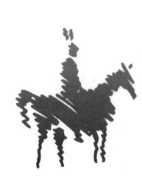

Suà is a Shoshone Indian word, derived from the Uto–Aztecna language, meaning "think." While much of the American Indian tradition focuses on oral communication, written languages have allowed American Indian perspectives and ideas to be understood by readers outside the American Indian culture. The writings of Leslie Marmon Silko, J. Scott Momaday, and Sherman Alexie have expressed important insights that all readers can consider.

Think of *suà*, and of how thinking can be communicated to others through writing, every time you begin to write. The power of writing allows you to express your own insights so that others can read them and perhaps benefit from knowing them. Explore your thoughts, sharpen your ideas, and remember the incredible power of the written word.

Applications   Chapter 7

KEY INTO YOUR LIFE
Opportunities to Apply What You Learn

 Evaluate Your Notes

Choose one particular class period from the last two weeks. Have a classmate photocopy his notes from that class period for you. Then evaluate your notes by comparing them with your classmate's. Think about:

- Do your notes make sense?
- How is your handwriting?
- Do the notes cover everything that was brought up in class?
- Are there examples to back up ideas?
- What note-taking system is used?
- Will these notes help you study?

Write your evaluation here: _____

_____

_____

_____

_____

_____

What ideas or techniques from your classmate's notes do you plan to use in the future?

_____

_____

_____

_____

_____

7.2 *Class vs. Reading*

Pick a class for which you have a regular textbook. Choose a set of class notes on a subject that is also covered in that textbook. Read the textbook section that corresponds to the subject of your class notes, taking notes as you go. Compare your reading notes to the notes you took in class.

Did you use a different system with the textbook or the same system as in class? Why? Which notes can you understand better? Why do you think that's true?

_____

_____

_____

_____

_____

What did you learn from your reading notes that you want to bring to your class note-taking strategy?

_____

_____

_____

_____

_____

7.3 *Prewriting*

Choose a topic you are interested in and know something about—for example, college sports, handling stress in a stressful world, our culture's emphasis on beauty and youth, health and illness experiences, or child rearing. Narrow your topic; then use the following prewriting strategies to discover what you already know about the topic and what you would need to learn if you had to write an essay about the subject for one of your classes. (If necessary, continue this prewriting exercise on a separate sheet of paper.)

Brainstorm your ideas: _____

_____

_____

_____

_____

Freewrite: _____

_____

_____

_____

_____

Ask journalists' questions: _____

_____

_____

_____

_____

7.4 *Writing a Thesis Statement*

Write two thesis statements for each of the following topics. The first statement should try to inform the reader, while the second should try to persuade. In each case, writing a thesis statement will require that you narrow the topic.

- *The rising cost of health care*

   Thesis with an informative purpose: _____

   _____

   _____

   Thesis with a persuasive purpose: _____

   _____

   _____

- *Taking care of your body and mind*

   Thesis with an informative purpose: _____

   _____

   _____

   Thesis with a persuasive purpose: _____

   _____

   _____

- *Career choice*

  Thesis with an informative purpose: _____

  _____

  _____

  Thesis with a persuasive purpose: _____

  _____

  _____

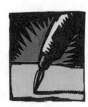

KEY TO SELF-EXPRESSION
Discovery Through Journal Writing

To record your thoughts, use a separate journal or the lined pages at the end of the chapter.

Your Relationship with Words

Some people love to work with words—writing them, reading them, speaking them—while others would rather do anything else. Do you enjoy writing in school, or does writing intimidate you? Do you write anything outside of school? Discuss how you feel about writing.

Name _____ Date _____

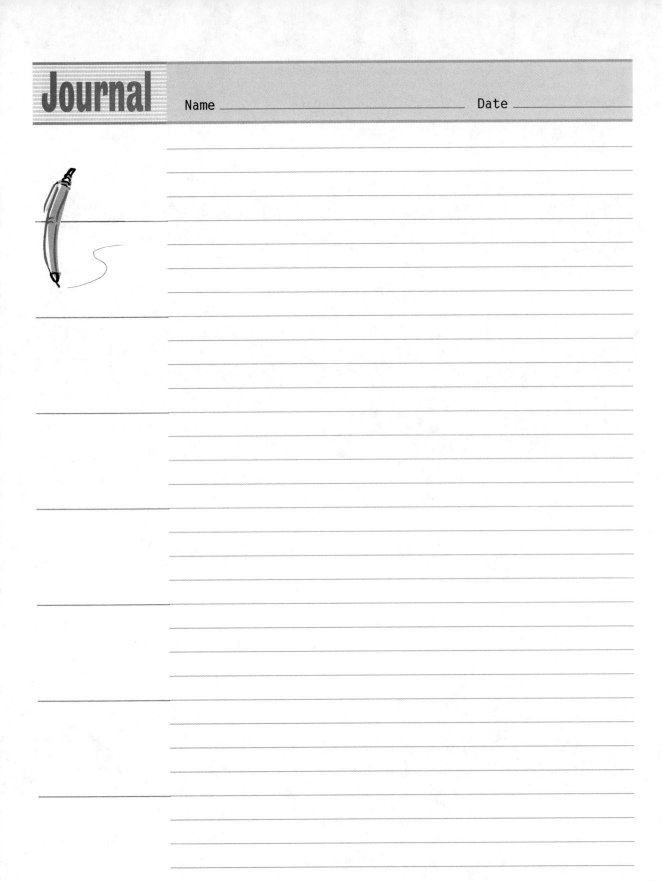

8

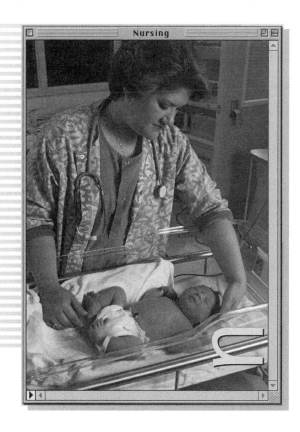

Nursing

Listening, Memory, and Test Taking

Taking In, Retaining, and Demonstrating Knowledge

College exposes you daily to facts, opinions, and ideas. It is up to you to take in, retain, and demonstrate knowledge of what you learn, for use in or out of school. You can accomplish these goals through active listening, focused use of your memory skills, and thorough preparation for taking tests.

Listening is one of the primary ways of taking in information and an essential skill for being a nurse. Listening is an important part of observation and assessment. Memory skills can help you retain what you've listened to so that you can recall it for a paper, a discussion, or a test. After you've listened and remembered, test taking is your key to demonstrating what you have learned to your instructor or others. In this chapter, you will learn strategies to improve your ability to take in, remember, and show knowledge of what you have learned.

In this chapter, you will explore answers to the following questions:

- How can you become a better listener?
- How does memory work?
- How can you improve your memory?
- How can tape recorders help you listen, remember, and study?
- How can preparation help improve test scores?
- What strategies can help you succeed on written tests?
- How can you learn from test mistakes?

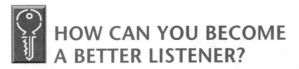

HOW CAN YOU BECOME A BETTER LISTENER?

The act of hearing isn't quite the same as the act of listening. While *hearing* refers to sensing spoken messages from their source, *listening* involves a complex process of communication. Successful listening results in the speaker's intended message reaching the listener. In school, and at home, poor listening results in communication breakdowns and mistakes, and skilled listening promotes progress and success.

Ralph G. Nichols, a pioneer in listening research, studied 200 students at the University of Minnesota over a nine-month period. His findings, summarized in Table 8-1, demonstrate that effective listening depends as much on attitude as on specific skills.[1]

Listening is a teachable—and learnable—skill. Improving your learning skills involves managing listening challenges and becoming an active listener. Although becoming a better listener will help in every class, it is especially important in subject areas that are difficult for you.

Manage Listening Challenges

Classic studies have shown that immediately after listening, students are likely to recall only half of what was said. This is partly due to particular listening challenges, including divided attention and distractions, the tendency to shut out the message, the inclination to rush to judgment, and partial hearing loss or learning disabilities.[2] To help create a positive listening environment, in both your mind and your surroundings, explore how to manage these challenges.

LISTENING IS HELPED BY . . .	LISTENING IS HINDERED BY . . .	TABLE 8-1
making a conscious decision to work at listening; viewing difficult material as a listening challenge.	caring little about the listening process; tuning out difficult material.	What helps and hinders listening.
fighting distractions through intense concentration.	refusing to listen at the first distraction.	
continuing to listen when a subject is difficult or dry, in the hope that one might learn something interesting.	giving up as soon as one loses interest.	
withholding judgment until hearing everything.	becoming preoccupied with a response as soon as a speaker makes a controversial statement.	
focusing on the speaker's theme by recognizing organizational patterns, transitional language, and summary statements.	getting sidetracked by unimportant details.	
adapting note-taking style to the unique style and organization of the speaker.	always taking notes in outline form, even when a speaker is poorly organized, leading to frustration.	
pushing past negative emotional responses and forcing oneself to continue to listen.	letting an initial emotional response shut off continued listening.	
using excess thinking time to evaluate, summarize, and question what one just heard and anticipating what will come next.	thinking about other things and, as a result, missing much of the message.	

Divided Attention and Distractions

Internal and external distractions often divide your attention. *Internal distractions* include anything from hunger to headache to personal worries. Something the speaker says may also trigger a recollection that may cause your mind to drift. In contrast, *external distractions* include noises (whispering, honking horns, screaming sirens) and even excessive heat or cold. It can be hard to listen in an overheated room that is putting you to sleep.

Your goal is to reduce distractions and focus on what you're hearing. Sitting where you can see and hear clearly will help you listen well. Dress comfortably and try not to go to class hungry or thirsty.

Shutting Out the Message

Instead of paying attention to everything the speaker says, many students fall into the trap of focusing on specific points and shutting out the rest of

"Women of that class have great opportunities and if they are intelligent may be well worth listening to. What instances, must pass before them of ardent, disinterested, self-denying attachment, of heroism, fortitude, patience, resignation; of all the conflicts and sacrifices that ennoble us most. A sick chamber may often furnish the worth of volumes."

JANE AUSTEN ON NURSE ROOK, PERSUASION

the message. Creating a positive listening environment includes accepting responsibility for listening. While the instructor communicates information to you, she cannot force you to listen. You are responsible for taking in that information. Instructors often cover material from outside the textbook during class and then test on that material. If you work to take in the whole message in class, you will be able to read over your notes later and think critically about what is most important.

The Rush to Judgment

People tend to stop listening when they hear something they don't like. If you rush to judge what you've heard, your focus turns to your personal reaction rather than the content of the speaker's message. Judgments also involve reactions to the speakers themselves. If you do not like your instructors or if you have preconceived notions about their ideas or cultural background, you may decide that their words have little value.

Work to recognize and control your judgments (see Chapter 5). Being aware of what you tend to judge will help you avoid putting up a barrier against incoming messages that clash with your opinions or feelings. Try to see education as a continuing search for evidence, regardless of whether it supports or negates your point of view.

Partial Hearing Loss and Learning Disabilities

Good listening techniques don't solve every listening problem. Students who have a partial hearing loss have a physical explanation for why listening is difficult. If you have some level of hearing loss, seek out special services that can help you listen in class. You may require special equipment or might benefit from tutoring. You may be able to arrange to meet with your instructor outside of class to clarify your notes.

Other diagnosed disabilities, such as attention deficit hyperactivity disorder (ADHD) or a problem with processing heard language, can cause difficulties with both focusing on and understanding that which is heard. People with such disabilities have varied ability to compensate for and overcome them. If you have or suspect you have, a disability, don't blame yourself for having trouble. Your counseling center, student health center, advisor, and instructors should be able to give you particular assistance in working through your challenges or information on getting tested.

 ## HOW DOES MEMORY WORK?

You need an effective memory in order to use the knowledge you take in throughout your life. Human memory works like a computer. Both have essentially the same purpose: to encode, store, and retrieve information.

During the *encoding stage*, information is changed into usable form. On a computer, this occurs when keyboard entries are transformed into electronic symbols and stored on a disk. In the brain, sensory information becomes impulses that the central nervous system reads and codes. You are encoding, for example, when you study a list of chemistry formulas.

During the *storage stage*, information is held in memory (the mind's version of a computer hard drive) for later use. In this example, after you complete your studying of the formulas, your mind stores them until you need to use them.

During the *retrieval stage*, memories are recovered from storage by recall, just as a saved computer program is called up by name and used again. In this example, your mind would retrieve the chemistry formulas when you had to take a test or solve a problem.

Memories are stored in three different storage banks. The first, called *sensory memory*, is an exact copy of what you see and hear, and it lasts for a second or less. Certain information is then selected from sensory memory and moves into *short-term memory*, a temporary information storehouse that lasts no more than 10 to 20 seconds. You are consciously aware of material in your short-term memory. While unimportant information is quickly dumped, important information is transferred to *long-term memory*—the mind's more permanent storehouse.

Having information in long-term memory does not mean that you will be able to recall it when needed. Particular techniques can help you improve your recall.

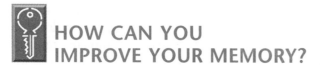 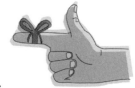

HOW CAN YOU IMPROVE YOUR MEMORY?

Your anatomy instructor is giving a test tomorrow on the parts of the brain. You feel confident, because you spent hours last week memorizing the material. Unfortunately, by the time you take the test, you may remember very little. That's because most forgetting occurs within minutes after memorization.

In a classic study conducted in 1885, researcher Herman Ebbinghaus memorized a list of meaningless three-letter words such as CEF and LAZ. Within one short hour, he measured that he had forgotten more than 50 percent of what he learned. After two days, he knew fewer than 30 percent. Although his recall of the syllables remained fairly stable after that, the experiment shows how fragile memory can be, even when you take the time and energy to memorize information.[3]

People who have superior memories may have an inborn talent for remembering. More often, though, they have mastered techniques for improving recall. Remember that techniques aren't a cure-all for memory difficulties, especially for those who may have learning disabilities. If you have a disability, the following memory techniques may help you but may not be enough. Seek specific assistance if you consistently have trouble remembering.

Memory Improvement Strategies

As a student, your job is to understand, learn, and remember information, from general concepts to specific details. The following suggestions will help improve your recall.

Develop a Will to Remember

Why can you remember the lyrics to dozens of popular songs but not the functions of the pancreas? Perhaps this is because you want to remember them, you connect them with a visual image, or you have an emotional tie to them. To achieve the same results at school or on the job, tell yourself that what you are learning is important and that you need to remember it. Saying these words out loud can help you begin the active, positive process of memory improvement.

Understand What You Memorize

Make sure that everything you want to remember makes sense. Something that has meaning is easier to recall than something that is gibberish. This basic principle applies to everything you study—from biology and astronomy to history and English literature.

Recite, Rehearse, and Write

When you *recite* material, you repeat it aloud in order to remember it. Reciting helps you retrieve information as you learn it and is a crucial step in studying (see Chapter 6). *Rehearsing* is similar to reciting, but is done in silence, in your mind. It involves the process of repeating, summarizing, and associating information with other information. *Writing* is rehearsing on paper. The act of writing solidifies the information in your memory.

Separate Main Points from Unimportant Details

If you use critical-thinking skills to select and focus on the most important information, you can avoid overloading your mind with extra clutter. To focus on key points, highlight only the most important information in your texts and write notes in the margins about central ideas. When you review your lecture notes, highlight or rewrite the most important information to remember.

Study During Short but Frequent Sessions

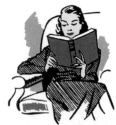

Research shows that you can improve your chances of remembering material if you learn it more than once, which is why "cramming" doesn't work. To get the most out of your study sessions, spread them over time. A pattern of short sessions followed by brief periods of rest is more effective than continual studying with little or no rest. Even though you may feel as though you accomplish a lot by studying for an hour without a break, you'll probably remember more from three 20-minute sessions. Try sandwiching study time into breaks in your schedule, such as when you have time between classes.

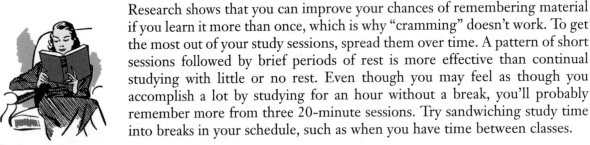

Separate Material into Manageable Sections

When material is short and easy to understand, studying it from start to finish may work. For longer material, you may benefit from dividing it into logical sections, mastering each section, putting all the sections together, and then testing your memory of all the material. Actors take this approach when learning the lines of a play, and it can work just as well for students.

Use Visual Aids

Any kind of visual representation of study material can help you remember. You may want to convert material into a think link or outline. Write material in any visual shape that helps you recall it and link it to other information.

Flashcards are a great visual memory tool. They give you short, repeated review sessions that provide immediate feedback. Make them from 3-by-5-inch index cards. Use the front of the card to write a word, idea, or phrase you want to remember. Use the back side for a definition, explanation, and other key facts. Figure 8-1 shows two flashcards for studying psychology.

Here are some additional suggestions for making the most of your flashcards:

- *Use the cards as a self-test.* Divide the cards into two piles: the material you know and the material you are learning. You may want to use rubber bands to separate the piles.

- *Carry the cards with you and review them frequently.* You'll learn the most if you start using cards early in the course, well ahead of exam time.

- *Shuffle the cards and learn information in various orders.* This will help avoid putting too much focus on some information and not enough on others.

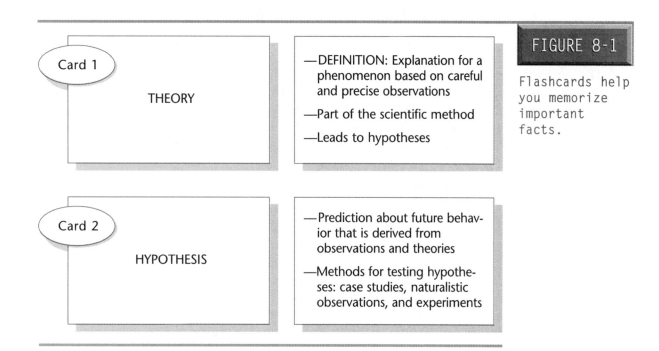

FIGURE 8-1

Flashcards help you memorize important facts.

Card 1

THEORY

—DEFINITION: Explanation for a phenomenon based on careful and precise observations

—Part of the scientific method

—Leads to hypotheses

Card 2

HYPOTHESIS

—Prediction about future behavior that is derived from observations and theories

—Methods for testing hypotheses: case studies, naturalistic observations, and experiments

■ *Test yourself in both directions.* First, look at the terms or ideas and provide definitions or explanations. Then turn the cards over and reverse the process.

Mnemonic Devices

Certain show business performers entertain their audiences by remembering the names of 100 strangers or flawlessly repeating 30 ten-digit phone numbers. These performers probably have superior memories, but genetics alone can't produce these results. They also rely on memory techniques, known as mnemonic devices (pronounced neh-MAHN-ick) to help them.

Mnemonic devices work by connecting information you are trying to learn with simpler information or information that is familiar. Instead of learning new facts by rote (repetitive practice), associations give you a hook on which to hang these facts and retrieve them. Mnemonic devices make information familiar and meaningful through unusual, unforgettable mental associations and visual pictures.

Here's an example to prove the power of mnemonics. Suppose you want to remember the names of the first six presidents of the United States. The first letters of their last names—Washington, Adams, Jefferson, Madison, Monroe, and Adams—together read W A J M M A. To remember them, you might add an "e" after the "J" and create a short nonsense word, "wajemma." To remember their first names—George, John, Thomas, James, James, and John—you might set the names to the tune of "Happy Birthday" or any musical tune that you know.

Visual images and acronyms are a few of the more widely used kinds of mnemonic devices. Apply them to your own memory challenges.

Create Visual Images and Associations

Visual images are easier to remember than images that rely on words alone. In fact, communication through visual images goes back to the prehistoric era when people made drawings, which still exist, on cave walls. It's no accident that the phrase "a picture is worth a thousand words" is so familiar. The best mental pictures often involve colors, three-dimensional images, action scenes, and disproportionate, funny, or ridiculous images. Especially for visual learners, turning information into mental pictures helps improve memory.

Create Acronyms

Another helpful association method involves the use of the acronym. The acronym "Roy G. Biv" often helps students remember the colors of the spectrum. Roy G. Biv stands for Red, Orange, Yellow, Green, Blue, Indigo, Violet. In history, you can remember the "big-three" Allies during World War II—Britain, America, and Russia—with the acronym BAR.

When you can't create a name like Roy G. Biv, create an acronym from an entire sentence, in which the first letter of each word in the sentence stands for the first letter of each memorized term. When science students want to remember the list of planets in order of their distance from the

---

TERMS

Mnemonic devices
Memory techniques that involve associating new information with information you already know.

"The true art of memory is the art of attention."
SAMUEL JOHNSON

TERMS

Acronym
A word formed from the first letters of a series of words, created in order to help you remember the series.

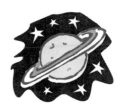

sun, they learn the sentence: My very elegant mother just served us nine pickles (Mercury, Venus, Earth, Mars, Jupiter, Saturn, Uranus, Neptune, and Pluto). In physiology and neurological nursing, remembering the cranial nerves is always a trick. Try this:

HOW TO REMEMBER THE TWELVE CRANIAL NERVES

On Old Olympus Treeless Top A Finn And German Viewed Some Hops

I Olfactory
II Optic
III Oculomotor
IV Trochlear
V Trigeminal
VI Abducens
VII Facial
VIII Acoustic
IX Glossopharyngeal
X Vagus
XI Spinal
XII Hypoglossal

Improving your memory requires energy, time, and work. In school, it also helps to master PQ3R, the textbook study technique that was introduced in Chapter 6. By going through the steps in PQ3R and using the specific memory techniques described in this chapter, you will be able to learn more in less time—and remember what you learn long after exams are over.

HOW CAN TAPE RECORDERS HELP YOU LISTEN, REMEMBER, AND STUDY?

The selective use of a tape recorder can provide helpful backup to your listening and memory skills and to your study materials. It's important, though, not to let tape recording substitute for active participation. Not all students like to use tape recorders, but if you choose to do so, here are some guidelines and a discussion of potential effects.

Guidelines for Using Tape Recorders

Ask the instructor whether he permits tape recorders in class. Some instructors don't mind, while others don't allow students to use them.

Use a small, portable tape recorder. Sit near the front for the best possible recording.

Participate actively in class. Take notes just as you would if the tape recorder were not there.

Use tape recorders to make study tapes. Questions on tape can be like audio flashcards. One way to do it is to record study questions, leaving ten to fifteen seconds between questions for you to answer out loud. Recording the correct answer after the pause will give you immediate feedback. For example, part of a recording for a writing class might say, "The three elements of effective writing are . . . (10–15 seconds) . . . topic, audience, and purpose."

Potential Positive Effects of Using Tape Recorders

- You can listen to an important portion of the lecture over and over again.
- You can supplement or clarify sections of the lecture that confused you or that you missed.
- Tape recordings can provide additional study materials to listen to when you exercise or drive in your car.
- Tape recordings can help study groups reconcile conflicting notes.
- If you miss class, you might be able to have a friend record the lecture for you.

Potential Negative Effects of Using Tape Recorders

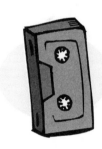

- You may tend to listen less in class.
- You may take fewer notes, figuring that you will rely on your tape.
- It may be time-consuming. When you attend a lecture in order to record it and then listen to the entire recording, you have taken twice as much time out of your schedule.
- If your tape recorder malfunctions or the recording is hard to hear, you may end up with very little study material, especially if your notes are sparse.

Think critically about whether using a tape recorder is a good idea for you. If you choose to try it, let the tape recorder be an additional resource for you instead of a replacement for your active participation and skills. Tape-recorded lectures and study tapes are just one study resource you can use in preparation for the tests that will often come your way.

 ## HOW CAN PREPARATION HELP IMPROVE TEST SCORES?

Many people don't look forward to taking tests. If you are one of those people, try thinking of exams as preparation for life. When you volunteer, get a job, or work on your family budget, you'll have to apply what you know. This is exactly what you do when you take a test.

Like a runner who prepares for a marathon by exercising, eating right, taking practice runs, and getting enough sleep, you can take steps to master your exams. Your first step is to study until you know the material that will be on the test. Your next step is to use the following strategies to become a successful test taker: Identify test type and material covered, use specific study skills, prepare physically, and conquer test anxiety.

Identify Test Type and Material Covered

Before you begin studying, try to determine the type of test and what it will cover:

- Will it be a short-answer test with true/false and multiple-choice questions, an essay test, or a combination?
- Will the test cover everything you studied since the semester began or will it be limited to a narrow topic?
- Will the test be limited to what you learned in class and in the text or will it also cover outside readings?
- Will the test be written or practical for a lab class?

Your instructors may answer these questions for you. Even though they may not tell you the specific questions that will be on the test, they might let you know what blocks of information will be covered and the question format. Some instructors may even drop hints throughout the semester about possible test questions. While some comments are direct ("I might ask a question on the subject of _____ on your next exam"), other clues are subtle. For example, when instructors repeat an idea or when they express personal interest in a topic ("One of my favorite theories is . . ."), they are letting you know that the material may be on the test.

Here are a few other strategies for predicting what may be on a test:

Use PQ3R to identify important ideas and facts. Often, the questions you write and ask yourself when you read assigned materials may be part of the test. In addition, any textbook study questions are good candidates for test material.

If you know people who took the instructor's course before, ask them about class tests. Try to find out how difficult the tests are and whether the test focuses more on assigned readings or class notes. Ask about instructor preferences. If you learn that the instructor pays close attention to detail such as facts or grammar, plan your work accordingly.

Examine old tests if instructors make them available in class or on reserve in the library. If you can't get copies of old tests, use clues from the class to predict test questions. After taking the first exam in the course, you will have a lot more information about what to expect in the future.

If the test is a practical lab exam find out if you can practice ahead of time. For instance, if you will be tested on plant identification, ask your instructor how to find samples for test preparation.

KRISTIN DUNPHY

Senior, University of Florida, Gainesville, Florida

Overall I've done well in my undergraduate studies, but memorization continues to be the most difficult part for me. In order to remember the material I have to be repetitive. In my pre-nursing courses, I could use short-term memory and memorize just what I needed to know for the test. But in nursing school you have to really know the information, such as laboratory values, because at some point you'll need to apply it. In core nursing courses you have to be able to demonstrate knowledge by using those facts.

Although I've not attended a study skills course, I've tried several study techniques on my own. In pharmacology, for example, I used note cards. I listed the drug on one side, with descriptions on the back. Then I'd quiz myself. I also try to relate the information to things I already know, instead of just memorizing them as random facts. My memory works much better when I can relate the information to a patient I see in my clinical rotation.

Another study area I would like to improve is textbook reading. Teachers often give overwhelming amounts to read. I find it easy to get lost in the details of the chapter so it's hard to pick out the key information I need to concen-

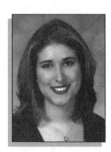

trate on. Also, my mind tends to wander when I'm reading more than a couple of pages at a time.

I have many strengths in regard to test taking, although essay tests are harder for me than multiple choice. With multiple choice questions you have more cues. I can eliminate the wrong answers and zero in on choosing the best answer. On essay tests, you must not only come up with the right answers, you must be able to expound on what you know.

I used to worry because my answers on essay tests were short and concise, but I've discovered that isn't really a problem. Professors are more interested in what you know than coming up with an elaborate, yet inaccurate explanation.

In the fall, I plan to begin a masters program in neonatal or midwifery, and I'm beginning to feel intimidated about it. I realize that masters level courses will be a step up from my undergraduate studies. I'm especially concerned about pharmacology because that involves straight memorization. You have to know more than just the basic drugs and their dosages. What can I do to improve my memorization skills so that I'll be better equipped to handle master level courses?

ARUNA CHANNAIAH RAMKARANSINGH, M.ED.

Coordinator of Student Enrollment and Advisement, Georgetown University School of Nursing, Washington, D.C.

I teach learning skills as part of an academic enrichment program called "Yes to Success! Transitions to Higher Excellence" at the Georgetown University School of Nursing. One of the main points we stress to students is that learning occurs over time. Therefore, repetition and application are key to memorization. Each experience you have with the content reinforces learning. Reviewing new material, even just ten minutes a day, is much more effective than cramming at the last minute. Daily rehearsal and organizing the material in your mind in ways that are meaningful to you usually lead to long-term memory.

When you are learning new material, create associations between novel information and things you already know. Categorize concepts in your mind. Start by picking out the main points and chunk them into parts. Next, wrap details around these ideas and facts as needed. Note cards are an excellent study tool because you can break up the content into manageable parts, and you can easily carry them around with you. You never know when or where you might have 10 extra minutes to review! Also, be sure to take 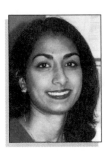 timely study breaks so that you return to your work refreshed.

Another effective memorization tool is mnemonic devices or memory tricks, which can take the form of acronyms, symbols, visual images, or stories. For example, when studying pharmacology, link a particular drug with a patient you may have cared for during one of your clinical experiences and his or her illness. You may also find it helpful to create a chart or diagram of what you're learning, especially if you're a visual learner. Graphical aids can help you condense and organize information into mental schemas, thus increasing your chances of remembering a concept or segment of information.

Essay questions are easier to manage if you prepare an outline of your response. You want your response to be organized and thorough, therefore, the outline should have an introduction and a conclusion with the key points you'd like to discuss falling in between. Also, be sure to develop smooth transitions that tie the key ideas in your essay together, thus giving the essay a coherent flow. Time is another problem that students often have with essay responses, because they can take longer to complete than multiple choice questions. Therefore, use the introduction to your advantage. In one or two sentences, state exactly what you plan to cover in your response. Even if you do run out of time, the professor can read what you planned to write down, which may increase your score for that question.

When you initially review your new textbooks, notice how the author organizes the material. Attempt to get the big picture first and then move on to details. Preview your syllabi and scan the assigned readings prior to class. This will prepare your mind for the lecture. Now, you're tackling the information from both a visual (the reading) and auditory (listening to the lecture) standpoint. As you read, look for typographical cues, which are usually underlined or in bold or italics. When you see them, realize that the author is saying, "This is important." This same rule applies to handouts distributed by your professor. Similarly, pay particular attention to verbal cues given by the instructor. These verbal cues highlight important information imparted in a lecture.

After reading a section in a chapter, go back and develop two or more study questions, depending on the complexity of the text. You can compile these questions as you read and use them for 15 minutes of review every day. If you don't prefer to create questions, write a summary of what you just read, restating it from memory in your own words.

Whether you are reading or listening, practice reacting to the material, instead of just passively letting the information pass by. Ask yourself, "Do I agree or disagree with what the professor is saying or what I am reading?" Also, If you can explain a concept or teach it to someone, that shows you really understand it. Another good self-test is to ask: "Can I come up with an example of this concept?" If you can't think of an example or are unable to explain the information to someone else, you probably don't fully grasp the concept. In that case, you should consult the professor or your textbooks for clarification. The take-home message here is that study strategies must be actively implemented on a daily basis over time in order for learning to occur.

Use Specific Study Skills

Certain study skills are especially useful for test taking. They include choosing study materials, setting a study schedule, critical thinking, and taking a pretest.

Choose Study Materials

Once you have identified as much as you can about the subject matter of the test, choose the materials that contain the information you need to study. You can save yourself time by making sure that you aren't studying anything you don't need to. Go through your notes, your texts, any primary source materials that were assigned, and any handouts from your instructor. Set aside any materials you don't need so that they don't take up your valuable time.

Set a Study Schedule

Use your time management skills to set a schedule that will help you feel as prepared as you can be. Consider all the relevant factors—the materials you need to study, how many days or weeks until the test date, and how much time you can study each day. If you establish your schedule ahead of time and write it in your date book, you will be much more likely to follow it.

Schedules will vary widely according to situation. For example, if you have only three days before the test and no other obligations during that time, you might set two 2-hour study sessions for yourself during each day. On the other hand, if you have two weeks before a test date, classes during the day, and work three nights a week, you might spread out your study sessions over the nights you have off work during those two weeks.

Prepare Through Critical Thinking

Using the techniques from Chapter 5, approach your test preparation critically, working to understand rather than just to pass the test by repeating facts. As you study, try to connect ideas to examples, analyze causes and effects, establish truth, and look at issues from different perspectives. Although it takes work, critical thinking will promote a greater understanding of the subject and probably a higher grade on the exam. Using critical thinking is especially important for essay tests. Prepare by identifying potential essay questions and writing your responses.

Take a Pretest

Use questions from the ends of textbook chapters to create your own pretest. Choose questions that are likely to be covered on the test, then answer them under testlike conditions—in quiet, with no books or notes to help you, and with a clock telling you when to quit. Try to duplicate the conditions of the actual test. If your course doesn't have an assigned text, develop questions from your notes and from assigned outside readings.

Prepare Physically

When taking a test, you often need to work efficiently under time pressure. If your body is tired or under stress, you will probably not think as clearly or perform as well. Avoid pulling an all-nighter. Get some sleep so that you can wake up rested and alert. If you are one of the many who press the snooze button in their sleep, try setting two alarm clocks and placing them across the room from your bed. That way you'll be more likely to get to your test on time.

Eating right is also important. Sugar-laden snacks will bring your energy up only to send it crashing back down much too soon. Similarly, too much caffeine can add to your tension and make it difficult to focus. Eating nothing will leave you drained, but too much food can make you want to take a nap. The best advice is to eat a light, well-balanced meal before a test. When time is short, grab a quick-energy snack such as a banana, some orange juice, or a granola bar. Sleep, protein, and carbs will help your recall. Being tired, or wired (on caffeine) will hinder recall.

Conquer Test Anxiety

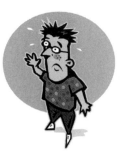

A certain amount of stress can be a good thing. Your body is on alert, and your energy motivates you to do your best. For many students, however, the time before and during an exam brings a feeling of near-panic known as *test anxiety*. Described as a bad case of nerves that makes it hard to think or remember, test anxiety can make your life miserable and affect how you do on tests. When anxiety blocks performance, here are some suggestions:

Prepare so you'll feel in control. The more you know about what to expect on the exam, the better you'll feel. Find out what material will be covered, the format of the questions, the length of the exam, and the percentage of points assigned to each question.

Put the test in perspective. No matter how important it may seem, a test is only a small part of your educational experience and an even smaller part of your life. Your test grade does not reflect the kind of person you are or your ability to succeed in life.

Make a study plan. Divide the plan into a series of small tasks. As you finish each one, you'll feel a sense of accomplishment and control.

Practice relaxation. When you feel test anxiety coming on, take some deep breaths, close your eyes, and visualize positive mental images related to the test, like getting a good grade and finishing confidently with time to spare.

Test Anxiety and the Returning Adult Student

If you're returning to school after five, ten, or even twenty years, you may wonder if you can compete with younger students or if your mind is still able to learn new material. To counteract these feelings of inadequacy, focus on how your life experiences have given you skills you can use. For example, managing work and a family requires strong time management, planning, and communication skills that can help you plan your study time, juggle school responsibilities, and interact with students and instructors.

In addition, your life experiences give you examples with which you can understand ideas in your courses. For example, your relationship experiences may help you understand concepts in a psychology course; managing your finances may help you understand math; and work experience may give you a context for learning teamwork. If you recognize and focus on your knowledge and skills, you may improve your ability to achieve your goals.

WHAT STRATEGIES CAN HELP YOU SUCCEED ON WRITTEN TESTS?

Even though every test is different, there are general strategies that will help you handle almost all tests, including short-answer and essay exams.

Write Down Key Facts

Before you even look at the test, write down any key information—including formulas, rules, and definitions—that you studied recently or even right before you entered the test room. Use the back of the question sheet or a piece of scrap paper for your notes (make sure it is clear to your instructor that this scrap paper didn't come into the test room already filled in!). Recording this information right at the start will make forgetting less likely.

Begin with an Overview of the Exam

Even though exam time is precious, spend a few minutes at the start of the test to get a sense of the kinds of questions you'll be answering, what kind of thinking they require, the number of questions in each section, and the point value of each section. Use this information to schedule the time you spend on each section. For example, if a two-hour test is divided into two sections of equal point value—an essay section with four questions and a short-answer section with sixty questions—you can spend an hour on the essays (fifteen minutes per question) and an hour on the short-answer section (one minute per question).

As you make your calculations, think about the level of difficulty of each section. If you think you can handle the short-answer questions in less than an hour and that you'll need more time with the essays, rebudget your time in a way that works for you.

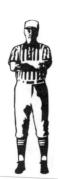

Know the Ground Rules

A few basic rules apply to any test. Following them will give you an advantage.

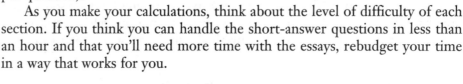

Read test directions. While a test made up of 100 true/false questions and one essay may look straightforward, the directions may tell you to answer eighty, or that the essay is a optional bonus. Some questions or sections may be weighted more heavily than others. Try circling or underlining key words and numbers that remind you of the directions.

Begin with the parts or questions that seem easiest to you. Starting with what you know best can boost your confidence and help you save time to spend on the harder parts.

Watch the clock. Keep track of how much time is left and how you are progressing. You may want to plan your time on a scrap piece of paper, especially if you have one or more essays to write. Wear a watch or bring a small clock with you to the test room. A wall clock may be broken, or there may be no clock at all! Also, take your time. Rushing is almost always a mistake, even if you feel you've done well. Stay till the end so you can refine and check your work.

Master the art of intelligent guessing. When you are unsure of an answer, you can leave it blank or you can guess. In most cases, guessing will benefit you. First eliminate all the answers you know—or believe—are wrong. Try to narrow your choices to two possible answers; then, choose the one that makes more sense to you. When you recheck your work, decide if you would make the same guesses again, making sure there isn't a qualifier or fact that you hadn't noticed before.

Follow directions on machine-scored tests. Machine-scored tests require that you use a special pencil to fill in a small box on a computerized answer sheet. Use the right pencil (usually a number 2) and mark your answer in the correct space. Neatness counts on these tests, because the computer can misread stray pencil marks or partially erased answers. Periodically, check the answer number against the question number to make sure they match. One question skipped can cause every answer following it to be marked incorrectly.

> **TERMS**
>
> Qualifier
> A word, such as *always*, *never*, or *often*, that changes the meaning of another word or word group.

Use Critical Thinking to Avoid Errors

When the pressure of a test makes you nervous, critical thinking can help you work through each question thoroughly and avoid errors. Following are some critical-thinking strategies to use during a test.

Recall facts, procedures, rules, and formulas. You base your answers on the information you recall. Think carefully to make sure you recall it accurately.

Think about similarities. If you don't know how to attack a question or problem, consider any similar questions or problems that you have worked on in class or while studying.

Notice differences. Especially with objective questions, items that seem different from what you have studied may indicate answers you can eliminate.

Think through causes and effects. For a numerical problem, think through how you plan to solve it and see if the answer—the effect of your plan—makes

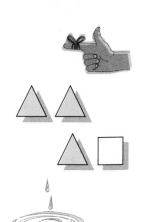

sense. For an essay question that asks you to analyze a condition or situation, consider both what caused it and what effects it has.

Find the best principle to match the example or examples given. For a numerical problem, decide what formula (principle) best applies to the example or examples (the data of the problem). For an essay question, decide what principle applies to, or links, the examples given.

Support principles with examples. When you put forth a principle, or idea, in an answer to an essay question, be sure to back up your idea with an adequate number of examples that fit.

Evaluate each test question. In your initial approach to any question, evaluate what kinds of thinking will best help you solve it. For example, essay questions often require cause and effect and principle to example thinking, while objective questions often benefit from thinking through similarities and differences.

The general strategies you have just explored also can help you address specific types of test questions.

Master Different Types of Test Questions

Although the goal of all test questions is to discover how much you know about a subject, every question type has its own way of asking what you know. Objective questions, such as multiple-choice or true/false, test your ability to recall, compare, and contrast information and to choose the right answer from among several choices. Subjective questions, usually essay questions, demand the same information recall but ask that you analyze the mind actions and thinking processes required, then organize, draft, and refine a written response. The following guidelines will help you choose the best answers to both types of questions.

Multiple-Choice Questions

Multiple-choice questions are the most popular type on standardized tests. The following strategies can help you answer these questions:

Read the directions carefully. While most test items ask for a single correct answer, some give you the option of marking several choices that are correct.

First read each question thoroughly. Then look at the choices and try to answer the question.

Underline key words and phrases in the question. If the question is complicated, try to break it down into small sections that are easy to understand.

Pay special attention to qualifiers such as *only, except,* **etc.** For example, negative words in a question can confuse your understanding of what the question asks ("Which of the following is *not* . . .").

If you don't know the answer, eliminate those answers that you know or suspect are wrong. Your goal is to narrow down your choices. Here are some questions to ask:

■ Is the choice accurate in its own terms? If there's an error in the choice— for example, a term that is incorrectly defined—the answer is wrong.

■ Is the choice relevant? An answer may be accurate, but it may not relate to the essence of the question.

■ Are there any qualifiers, such as *always, never, all, none,* or *every?* Qualifiers make it easy to find an exception that makes a choice incorrect. For example, the statement that "children *always* begin talking before the age of two" can be eliminated as an answer to the question, "When do children generally start to talk?"

■ Do the choices give you any clues? Does a puzzling word remind you of a word you know? If you don't know a word, does any part of the word (prefix, suffix, or root) seem familiar to you?

Look for patterns that may lead to the right answer, then use intelligent guessing. Test-taking experts have found patterns in multiple-choice questions that may help you get a better grade. Here is their advice:

■ Consider the possibility that a choice that is more *general* than the others is the right answer.

■ Look for a choice that has a middle value in a range (the range can be from small to large, from old to recent). This choice may be the right answer.

■ Look for two choices with similar meanings. One of these answers is probably correct.

Make sure you read every word of every answer. Instructors have been known to include answers that are right except for a single word.

When questions are keyed to a long reading passage, read the questions first. This will help you focus on the information you need to answer the questions.

Here are some examples of the kinds of multiple-choice questions you might encounter in a pharmacology course (the correct answer follows each question):

Interferon should be given with caution to clients with a previous history of

a. GI bleeding   c. asthma

b. hypertension   d. depression   *(correct answer is a)*

Amantadine (Symmetrel), when administered as an antiviral agent, is used to treat

a. herpes simplex   c. HIV

b. herpes zoster   d. influenza A   *(correct answer is d)*

You are administering oral tetracycline to a client. You will schedule the drug to be given

a. with milk   c. with antacids

b. one hour before meals   d. it doesn't matter when tetracycline
                              is administered

                                   (correct answer is b)

True/False Questions

True/false questions test your knowledge of facts and concepts. Read them carefully to evaluate what they truly say. Try to take these questions at face value without searching for hidden meaning. If you're truly stumped, guess (unless you're penalized for wrong answers).

Look for qualifiers in true/false questions—such as *all, only, always, because, generally, usually,* and *sometimes*—that can turn a statement that would otherwise be true into one that is false, or vice versa. For example, "The grammar rule, 'I before E except after C,' is *always* true" is *false*, whereas "The grammar rule, 'I before E except after C,' is *usually* true," is *true*. The qualifier makes the difference. The box below offers some examples of the kinds of true/false questions you might encounter in an Introduction to Psychology course (the correct answer follows each question).

Are the following questions true or false?

1. Alcohol use is always related to increases in hostility, aggression, violence, and abusive behavior. (False)

2. Marijuana is harmless. (False)

3. Simply expecting a drug to produce an effect is often enough to produce the effect. (True)

Essay Questions

An essay question allows you to use writing to demonstrate your knowledge and express your views on a topic. Start by reading the questions and deciding which to tackle (sometimes there's a choice). Then focus on what each question is asking, the mind actions you will have to use, and the writing directions. Read the question carefully, and do everything you are asked to do. Some essay questions may contain more than one part.

Watch for certain action verbs that can help you figure out what to do. Figure 8-2 explains some words commonly used in essay questions. Underline these words as you read any essay question and use them as a guide.

Next, budget your time and begin to plan. Create an informal outline or think link to map your ideas and indicate examples you plan to cite to support those ideas. Avoid spending too much time on introductions or flowery prose. Start with a thesis idea or statement that states in a broad way what your essay will say (see Chapter 7 for a discussion of thesis statements). As you continue to write your first paragraph, introduce the essay's points, which may be sub-ideas, causes and effects, or examples. Wrap it up with a concise conclusion.

Use clear, simple language in your essay. Support your ideas with examples, and look back at your outline to make sure you are covering everything. Try to write legibly. If your instructor can't read your ideas, it doesn't matter how good they are. If your handwriting is messy, try printing, skipping every other line, or writing on only one side of the paper.

Do your best to save time to reread and revise your essay after you finish getting your ideas down on paper. Look for ideas you left out and sentences that might confuse the reader. Check for mistakes in grammar, spelling, punctuation, and usage. No matter what subject you are writing about, having a command of these factors will make your work all the more complete and impressive.

Here are some examples of essay questions you might encounter in your Introduction to Physiology course. In each case, notice the action verbs from Figure 8-2.

1. Describe how different sense organs enable the body to obtain information about internal and external environments. Include specifics of taste, vision, hearing, touch, and smell.

2. What are the major glands of the endocrine system; what hormone(s) does each produce; and what are their affects on the body?

Analyze Break into parts and discuss each part separately.

Compare Explain similarities and differences.

Contrast Distinguish between items being compared by focusing on differences.

Criticize Evaluate the positive and negative effects of what is being discussed.

Define State the essential quality or meaning. Give the common idea.

Describe Visualize and give information that paints a complete picture.

Discuss Examine in a complete and detailed way, usually be connecting ideas to examples.

Enumerate/List/Identify Recall and specify items in the form of a list.

Explain Make the meaning of something clear, often by making analogies or giving examples.

Evaluate Give your opinion about the value or worth of something, usually by weighing positive and negative effects, and justify your conclusion.

Illustrate Supply examples.

Interpret Explain your personal view of facts and ideas and how they relate to one another.

Outline Organize and present the sub-ideas or main examples of an idea.

Prove Use evidence and argument to show that something is true, usually by showing cause and effect or giving examples that fit the idea to be proven.

Review Provide an overview of ideas, and establish their merits and features.

State Explain clearly, simply, and concisely, being sure that each word gives the image you want.

Summarize Give the important ideas in brief.

Trace Present a history of the way something developed, often by showing cause and effect.

FIGURE 8-2

Common action verbs on essay tests.

HOW CAN YOU LEARN FROM TEST MISTAKES?

The purpose of a test is to see how much you know, not merely to achieve a grade. The knowledge that comes from attending class and studying should allow you to correctly answer test questions. Knowledge also comes when you learn from your mistakes. If you don't learn from what you get wrong on a test, you are likely to repeat the same mistake again on another test and in life. Learn from test mistakes just as you learn from mistakes in your personal and business life.

Try to identify patterns in your mistakes by looking for:

- *Careless errors*—In your rush to complete the exam, did you misread the question or directions, blacken the wrong box, skip a question, or use illegible handwriting?

- *Conceptual or factual errors*—Did you misunderstand a concept or never learn it in the first place? Did you fail to master certain facts? Did you skip part of the assigned text or miss important classes in which ideas were covered?

You may want to rework the questions you got wrong. Based on the feedback from your instructor, try rewriting an essay, recalculating a math problem, or redoing the questions that follow a reading selection. As frustrating as they are, remember that mistakes show that you are human, and they can help you learn. If you see patterns of careless errors, promise yourself that next time you'll try to budget enough time to double-check your work. If you pick up conceptual and factual errors, rededicate yourself to better preparation.

When you fail a test, don't throw it away. First, take comfort in the fact that a lot of students have been in your shoes and that you are likely to improve your performance. Then recommit to the process by reviewing and analyzing your errors. Be sure you understand why you failed. You may want to ask for an explanation from your instructor. Finally, develop a plan to really learn the material if you didn't understand it in the first place.

ཤེམས་མ་ཡེང་ཤེན།

In Sanskrit, the written language of India and other Hindu countries, the characters above read *sem ma yeng chik*, meaning, "do not be distracted." This advice can refer to focus for a task or job at hand, the concentration required to critically think and talk through a problem, or the mental discipline of meditation.

Think of this concept as you strive to improve your listening and memory techniques. Focus on the task, the person, or the idea at hand. Try not to be distracted by other thoughts, other people's notions of what you should be doing, or any negative messages. Be present in the moment to truly hear and remember what is happening around you. Do not be distracted.

Applications   Chapter 8

KEY INTO YOUR LIFE
Opportunities to Apply What You Learn

 8.1   *Optimum Listening Conditions*

Describe a recent classroom situation in which you had an easy time listening to the instructor:

Where are you? _____

What is the instructor discussing? _____

Is it a straight lecture, or is there give-and-take between instructor and students? _____

_____

What is your state of mind? (List factors that might affect your ability to listen.) _____

_____

_____

_____

_____

Are there any external barriers to communication? If yes, what are they, and how do they affect your concentration? _____

_____

_____

_____

_____

Now describe a situation where you have found it more difficult to listen.

Where are you? _____

What is the instructor discussing? _____

Is it a straight lecture, directions for a lab, or is there give-and-take between instructor and students? _____

_____

What is your state of mind? (List factors that might affect your ability to listen.) _____

_____

_____

_____

_____

Are there any external barriers to your hearing, physical or environmental? If yes, what are they, and how do they affect your concentration? _____

_____

_____

_____

_____

Examine the two situations. Based on your descriptions, name three conditions that are crucial for you to listen effectively.

1. _____

2. _____

3. _____

What steps can you take to re-create these conditions in more difficult situations like the second one you described? _____

_____

_____

_____

8.2   *Create a Mnemonic Device*

Look back at all the memory principles examined in this chapter. Using what you learned about mnemonic devices, create a mnemonic that allows you to remember these memory principles quickly. You can create a mental picture or an acronym. If you are using a mental picture, describe it here; if you are using an acronym, write it and then indicate what each letter stands for.

_____

_____

_____

_____

_____

Think of other situations in which you used a mnemonic device to remember something. What was the device? How effective was it in helping you remember the information?

_____

_____

_____

_____

_____

_____

8.3   *Learning from Your Mistakes*

For this exercise, use an exam on which you made one or more mistakes.

■ Why do you think you answered the question(s) incorrectly?

_____

_____

_____

■ Did any qualifying terms, such as *always, sometimes, never, often, occasionally, only, no,* and *not,* make the question(s) more difficult or confusing? What steps could you have taken to clarify the meaning?

_____

_____

_____

■ Did you try to guess the correct answer? If so, why do you think you made the wrong choice?

_____

_____

_____

■ Did you feel rushed? If you had had more time, do you think you would have gotten the right answer(s)? What could you have done to budget your time more effectively?

_____

_____

_____

- If an essay question was a problem, what do you think went wrong? What will you do differently the next time you face an essay question on a test?

_____

_____

_____

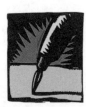

KEY TO SELF-EXPRESSION
Discovery Through Journal Writing

To record your thoughts, use a separate journal or the lined pages at the end of the chapter.

Write about how you feel about tests and how you generally perform when you take them.

As you walk into a room for a test, does your heart race or your mind go blank? Do you feel apprehensive? Does your performance on tests accurately reflect what you know or do your tests scores fall short of your knowledge? If there is a gap between your knowledge and your scores, why do you think this gap exists? What can you do to work through any test anxiety you have?

Name _____ Date _____

9

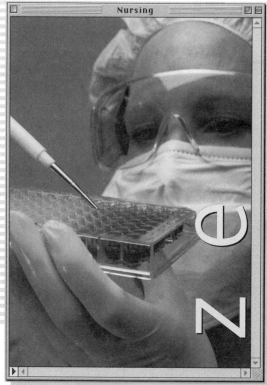

Nursing

Working in the Laboratory

Safe Science in Action

O n your way to becoming a nurse, you will take many prerequisite science courses, and most science courses involve labs. Basically, there are two types of labs. One type, confirmatory, gives you the chance to better understand, or confirm, concepts you are studying in the classroom. You will do predetermined experiments that let you see for yourself evidence that confirms theories (also known as deductive). The second, original inquiry, gives you the opportunity to learn skills needed to set up an experiment to answer original questions. In either case, experiments done in undergraduate labs involve doing research by learning methods for collecting data to test theories, confirm hypotheses, or answer questions, raised by a nurse researcher.

This chapter will help prepare you for your lab classes, and if you are a returning student who hasn't been in a lab class for some time, familiarize you with the basic do's and don'ts for safe labs. Inquiry-based lab science will be explored along with the practical considerations such as credit hours and equipment.

In this chapter, you will explore the answers to the following questions:

- What is inquiry-based research?
- What equipment will you need in the lab?
- How do credit hours translate into lab time?
- What can you do to boost your chances for success?
- Why is it important to practice safe lab science?
- What skills does lab work give you?

WHAT IS INQUIRY-BASED RESEARCH?

When the answers are not known you may take on the role of a researcher. Inquiry is just as it sounds, an inquiry, or exploration, into something you desire to know.

The *American Heritage College Dictionary* defines inquiry as follows:

1. The act of inquiring.
2. A question; a query.
3. A close examination of a matter in a search for information or truth.

> "Twinkle, twinkle little star I don't wonder what you are For by spectroscopic ken I know that you are hydrogen."
>
> ANONYMOUS

As the definition states, inquiry is about asking questions and carefully examining evidence that helps you answer the questions. This is usually done by forming a hypothesis and then deciding how to test your hypothesis.

A hypothesis is like an assumption, or a likely explanation to your question. If you are wondering about the effect of alcohol consumption during pregnancy, you might ask the question, "Do women who drink alcohol during pregnancy have infants that are small and poorly developed?" From this you develop a testable hypothesis:

Birth weight is lower among infants of alcoholic women than among infants of nonalcoholic women.

To test this directly you would have to have access to patient charts so you could look for alcoholic women who drank during their pregnancy and nonalcoholic women who didn't and then look for the weights of their infants and compare. Were the infants of women who drank smaller than those whose women didn't drink? In the lab you could devise an experiment to see if alcohol affects individual cell development.

Often the answers to your questions are not known. This gives you an opportunity, in the lab or in the field, to take on the role of the researcher. You will learn how to:

1. Ask questions
2. Form ways to answer your questions, either experimentally or through observation.
3. Collect information and record it for later use or analysis.

Qualities of a Researcher

Labs, especially those based on inquiry, teach you many qualities, including creativity, patience, and persistence.

Creativity. You have to find different ways to answer your questions, which requires looking at things from different viewpoints, understanding your own biases, and letting your mind wander; daydreaming can be an important aspect of the creative process.

Patience. You must possess, or learn to possess, a willingness to not have clear answers right away. Very little in science or nursing is black and white, yes or no. You need to tolerate some degree of ambiguity, or uncertainty. Research requires time, repeating your work, and meticulous attention to detail.

Persistence. Because the questions and answers are often not immediately clear, you must be able to continue searching, experimenting, and observing even when you are not getting results right away. Florence Nightingale, for instance, spent years analyzing her data from her work in the Crimea. She was the first biostatistician.

Levels of Inquiry

In the lab you will really begin to learn about science by practicing science. The key to success in the lab is learning to think for yourself. There are three levels of inquiry and going through them will help lead you toward learning to think for yourself.

You will start in middle school, high school, and often as an undergraduate, with the first level, or "recipe lab" science. This is when you are given exact instructions, like a recipe, on how to do the lab and what your results should look like. This is good for learning how to follow instructions, use the equipment, and compare your results to a known standard.

The next level is guided inquiry. At this level the instructor knows the answers to predetermined questions. The instructor helps you find the methods needed to answer the question. You begin to think for yourself and to make some choices about how to proceed in your experiments.

At the third level, the student does it all. You decide what questions to ask, you develop a hypothesis, and you choose and decide upon methods for answering those questions.

Inquiry, according to research scientist Sylvia Oliver, Ph.D., is what makes everybody a scientist. "From the time you wake up in the morning," she says, "until you go to sleep at night, you ask questions about the world around you." Inquiry is simply observation sparking questions that lead to assumptions and eventually to decisions on what steps to take to answer the question, or test the truth of your assumption. This process requires that you do not accept what you hear, read, or even see, as fact. You must always ask "why," and when you learn to do this, you will be on your way to becoming a creative nurse and nurse researcher.

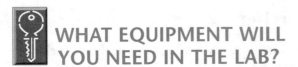

WHAT EQUIPMENT WILL YOU NEED IN THE LAB?

You probably already know the basic equipment needed for any lab:

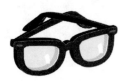

Lab coat to protect your clothing

Safety eyeglasses to protect your eyes

Latex or nonlatex (if you are sensitive or allergic to latex) gloves

Lab books, notebooks to record data

Other equipment needed for labs will vary from course to course. Most will require an additional lab fee to cover the costs of materials. Some equipment you use will be very complex and technical, such as that used for electrophoresis, and others will be more simple, such as test tubes and agar plates.

Check the course syllabus to see what you need to buy. Usually, any required equipment will be available in the school's bookstore. Borrowing equipment is a possible way to cut costs, as long as the equipment is in good condition. If you can find students in your other classes who have previously taken the course, ask if you can borrow or buy their used equipment.

HOW DO COURSE CREDIT HOURS TRANSLATE INTO LAB TIME?

Knowing how many hours per week you will be in lab helps you plan your time. Usually the number of course credit hours you take equals the number of hours per week you spend in the classroom. If you attend a school that breaks the year into semesters, each credit means one hour per week spent in class. If you take a three-credit class, you spend three hours a week attending class. However, for a lab, the number of hours spent in the lab is usually at least doubled. For a two-credit lab course, you may spend four to six hours a week in the lab.

The reason you are given more time in the lab is that unlike lectures, where large amounts of information can be conveyed in a short time, lab work requires longer to see results. If you are coming into college directly out of high school, this is not a new concept for you. If, however, you are returning to school to pursue a second career, it may have been some time since you took a lab course. Labs require preparation time before each session, scheduled lab time, and time after the lab to write up your work.

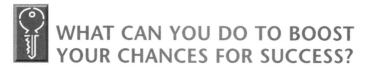

WHAT CAN YOU DO TO BOOST YOUR CHANCES FOR SUCCESS?

Four keys to success in the lab are:

1. Preparation: Taking time to prepare before each lab.
2. Attendance: Showing up at every lab.
3. Writing: Taking the time during and immediately after the lab to write up your work. In other words, don't rely on your memory.
4. Curiosity: Learning to ask why.

Preparation

Instructors will tell you that preparation is the key to success in the lab. Why? Because you must know what you will be doing before you do it; think of it as rehearsing for a play, a concert, a speech, or any other kind of performance. Preparation is time well spent because it will save you time once you are in the lab, allowing time to actually perform the experiments instead of reading the instructions.

Another important outcome of good preparation is that you will get better results if you know beforehand what you are going to do and how you are going to do it; that's the rehearsal part. "Always be prepared" is a good motto for lab classes.

TO PREPARE:

- Read through the lab at least once.
- Picture the lab step-by-step all the way through to the results. This is a mental rehearsal, done just like a downhill skier, snow boarder, or any other competitor who visualizes and memorizes the course before they are on it.
- Write one or two pages about the lab and highlight any questions you may have. Make these "what would happen if" questions to discuss with your lab instructor (often a graduate student) during or after class.

Attendance

Labs are more difficult to make up than lectures, and you will want to make up any missed labs. If you know you will be unable to attend a lab session, you must contact the instructor beforehand, either by phone, e-mail, or in person, to let them know. When you talk to them, be sure to discuss how you can make up the lab. If a sudden emergency occurs, so that you cannot contact the instructor before the missed lab, contact them as soon as you are able. It shouldn't be necessary to make long explanations. Simply tell them in a sentence or two that you will not be at the lab and why. If your reasons are legitimate, there is no need to apologize, plead, or complain in any way. Simply state the facts.

Writing

Although most of your lab time will be spent on preparation and doing the actual lab work, you are required to write up your work. The purpose for this is to show others what you did. This is a basic tenet of the research process: leaving a trail that can be followed and repeated. This is how research findings are verified. Repetition of studies and research methods is done to examine the appropriateness and accuracy of a study's results. This skill will be very useful when you become a nurse and document patient care and management.

There are many formats for lab write-ups, and it is certain that your instructors will tell you what is expected in their courses. This means that from lab course to lab course you may change write-up formats, but essentially the information you include will be the same. Figure 9-1 is an example of a lab write-up for a microbiology course; look for format and required components.

Curiosity

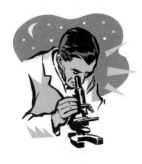

You are working in the microbiology lab observing bacteria cells you cultured the day before. They appear healthy and thriving, except that on closer inspection you notice an area without cell growth. You try to remember preparing the culture, and wonder if you accidentally contaminated the plate. This starts a string of questions beginning with, "Is something contaminating the plate that inhibited bacterial growth?" You are familiar with serendipity, and although you consider it unlikely that you will make a major discovery in sophomore microbiology class, you are curious about the phenomenon you are observing.

Curiosity is the desire to make further inquiry. It means being inquisitive about new observations, new situations, and new questions. It also means not taking everything you see, or are told, as fact. Questioning is the outcome of curiosity, and questions are at the root of hypothesis and, therefore, research science. How did anyone decide to check out if the earth was really flat? They considered their observation of the curved horizon and then asked: "What if the earth could be curved, or even round?" To test this idea, they hypothesized that the earth was round and proposed sailing to the edge to test their hypothesis. This took courage as well as curiosity.

WHY IS IT IMPORTANT TO PRACTICE SAFE LAB SCIENCE?

No doubt in high school you were thoroughly drilled about lab safety, but again, if you haven't been in school for a while, a refresher helps. Instructors are always passionate about lab safety. Why? Because there are many things that can go wrong, leading to injury, equipment damage, or a failed experiment (which equals wasted time).

Laboratories are full of expensive and delicate equipment, and potential hazards: electronics, glassware, caustic chemicals, flammable chemicals and gases, sensitive measurement instruments, bacteria and viruses, automated machinery, potentially slippery floors, and most of all, human bodies. Squirting liquids or moving objects can easily find their way into eyes. Toxic fumes from burning or evaporation can find their way into nostrils and mouths, leading to the tender bronchus, lung tissue, and alveoli.

The list could go on indefinitely, but as you know, everything you do has risk. The important thing is to minimize the risk to yourself and to others by following the lab rules. Again, as a nurse, safety for yourself and your clients is always a priority.

FIGURE 9-1   Microbiology lab write-up.

Bacterial Conjugation   F-duction in *"E. Coli"*   7/11/00

Following protocol, the F+/F− mix was placed in the 37 degree C incubation at 1:44 PM.

3:45 PM: Began streaking plates as per protocol on the control plates. All the streaks were completed and placed in the 37 degree C incubator at 3:59 PM.

MacConkey agar used (Beta − gal+ colonies will be red).

To be incubated overnight.

July 12/00 1:00 PM

	Plate	Presence of colonies	Colony color	Lac+ Lac−	Strep resistance Strep sensitive
Controls *with* Streptomycin	F+ (male)	none	___	___	Sensitive
	F− (female)	Yes	cream	Lac−	Resistant
Controls *without* Streptomycin	F+	Yes	red	Lac+	___
	F−	Yes	cream	Lac−	___
Mated		Yes	red &	Lac+	Resistant
			cream	Lac−	Resistant

Conclusions: The mated plate produced the colonies we expected. The cream-colored colonies would be F− bacteria that were not conjugated and due to their Strep resistance can still grow. The red colonies were evidence of successful conjugation: F− bacteria with Strep resistance having received Lac+ from the F+ strain. These results assume that the information given on F+, or F−, was accurate.

CRYSTAL JOHNSON

Senior, Emory University, Atlanta, Georgia

Even though I'm in my last rotation of nursing clinicals, I have a lot of apprehension about beginning my career as a nurse. I still feel fuzzy about what to expect, and I don't think I'm alone in the way I feel. I've talked to many other nursing students and they also feel nervous about starting their first real job. I mean, it's one thing to be a student but it's something else to be a nurse on the floor. In about six months I'll be a professional and that's scary.

I think part of the reason I feel less than confident is because I don't see how the theory I'm learning in class applies to clinical work. What I've learned in the textbooks sometimes doesn't seem practical in real-life situations. Maybe I'm looking at it the wrong way, but the two often appear incompatible. For example, I've learned about family centered care, which is a theory that says to keep the patient at the center by allowing the patient to have input in their treatment. But

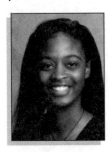

in my clinical experience, I've noticed that few nurses seem to follow that procedure. Most nurses tell the patient what to do without inviting feedback. Seeing these inconsistencies leaves me feeling a little confused about my future role as a nursing professional. What is the importance of theory for clinical practice?

BARBARA ANDRE, R.N., C.C.R.N, C.R.N.A.

Retired. Westlake Community Hospital, Melrose Park, Illinois

Your question about theory versus the real world is a good one. Theory is essential to providing quality patient care. You need to know the theory behind nursing practices in order to set your own goals for what kind of nurse you want to be. Theory gives you the ideal situation. Of course, we all know there are few ideal situations in the real world! As a nurse, you will create your own method of doing things, and your motives should be to aim for the ideal.

You do want to communicate with your patients and involve them in their own health care. For instance, if they are reluctant to learn

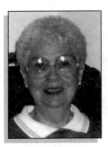

how to give their own inhalation treatments, you could give them the option of doing it while sitting up in a chair or waiting until they go back to bed. This may help them feel a little more in charge and motivate them. However, you may be very busy with other more critical patients, making it necessary for you to give the treatment when you have a free moment. But your goal will be to try your best to work it into your schedule because you know how important it will be for your patients to follow-through on their own when they get home. You want them to become self-motivated.

Feeling comfortable communicating with and involving patients in their care comes with experience. I have found that older nurses are very willing to share their knowledge and experience with new graduates—if they ask. I worked with one new graduate who pretended she knew everything. She isolated herself and made mistakes. The first lesson to learn on any new job is to ask questions. Most hospitals provide training programs that introduce new nurses to the job. The theory you are learning in school can help you to understand why certain situations have been adapted or altered to fit a particular hospital setting.

Therefore, if you are taught to do something one way in school but then asked to do it another way in clinicals, find out why. There is probably a good reason for the change. A bruised ego is easier to heal than a reprimand for doing it wrong. The safety of the patient always comes before pride, not only in theory but in practice. Occasionally you may discover an error in another nurse's judgment. Or your theory may reveal a better way to carry out a procedure. Other nurses are more likely to listen to you if you submit your ideas to them humbly.

It's perfectly normal to feel apprehensive about your future role as a nurse, but rest assured that gradually you'll grow in confidence and professionalism. The theory you are learning in class coupled with practical work experience will help you succeed in your nursing career.

BASIC LAB RULES

- Know where the chemical shower and eye wash are located and how to use them.
- Have all the equipment ready before you start the lab.
- Follow the instructions.
- Understand the fire safety rules.
- Pay attention to what is going on around you.

 WHAT SKILLS DOES LAB WORK GIVE YOU?

Lab work gives you the chance to practice and improve on many skills, not just the skills needed to carry out the experiment. You will learn how to use the equipment and set up experiments; you will learn how to work as part of a team, think creatively and analytically, be precise and write objectively; and you will learn how to communicate effectively.

Communication Skills

Can you write a clear, concise, and persuasive cover letter for a job interview, for a grant proposal, or for a scholarship application? Can you articulate the nature of your pursuit in science to people who know nothing about your subject, as well as to experts in your field? Communication skills are an integral part of nursing, and you will practice them in the lab setting during your classes when you work with your lab partners, talk to your professor, write up your lab findings, and present lab results to your peers.

The need for communication competence cannot be stressed enough. Nurses must have outstanding communication skills from listening to speaking, from writing to reading. The workplace is busy and complex requiring you to interact with a variety of people in a variety of professions. You must be able to speak and write clearly and coherently about the work you are doing and you must do so to many different people. For instance, you may be required to justify the importance of your work to your supervisor or present your work to a congressional panel or to public, private, or professional groups. Your skills in communicating may make the difference between gaining or losing funding for your work. Procuring funding for your work will always be a challenge and having optimal communication skills will benefit you in this area.

Teamwork Skills

Your lab classes will be done in small groups, or with a partner. A good team worker is something all employers are looking for, not only in research, but in all areas of nursing. Spending time in meetings to share results, strategize, make decisions, and plan budgets is something everyone does in the sciences. Writing scientific papers or preparing presentations also involves teamwork. Your science labs offer you an excellent opportunity to practice team skills.

Research is often done in teams with one person designated as the principal investigator, or leader, of the team. In universities your professors may be doing their own research, in which case he or she would be the principal investigator. Graduate students often make up the research team members. To gain more experience in research, and to practice team skills, you may be able to volunteer, or even find a work-study job in a professor's lab.

Critical-Thinking Skills

In the lab, especially as an undergraduate, you will most often be following a set of instructions to reach a specific result (confirmatory lab). Use your natural curiosity and inquisitiveness to practice critical thinking skills in these labs. Here are steps you can take to hone your thinking skills and add challenge to your labs:

- Read all lab instructions.
- Picture yourself doing each step of the lab and checking your results.
- Write several pages describing the lab.
- Write down questions that come to mind while studying.

For instance, in a histology lab you would be studying different types of tissue cells. Preparing for the lab may be very straightforward, but that does not keep you from asking questions that begin with the query, "What would happen if . . ." These are the types of questions research is based on. You can discuss your questions with the lab instructor or do research in the library on your own to begin finding answers to your questions. This process of asking questions and seeking answers is fundamental to improving your critical-thinking skills, and thus to becoming a better researcher and nurse.

Technical Skills

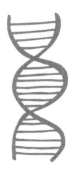

Technology is changing every day, and working in a lab is an opportunity to learn how new technology can be used to better understand old questions. Technology can also be used to begin asking new questions not considered in the past because the means for answering them did not exist.

Genetics and biotechnology is an example. The field of genetics has been around for over a century, beginning with recognizing inherited phenomena observable with the human eye (phenotype). Gregor Mendel did the first groundbreaking work in genetics by observing peas and their variations through breeding. Although Mendel wondered what caused these differences to occur, it wasn't until technology provided the means to discover them that genes controlling the visible pea traits were known.

As technology has helped us gain new knowledge in genetics, research such as the international Human Genome Project is well on the way to mapping the entire human genome. Learning how genes control disease is leading to advances in gene therapy research and the hope that someday genetic diseases may be treated or prevented.

A Summary for Lab Success

BE PREPARED BEFORE YOU ATTEND LAB:

- Read and reread the instructions.
- Picture yourself doing each step.
- Picture the results.
- Write one to two pages about the lab.
- Ask further questions.
- Be familiar with the purpose and goal of the lab.

FOLLOW INSTRUCTIONS:

- Follow lab instructions carefully.
- During lab, write down everything you do.
- Don't prejudge; nothing is insignificant.

LEARN SKILLS:

- Practice technical skills.
- Practice communication in the lab.
- Work in teams by cooperating with others.
- Sharpen math skills used in data analysis, volume conversions, measurement.
- Use precision and observation skills.
- Record events objectively and accurately.

  And don't forget: attendance is crucial to your success.

Docendo Discimus

This Latin phrase means "we learn by teaching." As a student you may think that you are doing all the learning and your instructors all the teaching. But, you teach when helping other students in laboratories and in study groups and you teach your instructors through inquiring questions, thoughtful answers, and interesting life experiences. The concept that everyone learns as they teach emphasizes the cyclical and ongoing nature of education.

Applications   Chapter 9

KEY INTO YOUR LIFE
Opportunities to Apply What You Learn

 Inquiry in Action

Read the following nursing research situation from *Reflection*.[1] (Reprinted with permission from *Reflection*, copyright © 1999.)

THE PAIN

by Susan Beck

SALT LAKE CITY, August 1999—The suffering that results from cancer pain is unnecessary. In fact, according to the World Health Organization, implementation of existing knowledge of pain and symptoms can achieve critical improvements in the quality of life for cancer patients and their families (WHO, 1996). The Agency for Health Care Policy and Research (a United States government body) rigorously reviewed existing knowledge related to pain management resulting in the 1994 publication of an evidence-based *Clinical Practice Guideline on Management of Cancer Pain* (Jacox et al., 1994). The translation of this knowledge into practice is slow.

Inadequate treatment of pain is recognized as an international health problem. However, certain groups may be at higher risk. Studies in the United States indicate that minority patients and the elderly are less likely to receive adequate pain treatment. In my own research in South Africa, nonwhites had significantly higher pain levels than whites. From a health policy perspective, countries that still do not allow the manufacture or importation of opioids lack the basic tools to provide analgesia.

Studies of cancer pain prevalence indicate that approximately 30 to 50 percent of patients receiving cancer treatment experience pain. The prevalence may approach 70 to 90 percent in patients with advanced cancer.

In patients with breast cancer, two types of pain predominate (Miaskowski & Dibble, 1995). Many women suffer from a neuropathic pain syndrome following surgery for breast cancer. This type of pain is neuropathic in origin; the patient describes it as a tight, constrictive burning pain in the anterior axilla or anterior chest wall. The other common type of pain is due to metastasis to the bones. This type of pain is usually localized and is described as dull and achy. One patient aptly described it as a "tooth-ache in my bones."

This type of pain is also common in men with prostate cancer, as bone is the most common site of metastasis. Growth of prostate tumors within the pelvis can also cause pain in the back, pelvis, and lower extremities (Payne, 1993).

For persons with cancer and their family-caregivers, pain can be overwhelming as it negatively influences the quality of lives. Pain may cause or enhance the intensity of other distressing physical symptoms, such as sleep disturbances and fatigue. Pain limits an individual's ability to carry out responsibilities at home, work, and in the community. Pain causes emotional distress and has been associated with changes in mood states, including depression, anxiety and anger. Some patients may choose discontinuation of treatment, or even consider assisted suicide, because of unrelieved pain.

Individuals caring for patients in pain describe feelings of helplessness, frustration, isolation, futility and anger. As one caregiver explains, "It's just difficult

. . . you're helpless. You have to watch somebody agonize, and you can't help them" (Ferrell et al., 1993).

Therapies for pain must be integrated into the overall management of the patient. If possible, the first approach to pain management is to eliminate the cause. Thus, treatments such as radiation therapy, chemotherapy, hormonal agents, biological response modifiers and surgery may be useful, depending on the type of cancer.

The mainstay of cancer pain relief is pharmacologic management. A simple method to guide pharmacological management has been developed by the World Health Organization. Three steps are summarized:

WHO Analgesic Ladder, 1996

Step 1: Use non-opioid analgesics, including acetaminophen (paracetamol) and the nonsteroidal anti-inflammatory drugs for mild pain.

Step 2: When pain persists or increases, add an opioid conventionally used orally for mild to moderate pain, including codeine, oxycodone, hydrocodone or dihydrocodeine.

Step 3: When pain is persistent, or moderate to severe at the outset, use adequate doses of a strong opioid, including morphine, hydromorphone, oxycodone (as a single entity), levorphanol, methadone or fentanyl.

Adjuvant drugs to enhance the analgesic effect or manage concurrent symptoms, such as nausea or constipation, should be added at any stage as needed. Because each patient responds differently to medications, it is essential to individualize the approach. Carefully and regularly assess the patient's response, and make adjustments as needed.

Medications for cancer pain are highly effective in the oral form and can usually be administered orally unless the patient is vomiting, cannot swallow, or is not absorbing. Medications *should not* be given as needed but should be administered on a regular around-the-clock schedule with additional doses as needed. This approach maintains a consistent level of analgesic in the body and helps to prevent pain. Sudden escalations in the use of supplemental doses for "break-through pain" may indicate a need for a higher dosage around-the-clock. The simplest approaches and schedules should be used first.

Is has been estimated that pharmacologic interventions currently available are adequate to treat 90 percent of cancer pain when used in the correct dose, route, and combination. In addition, there are numerous interventions that nurses or patients can use to augment pain relief. Most are relatively inexpensive and fairly easy to implement. Many of these types of interventions provide a distraction from the pain experience. As one patient who found music therapy to be effective described, "I was concentrating on the music and not on how I was hurting."

Effective management of cancer pain requires an integrated approach of primary therapy (i.e., treatment of the tumor itself) and pharmacologic and nonpharmacologic analgesic strategies. The nurse is usually on the frontline in pain management and must advocate for adequate drug therapy and use complementary therapies to augment pain relief.

Dr. Susan Beck's cancer work in South Africa

Although health services in South Africa have been plagued by inequity and inadequate resources, new health policies have set a path to ensure universal access to health care, including palliative care for cancer. Dr. Beck's research has been distributed to governmental bodies.

Her 1998 and 1999 research validated the importance of cultural beliefs and practices for understanding cancer pain and how it is managed.

In several studies conducted to help alleviate suffering, Dr. Beck examined pain treatment to support South African efforts to improve care. Her findings showed management of pain varied by provider and setting, with major problems for access to care in the rural areas.

In African cultures, views about cancer are thought to prevent patients from seeking treatment, including for pain. Without a uniform concept of cancer as an entity, Africans have historically denied that cancer is a community problem. One resident explained, "Cancer is only for whites." In a study of 426 patients in multiple settings, nearly one-third of the cancer patients experienced pain of severe intensity. Thirty percent were not treated with adequate drugs, according to the WHO Analgesic Ladder.

References

Beck, S. L. (1998). A systematic review of opioid availability and use in the Republic of South Africa. Journal of Pharmaceutical Care in Pain and Symptom Control, 6(4), 5–22.

Beck, S. L. (1999). Health policy, health services, and cancer pain management in the new South Africa. Journal of Pain and Symptom Control, 17(1), 16–26.

Beck, S. L. (In Press). Factors influencing cancer pain management in South Africa. Cancer Nursing.

Ferrell, B. R., Johnston Taylor, E., Sattler, G., Fowler, M., & Cheyney, B. L. (1993). Searching for the meaning of pain. Cancer Practice 1(3), 185–194.

Jacox, A., Carr, D. B., Payne, R., et al. (1994). Management of Cancer Pain: Clinical Practice Guideline (No. 9 AHCPR Publication No. 94–0592). Rockville, MD: Agency for Health Care Policy and Research, U. S. Department of Health and Human Services, Public Health Service.

Miaskowski, C., Dibble, S. L. (1995). The problem of pain in outpatients with breast cancer. Oncology Nursing Forum 22(5), 791–797.

Payne, R. (1993). Pain management in the patient with prostate cancer. Cancer 71(3) suppl. 1131–1137.

World Health Organization. (1996). WHO Expert Committee on Cancer Pain Relief and Active Supportive Care. Cancer Pain Relief: With a Guide to Opioid Availability (2nd edition). Geneva: WHO Technical Reports.

Using the article above, answer the following questions.

1. Identify a problem, and write a research question that could be used to direct research to help fill a "major gap in knowledge." _____

_____

_____

_____

_____

2. What lab experiments could be conducted to answer your question? What lab equipment would you need? _____

_____

_____

_____

_____

3. What field studies could be conducted and what equipment would you need? _____

_____

_____

_____

_____

4. What is the logic behind doing research on pain? _____

   a. _____

   b. _____

   c. _____

9.2   *Using World Wide Web Science Sites*

> "If only I can get through the first three years of nursing school (if I am accepted), I can go out and nurse in the West... Colorado for instance."
>
> MARGARET SANGER

Using the Internet, go to one of the following sites and, using information found there, write several questions of your own that could be developed into experiments. Write them in the space on the following page, and be sure to include which site you visited.

www.nursingworld.org

http://uga.edu/~protozoa

www.science.news.com

www.discover.com

www.utdallas.edu/research/issues

http://pao.gsfc.nasa.gov/gsfc/newsroom/flash/flash.htm

www.4woman.org

www.researchpaper.com

www.nsf.org

www.sHi.org

1. _____

2. _____

3. _____

4. _____

5. _____

Site: _____

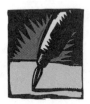

KEY TO SELF-EXPRESSION
Discovery Through Journal Writing

To record your thoughts, use a separate journal or the lined pages at the end of the chapter.

Writing Questions

Think of at least one science topic that interests you. Write one or two sentences that sums up a problem in that topic area. Now, using that problem, write questions you could use to design experiments to answer them. Just brainstorm and let your mind "think up" whatever problems and questions you can.

Journal

Name _____   Date _____

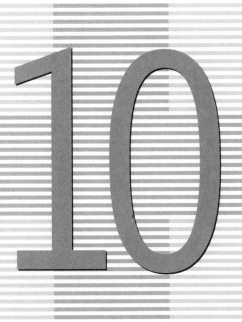

10

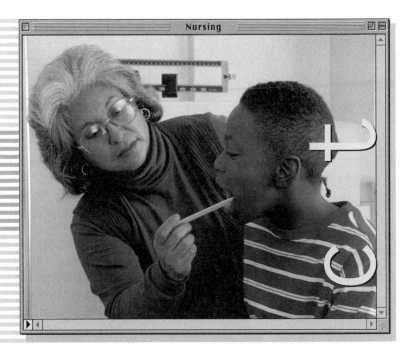

Relating to Others

Appreciating Your Diverse World¶

The greater part of your waking life involves interaction with people—family and friends, peers, fellow students, coworkers, instructors, and many more. When you put energy into your relationships and open the lines of communication, you can receive much in return. Having a strong network of relationships can help you grow and progress toward your goals.

This chapter will explore the issues of diversity that can hinder or help how you perceive others and relate to them. You will also explore communication styles, personal relationships, and the roles you can play in groups and on teams. Finally, you will read about various kinds of conflict and criticism, examining how to handle them so they benefit you instead of setting you back.

In this chapter, you will explore answers to the following questions:

- How can you understand and accept others?
- How can you express yourself effectively?
- How do your personal relationships define you?
- How can you handle conflict and criticism?
- What role do you play in groups?

HOW CAN YOU UNDERSTAND AND ACCEPT OTHERS?

Human interaction is an essential element of life. In a diverse world, many people are different from what you are familiar with and perceive as "normal." In this section you will explore diversity in your world, the positive effects of accepting diversity, and how to overcome barriers to understanding. The first requirements for dealing with differences are an open mind and a willingness to learn.

Diversity in Your World

For centuries, travel to different countries was seen as part of a complete education. Edith Wharton, a nineteenth-century author, wrote a story called "False Dawn" in which a character named Mr. Raycie recommends travel to his son: "A young man, in my opinion, before setting up for himself, must see the world; form his taste; fortify his judgment. He must study the most famous monuments, examine the organization of foreign societies, and the habits and customs of those older civilizations . . . I believe he will be able to learn much."[1] When cultures were so separated, learning about differences was best accomplished through travel.

Today, although traveling is still a valuable way to learn, different places and people often come to you. More and more, diversity is part of your community, on your television, on your Internet browser, at your school, in your workplace, and in your family. It used to be that most people lived in societies with others who seemed very similar to them. Now, differences are often woven into everyday life.

You may encounter examples of diversity like these:

- Communities with people from different stages of life
- Coworkers who represent a variety of ethnic origins
- Classmates who speak a number of different languages

> **TERMS**
>
> **Diversity**
> The variety that occurs in every aspect of humanity, involving both visible and invisible characteristics.

- Social situations featuring people from various cultures, religions, and sexual orientations
- Individuals who marry a person or adopt a child from a different racial or religious background
- Diverse restaurants, services, and businesses in the community
- Neighborhoods with immigrants from a variety of social/class backgrounds
- Different lifestyles as reflected in books, magazines and newspapers, television, movies, music, the Internet, and other forms of popular culture
- People in the workplace who have a variety of disabilities—some more obvious than others

Each person has a choice about how to relate to others—or *whether* to relate to them. No one can force you to interact with any other person, or to adopt a particular attitude as being "right." Considering two important responsibilities may help you sort through your options.

Your responsibility to yourself lies in being true to yourself, in taking time to think through your reactions to other people. When you evaluate your thoughts, try to also consider their source: Have you heard these ideas from other people or organizations or the media? Do you agree with them, or does a different approach feel better to you? Through critical thinking you can arrive at decisions about which you feel comfortable and confident.

Your responsibility to others lies in treating people with tolerance and respect. No one will like everyone he or she meets, but acknowledging that others deserve respect and have a right to their opinions will build bridges of communication. The more people accept one another, the more all kinds of relationships will be able to thrive.

The Positive Effects of Diversity

More than just "a nice thing to do," accepting diversity has very real benefits to people in all kinds of relationships. Acceptance and respect form the basis for any successful interaction. As more situations bring diverse people into relationships, communication will become more and more dependent upon acceptance and mutual understanding.

Consider how positive relationships with diverse people may contribute to success. Relationships among family, friends, and neighbors affect personal life. Relationships among students, instructors, and other school personnel affect student life. Relationships among coworkers, supervisors, and customers/clients affect work life. Understanding and communication in these relationships can bring positive effects such as satisfying relationships, achievement, and progress. Failure to understand and communicate well can have negative effects.

For example, examine the potential effects of reactions to diversity in the following situations. Although each of these situations focuses on the reaction of only one person, it's important to note that both parties need to work together to establish mutual trust and openness.

> "Minds are like parachutes. They only function when they are open."
>
> SIR JAMES DEWAR

A male Hispanic employee has a female African-American supervisor. If the employee believes negative stereotypes about women or African-American people and resists taking directions from the supervisor, he may lose his job or be viewed as a liability. On the other hand, if the employee can respect the supervisor's authority and consider any different methods or ideas she has, their relationship is more likely to become supportive and productive. He may then be more likely to feel comfortable, perform well, and move up at work.

A learning-disabled student has an Asian-American instructor. If the student assumes that Asian-American people are superior and intimidating, letting that opinion lead her to resist the advice and directions her instructor gives her, she may do poorly in the class or drop the course. On the other hand, if the student stays open to what the instructor has to offer, the instructor may feel respected and may be more encouraging. The student may then be more likely to pay attention in class, work hard, and advance in her education.

A Caucasian man has a sister who adopts a biracial child. If the man cuts off contact with his sister because he fears racial differences and doesn't approve of racial mixing, he may deny himself her support and create a rift in the family. On the other hand, if the man can accept the new family member and respect his sister's choice, she may feel more supported and continue to support him in turn. The situation may help to build a close and rewarding family relationship.

Accepting others isn't always easy, and it's common to let perceptions about people block your ability to communicate. Following are some barriers that can hinder your ability to accept and understand others, and suggestions for how to overcome them.

Barriers to Understanding

You deserve to feel positive about who you are, where you come from, what you believe, and the others with whom you identify. However, problems arise when people use the power of group identity to put others down or cut themselves off from others. Table 10-1 shows how an open-minded approach can differ from an approach that is characterized by barriers.

Stereotypes, prejudice, discrimination, and fear of differences can form barriers to communication.

Stereotypes

As you learned in Chapter 5, an assumption is an idea that you accept without looking for proof. A stereotype occurs when an assumption is made about a person or group of people based on one or more characteristics. You may have heard stereotypical assumptions such as these: "Women are too emotional for business." "African-Americans can run fast and sing well." "Hispanics are Catholic and have tons of kids." "White people are cold-hearted and power-hungry." "Gay people sleep around." "Learning-disabled people can't hold down jobs." "Older people can't learn new things." Stereotypes are as common as they are destructive.

TERMS

Stereotype
A standardized mental picture that represents an oversimplified opinion or uncritical judgment.

| TABLE 10-1 | A closed-minded approach vs. an open-minded approach. |

YOUR ROLE	SITUATION	CLOSED-MINDED APPROACH	OPEN-MINDED APPROACH
Team member the pediatric unit	A coworker from India observes a Hindu religious ritual at lunchtime.	You stare at the religious ritual, thinking it weird. You feel that this coworker should just blend in and act like everyone else.	You observe the ritual, on respecting how the person expresses religious beliefs. You look up Hindu religion in your spare time to learn more.
Fellow student	For an assignment, you are paired up with a student old enough to be your mother.	You figure that the student will be closed off to the modern world. You think that she might also act like a parent and preach to you about how to do the assignment.	You avoid thinking that this student will act like your parents and get to know her as an individual. You stay open to what you can learn from her experiences and knowledge.
Friend	You are invited to dinner at a friend's house for the first time. When he introduces you to his partner, you realize that he is gay.	You are turned off by the idea of two men in a relationship and by gay culture in general. You are uncomfortable and make an excuse to leave early. You avoid your friend from then on.	You have dinner with your friend and his partner. You learn that they have a committed, supportive relationship. You take the opportunity to learn more about who they are and what their lives are like.
Employee	Your new nurse manager is Japanese-American, hired from a competing hospital.	You assume that your new supervisor is very hard-working, expecting unrealistic things from you and your coworkers. You assume she doesn't take time to socialize.	You rein in your assumptions, knowing they are based on stereotypes, and approach your new supervisor with an open mind.

Why might people stereotype? The list below offers a few reasons.

People seek patterns and logic. Trying to make sense of a complex world is part of human nature. People often try to find order by using the labels and categories that stereotypes provide.

Stereotyping is quick and easy. Stereotyping is something nurses know about! Think about your image of a nurse. Is the nurse female, white, in a white dress and cap? Making an assumption about a person from observing an external characteristic is easier than working to know a person as a unique individual. Labeling a group of people based on a characteristic they seem to have in common takes less time and energy than exploring the differences and unique qualities within the group.

Movies, magazines, and other media encourage stereotyping. The more people see stereotypical images—the unintelligent blonde nurse looking for a doctor to marry, the funny overweight person, the evil white businessman, the person on welfare as lazy—the easier it is to believe that such stereotypes are universal.

The ease of stereotypes comes at a high price. First and foremost, stereotypes can perpetuate harmful generalizations and falsehoods about others. These false ideas can promote discrimination. For example, if an employer believes that Vietnamese people cannot speak English well, he might not even bother to interview them. Secondly, stereotypes also communicate the message that you don't care about or respect others enough to discover who they really are. This may encourage others to stereotype you in return. Others may not give you a chance if they feel that you haven't given them a chance.

Addressing stereotypes. Recall from the critical-thinking material in Chapter 5 the questions you can ask about an assumption in order to examine its validity. Apply these questions to stereotypes:

1. In what cases is this stereotype true, if ever? In what cases is it not true?
2. Has stereotyping others benefited me? Has it hurt me? In what ways?
3. If someone taught me this stereotype, why? Did that person think it over or just accept it?
4. What harm could be done by always accepting this stereotype as true?

Using these steps, think through the stereotypes you assume are true. When you hear someone else use a stereotype and you know some information that disproves it, volunteer that information. Encourage others to think through stereotypes and to reject them if they don't hold up under examination.

Give others the benefit of the doubt. Thinking beyond stereotypes is an important step toward more open lines of communication.

Prejudice

Prejudice occurs when people "prejudge," meaning that they make a judgment before they have sufficient knowledge upon which to base that judgment. People often form prejudiced opinions on the basis of a particular characteristic—gender, race, culture, abilities, sexual orientation, religion, and so on. You may be familiar with the labels for particular kinds of prejudice, such as *racism* (prejudice based on race) or *ageism* (prejudice based on age). Any group can be subjected to prejudice, although certain groups have more often been on the receiving end of such closed-minded attitudes. Prejudice can lead people to disrespect, harass, and put down others. In some cases, prejudice may lead to unrealistic expectations of others that aren't necessarily negative, such as if someone were to judge all Jewish people as excelling in business.

Prejudice can have one or more causes. Some common causes include the following.

TERMS

Prejudice
A preconceived judgment or opinion, formed without just grounds or sufficient knowledge.

People experience the world through the lens of their own particular identity. You grow up in a particular culture and family and learn their attitudes. When you encounter different ideas and ways of life, you may react by categorizing them. You may also react with ethnocentrism—the idea that your group is better than anyone else's.

When people get hurt, they may dislike or blame anyone who seems similar to the person who hurt them. Judging others based on a bad experience is human, especially when a particular characteristic raises strong emotions.

Jealousy and fear of personal failure can lead a person to want to put others down. When people are feeling insecure about their own abilities, they might find it easier to devalue the abilities of others rather than to take risks and try harder themselves.

The many faces of prejudice often appear on college campuses. A student may not want to work with an in-class group that contains people of another race. Campus clubs may tend to limit their membership to a particular group and exclude others. Religious groups may devalue the beliefs of other religions. Groups that gather based on a common characteristic might be harassed by others. Women or men may find that instructors or fellow students judge their abilities and attitudes based on their gender. All of these attitudes severely block attempts at mutual understanding.

Addressing prejudice. Being critical of people who are different cuts you off from all kinds of perspectives and people that can enhance the quality of your life. Critical thinking is your key to changing prejudicial attitudes. For example, suppose you find yourself thinking that a certain student in your class isn't the type of person you want to get to know. Ask yourself: Where did I get this attitude? Am I accepting someone else's judgment? Am I making judgments based on how this person looks or speaks or behaves? How does having this attitude affect me or others? If you see that your attitude needs to change, have the courage to activate that change by considering the person with an open, accepting mind.

Another tactic, and often an extremely difficult yet important one, is to confront people you know when they display a prejudicial attitude. It can be hard to stand up to someone and risk a relationship or, if the person is your employer, even a job. On the other hand, your silence implies that you agree. Evaluate the situation and decide what choice is suitable and true to your values. Ask yourself if you can associate with a person if he or she thinks or behaves in a way that you do not respect.

You have a range of choices when deciding whether to reveal your feelings about someone's behavior. You can decide not to address it at all. You may drop a humorous hint and hope that you make your point. You may make a small comment to "test the waters" and see how the person reacts, hoping that later you can have a more complete discussion about it. Whatever you do, express your opinion respectfully. Perhaps the other person will take that chance to rethink the attitude; perhaps he or she will not. Either way, you have taken an important stand.

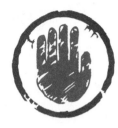

Discrimination

Discrimination occurs when people deny others opportunities because of their perceived differences. Prejudice often accompanies discrimination. Discrimination can mean being denied jobs or advancement, equal educational opportunities, equal housing opportunities, services, or access to events, people, rights, privileges, or commodities.

Discrimination happens in all kinds of situations, revolving around gender, language, race, culture, and other factors. A 32-year-old married woman may not get a job because the interviewer assumes that she will become pregnant. A Russian person may be fired from a restaurant job because his English is heavily accented. Sheryl McCarthy, an African-American columnist for *New York Newsday*, sees it on the street. "Nothing is quite so basic and clear as having a cab go right past your furiously waving body and pick up the white person next to you," she says in her book, *Why Are the Heroes Always White?*[2] "Sometimes you can debate whether racism was the motivating factor in an act; here there is no doubt whatsoever." Even so-called majority populations may now experience the power of discrimination. For example, a qualified white man may be passed up for a promotion in favor of a female or minority employee.

The disabled are often targets of discrimination because people may believe that they are depressed and incapacitated. John Hockenberry, a wheelchair-using paraplegic who travels the world in his work as an award-winning journalist, challenges the idea that disabled people lead lives of unproductive misery. "My body may have been capable of less, but virtually all of what it could do was suddenly charged with meaning. This feeling was the hardest to translate to the outside, where people wanted to believe that I must have to paint things in this way to keep from killing myself," he says in his memoir *Moving Violations.*[3]

Obesity can invite discrimination as well. People who are overweight may have trouble winning jobs or moving up at work. Even shopping for clothing can present limited options. Only in recent years have certain brand-name designers begun to create clothing in women's sizes above 12, and many designers still discriminate.

Addressing discrimination. U. S. federal law states that it is unlawful for you to be denied an education, work, or the chance to apply for work, housing, or basic rights based on your race, creed, color, age, gender, national or ethnic origin, religion, marital status, potential or actual pregnancy, or potential or actual illness or disability (unless the illness or disability prevents you from performing required tasks, and unless accommodations for the disability are not possible). Unfortunately, the law is frequently broken, with the result that incidents go unnoticed. Many times people don't report incidents, fearing trouble from those they accuse. Sometimes people don't even notice their attitudes seeping through, such as in an interview situation.

First and foremost, be responsible for your own behavior. Never knowingly participate in or encourage discrimination. When you act on prejudicial attitudes by discriminating against someone, the barrier to communication this discrimination causes hurts you as well as anyone else involved. A person who feels denied and shut out may be likely to do the same to you, and may even encourage others to do so.

Second, if you witness a discriminatory act or feel that you have been discriminated against, decide whether you want to approach an authority about it. You may want to begin by talking to the person who can most directly affect the situation—an instructor, your supervisor, a housing authority. Don't assume that people know when they hurt or offend someone. For example, if you have a disability and you find that accommodations haven't been made for you at school, speak up. Meet with an advisor to discuss your needs for transport, equipment, or a particular schedule.

If you don't find satisfaction and change at that level, try the next level of authority (an administrator, your supervisor's boss, a government official). If that doesn't produce results, you can take legal action, although legal struggles can take a lot of time and drain a great deal of money out of your pocket. At each decision stage, weigh all the positive and negative effects and evaluate whether the action is feasible for you. Although keeping quiet may not bring change, you may not be able to act right away. In the long run, if you are able to stand up for what you believe, your actions may be worthwhile.

Fear of Differences

It's human instinct to fear the unknown. Many people stop long before they actually explore anything unfamiliar. They allow their fear to prevent them from finding out anything about what's outside their known world. As cozy as that world can be, it also can be limiting, cutting off communication from people who could enrich that world in many different ways.

The fear of differences has many effects. A young person who fears the elderly may avoid visiting a grandparent in a nursing home. A person of one religion might reject friendships with those of other religions out of a fear of different religious beliefs. Someone in a relationship may fear the commitment of marriage. A person might turn down an offer to buy a house in a neighborhood that is populated with people from a different ethnic group. In each case, the person may deny him or herself a chance to learn a new perspective, communicate with new individuals, and grow from new experiences.

Addressing fear of differences. Differences don't mean that you have to feel comfortable with everyone or agree with what everyone else believes. The fear of differences, though, can keep you from discovering anything outside your own world. Challenge yourself by looking for opportunities to expose yourself to differences. Today's world increasingly presents such opportunities. You can choose a study partner in class who has a different ethnic background. You can expand your knowledge with books or magazines. You can visit a museum or part of town that introduces a culture new to you. You can attend an unfamiliar religious service with a friend. Gradually broaden your horizons and consider new ideas.

If you think others are uncomfortable with differences, encourage them to work through their discomfort. Explain the difference so that it doesn't seem so mysterious. Offer to help them learn more in a setting that isn't threatening. Bring your message of the positive effects of differences to others.

"MOTHERS
Can you afford to have a large family?
Do you want any more children?
If not, why do you have them?
DO NOT KILL. DO NOT TAKE LIFE, BUT PREVENT.
Safe harmless information can be obtained at
Nurses
46 Amboy Street
Near Pitkin Ave.—Brooklyn
Tell your friends and neighbors. All mothers welcome. A registration fee of 10 cents entitles any mother to this information."
MARGARET SANGER, 1916

LIDUVINA PEREZ

Senior, Arizona State University, Tempe, Arizona

I've been a translator for as long as I can remember. My mother suffered from heart disease, and she didn't speak English. Since I knew both English and Spanish, I served as the interpreter for my mother and explained what the doctors and nurses said. Every other Tuesday I would have to miss school so that I could go with my mother to the clinic and translate for her. It became routine for me to fall behind in school, but I worked hard to stay caught up.

When you're only six-years-old it's difficult to translate medical terms and procedures correctly, so I'm sure I made mistakes at times. This role put me under a lot of pressure, but I also felt good about helping my mom. Not long after she had a pacemaker put in, my mother died of a heart attack. I was twelve-years-old. After that I went to live with my godparents, and they encouraged me to pursue an education. Taking care of my mother is the main reason I decided to train for a career in nursing.

Now that I'm in clinicals, I see many non-English speaking patients struggle, as my mother did, to grasp what is happening to them. For instance, during my medical-surgical rotation I had a Mexican patient with tuberculosis. He didn't understand his disease or how to help himself recover. There are many patients like him, and I see fear and confusion on their faces, too. We have a large Hispanic population in

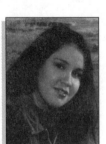

Arizona, and I can tell it really helps when I step in and explain things to them in their language.

During my community health rotation I saw a little Asian girl begin her eye screening test with a school nurse, but the child didn't know English. Then the nurse did something that I thought was very smart and sensitive. She pulled out picture cards which showed children doing different things related to an eye exam. The nurse pointed to the cards to demonstrate what she wanted the little girl to do. The child did it, and the eye exam was successfully completed. I found that very inspiring.

I will be the first person in my family to graduate from college. I'm also considering graduate school to become a nurse practitioner. As I prepare to enter the diverse world of nursing, what can I do to fulfill my role as a bilingual professional?

ELDA G. RAMIREZ

Assistant Professor of Clinical Nursing, University of Texas Health Science Center, Houston, Texas

I can certainly appreciate your question because I grew up in a barrio near the border of Mexico. Some of us spoke better English than others, but there was a barrier even more profound than language: the barrier of social class. When I revisit my old neighborhood, I see barefoot kids play outside even on cold days, and they live in houses that are not up to building code. Yet these same children have the latest toys and their parents drive new cars. The dichotomy is almost unbeliev-

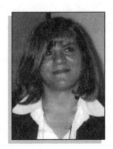

able as I watch these families struggle to fit into the American way of life.

When I was thirteen I volunteered in emergency care at the local hospital, so I've had the desire to be a nurse for a long time. I didn't grow up experiencing prejudice because I was only around my own people, and I never thought much about ethnicity. But when I arrived in Houston to attend college, all of a sudden I was referred to as "this Mexican girl." When people met me, my being Hispanic seemed to be at the forefront of their mind.

When I started seeing Hispanic patients during my clinical rotations, I was angry because they weren't taking care of themselves. They came in with conditions that should have been taken care of a long time ago. Many of these patients had put off their health care needs in order to avoid interacting with people who don't speak their language. I criticized, and even yelled, at them for eating menudo and corn tortillas. At this point I began to face an identity crisis. I realized I had been educated by a westernized force of knowledge that didn't fit my people.

A personal breakthrough occurred when I met Dr. Dalhia Rojas, and she became my mentor. She asked me two questions: "What are you doing for your people, and do you like who you are becoming?" She also asked me if I was condescending to the very people I was trying to help. Thinking through these questions prompted me to choose a direction for my career. For my undergraduate community experience project, I decided to work at an impoverished apartment complex where several Hispanic families lived. When I walked into that community I found myself. Today I feel privileged to be highly educated, and I also feel privileged to be Hispanic. I am them and they are me.

My suggestion to you is to find out what you love and what you believe in. Also, I think it's important to understand that when you change one person you really do change the world. With my patients and my students I try to break the stereotypical visions they have of other cultures. If you attack the patient's inner self, they become defensive. But when you identify with them, perhaps by saying, "I like that food too, but I've tried this as an alternative," you become the strongest tool to better that society. Being a bilingual professional is about embracing the culture and incorporating health care knowledge into that tradition.

One final piece of advice. As a nursing professional, it's easy to become overwhelmed. When I find myself getting off balance I go back to my roots by refocusing on the three things that matter most to me: Family, God, and self. You need to take care of yourself, too. You can't give something away that you don't have. Providing health care isn't only about healing the physical. True healing is what you give of yourself to your patients: a smile, reassuring words, a hug when they leave. My patients often bless me by expressing their thanks or by saying, "God bless you for what you've done for me." We touch people when we keep the whole person in mind.

Accepting and Dealing with Differences

Successful interaction with the people around you benefits everyone. The success of that exchange depends upon your ability to accept differences. How open can you be? Your choices range from rejecting all differences to freely celebrating them, with a range of possibilities in between. Ask yourself important questions about what course of action you want to take. Realize that the opinions of family, friends, the media, and any group with which you identify may sometimes lead you into perspectives and actions that you haven't thought through completely. Do your best to sort through outside opinions and make a choice that feels right.

At the forefront of the list of ways to deal with differences is mutual respect. Respect for yourself and others is essential. Admitting that other people's cultures, behaviors, races, religions, appearances, and ideas deserve as much respect as your own promotes communication and learning.

What else can you do to accept and deal with differences?

Avoid judgments based on external characteristics. These include skin color, weight, facial features, or gender.

Cultivate relationships with people of different cultures, races, perspectives, and ages. Find out how other people live and think, and see what you can learn from them.

Educate yourself and others. "We can empower ourselves to end racism through massive education," say Tamara Trotter and Joycelyn Allen in *Talking Justice: 602 Ways to Build and Promote Racial Harmony*.[4] "Take advantage of books and people to teach you about other cultures. Empowerment comes through education. If you remain ignorant and blind to the critical issues of race and humanity, you will have no power to influence positive change." Read about other cultures and people.

Be sensitive to the particular needs of others at school and on the job. Think critically about their situations. Try to put yourself in their place by asking yourself questions about what you would feel and do if you were in a similar situation.

Work to listen to people whose perspectives clash with or challenge your own. Acknowledge that everyone has a right to his or her opinion, whether or not you agree with it.

Look for common ground—parenting, classes, personal challenges, interests.

Help other people, no matter how different they may be. Sheryl McCarthy writes about an African-American man who, in the midst of the 1992 Los Angeles riots, saw a man being beaten and helped him to safety. "When asked why he risked grievous harm to save an Asian man he didn't even know, Williams said, 'Because if I'm not there to help someone else, when the mob comes for me, will there be someone there to save me?'"[5] Continue the cycle of kindness.

Explore your own background, beliefs, and identity. Share what you learn with others.

Cultivate your own personal diversity. You may be one of the growing population of people who have two, three, or ten different cultures in your background. Perhaps your father is Native American and Filipino and Scottish and your mother is Creole (French, Spanish, and African-American). Respect and explore your heritage. Even if you identify only with one group or culture, there are many different sides of you.

Take responsibility for making changes instead of pointing the finger at someone else. Avoid blaming problems in your life on certain groups of people.

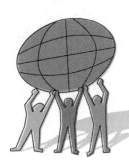

Learn from the atrocities of history like slavery and the Holocaust. Cherish the level of freedom you have. Seek continual improvement at home and elsewhere in the world without forgetting the importance of past events and their effect on your life today.

Teach your children about other cultures. Impress upon them the importance of appreciating differences while accepting that all people have equal rights.

Recognize that people everywhere have the same basic needs. Everyone loves, thinks, hurts, hopes, fears, and plans. People are united through their essential humanity. When you become a nurse and begin working with people, this idea will become very clear to you.

Expressing your ideas clearly and interpreting what others believe are crucial keys to communicating within a diverse world. The following section examines how you can communicate most effectively with the people around you.

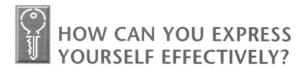

HOW CAN YOU EXPRESS YOURSELF EFFECTIVELY?

The only way for people to know each other's needs is to communicate as clearly and directly as possible. Successful communication promotes successful school, work, and personal relationships. Nurses work with other health professionals as part of a team. Nurses often act as the team member who acts as liaison between the client and all others participating in the client's case. Exploring communication styles, addressing communication problems, and using specific success strategies will help you express yourself effectively.

Adjusting to Communication Styles

Communication is an exchange between two or more people. The speaker's goal is for the listener (or listeners) to receive the message exactly as the speaker intended. Different people, however, have different styles of communicating. Problems arise when one person has trouble "translating" a message that comes from someone who uses a different style. There are at least four communication styles into which people tend to fit: the Intuitor, the Senser, the Thinker, and the Feeler. Of course, people may shift around or possess characteristics from more than one category, but for most people one or two styles are dominant. Recognizing specific styles in others will help you communicate more clearly. Research by the linguist and author Deborah Tannen also shows differences in communication style between men and women. For more on this relevant topic: *Talking from 9 to 5: Women and Men in the Workplace.*[6]

The Styles

The following are characteristics of each communication style.

> A person using the *Intuitor* style is interested in ideas more than details, often moves from one concept or generalization to another without referring to examples, values insight and revelations, talks about having a vision, looks toward the future, and can be oriented toward the spiritual.

> A person showing the style of *Senser* prefers details or concrete examples to ideas and generalizations, is often interested in the parts rather than the whole, prefers the here and now to the past or future, is suspicious of sudden insights or revelations, and feels that "seeing is believing."

> A person using the *Thinker* style prefers to analyze situations, likes to solve problems logically, sees ideas and examples as useful if they help to figure something out, and becomes impatient with emotions or personal stories unless they have a practical purpose.

> A person showing the style of *Feeler* is concerned with ideas and examples that relate to people, often reacts emotionally, is concerned with values and their effects on people and other living things, doesn't like "cold logic" or too much detail.

Many nurses fit into the Senser or Feeler styles of communication. You can benefit from shifting from style to style according to the situation, particularly when trying to communicate with someone who prefers a style different from yours. Shifting, however, is not always easy or possible. The most important task is to try to understand the different styles and to help others understand yours. In general, no one style is any better than another. Each has its own positive effects that enhance communication and negative effects that can hinder it, depending on the situation.

Identifying Your Styles

These four styles are derived from the Myers-Briggs Type Indicator (MBTI). Because the learning style assessments are also in part derived from the MBTI, you will notice similarities between those assessments and these communication styles. Table 10-2 shows how some learning styles may correspond loosely to the communication styles. Not all individual learning styles within the assessments are mentioned, and the styles that are noted may correspond with different styles in different situations, but these matchups depict the most common associations. Finding where your learning styles fit may help you to determine your dominant communication style or styles. Try this website for a Myers-Briggs temperment test and score: http://Keirsey.com.

Adjusting to the Listener's Style

When you are the speaker, you will benefit from an understanding of both your own style and the styles of your listeners. It doesn't matter how clear you think you are being if the person you are speaking to can't "translate" your message by understanding your style. Try to take your listener's style into consideration when you communicate.

Following is an example of how adjusting to the listener can aid communication.

An intuitor-dominant instructor to a senser-dominant student: "Your writing isn't clear." The student's reply: "What do you mean?"

TABLE 10-2 Learning styles and communication styles.

COMMUNICATION STYLE	LEARNING STYLES INVENTORY	PATHWAYS TO LEARNING (MULTIPLE INTELLIGENCES)	PERSONALITY SPECTRUM
Intuitor	Theoretical, Holistic	Intrapersonal	Adventurer
Senser	Factual	Bodily-Kinesthetic	Organizer
Thinker	Linear	Logical-Mathematical	Thinker
Feeler	Reflective	Interpersonal	Giver

- *Without adjustment:* If the intuitor doesn't take note of the senser's need for detail and examples, he or she may continue with a string of big-picture ideas that might further confuse and turn off the senser. "You need to elaborate more. Try writing with your vision in mind. You're not considering your audience."

- *With adjustment:* If the intuitor shifts toward a focus on detail and away from his or her natural focus on ideas, the senser may begin to understand, and the lines of communication can open. "You introduced your central idea at the beginning but then didn't really support it until the fourth paragraph. You need to connect each paragraph's idea to the central idea. Also, not using a lot of examples for support makes it seem as though you are writing to a very experienced audience."

Adjusting to the Communicator's Style

As a facet of communication, listening is just as important as speaking. When you are the listener, try to stay aware of the communication style of the person who is speaking to you. Observe how that style satisfies, or doesn't satisfy, what a person of your particular style prefers to hear. Work to understand the speaker in the context of his or her style and translate the message into one that makes sense to you.

Following is an example of how adjusting to the communicator can boost understanding.

A feeler-dominant employee to a thinker-dominant supervisor: "I'm really upset about how you've talked down to me. I don't think you've been fair. I haven't been able to concentrate since our discussion and it's hurting my performance."

- *Without adjustment:* If the thinker becomes annoyed with the feeler's focus on emotions, he or she may ignore them, putting up an even stronger barrier between the two people. "There's no reason to be upset. I told you clearly and specifically what needs to be done. There's nothing else to discuss."

- *With adjustment:* If the thinker considers that emotions are dominant in the feeler's perspective, he or she could respond to those emotions in a way that still searches for the explanations and logic the thinker understands best: "Let's talk about how you feel. Please explain to me what has caused you to become upset, and we'll discuss how we can improve the situation."

Overcoming Communication Problems

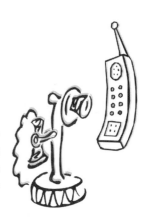

Communication problems may occur when information is not clearly presented, or when those who receive information filter it through their own perspectives and interpret it in different ways. A few of the most common communication problems follow, along with strategies to help you combat them.

Problem: Unclear or Incomplete Explanation
Solution: Support Ideas with Examples

When you clarify a general idea with supporting examples that illustrate how it works and what effects it causes, you will help your receiver understand what you mean and therefore have a better chance to hold his or her attention.

For example, if you tell a friend to take a certain class, that friend might not take you seriously until you explain why. If you then communicate the positive effects of taking that class (progress toward a major, an excellent instructor, friendly study sessions), you may get your message across. The same principle applies to your attitude toward this course. If others communicate to you specific examples of how your work in the course will benefit your education, career, and personal life, you may be more likely to apply yourself.

Work situations benefit from explanation as well. As a supervisor, if you assign a task without explanation, you might get a delayed response or find mistakes in your employee's work. If, however, you explain the possible positive effects of the task, you'll have better results. In nursing school and the nursing profession this concept is a key to success. You *must* use evidence or examples to support your assessments, actions, and evaluations.

Problem: Attacking the Receiver
Solution: Send "I" Messages

When a conflict arises, often the first instinct is to pinpoint what someone else did wrong. "You didn't lock the door!" "You never called last night!" "You left me out!" Making an accusation, especially without proof, puts the other person on the defensive and shuts down the lines of communication.

Using "I" messages will help you communicate your own needs rather than focusing on what you think someone else did wrong or should do differently. "I felt uneasy when I came to work and the door was unlocked." "I became worried about you when I didn't hear from you last night." "I felt disappointed when I realized that I couldn't join the party." "I" statements soften the conflict by highlighting the *effects* that the other person's actions have had on you, rather than the person or the actions themselves. When you focus on your own response and needs, your receiver may feel more free to respond, perhaps offering help and even acknowledging mistakes.

If you often feel dissatisfied and tense after an exchange, you may benefit from focusing more on your own needs when you communicate. Translate your anger into an "I" statement before speaking. Ask the other person, "Can we decide together how to improve this situation? Here's how I feel about what has happened." Using "I" statements will bring better results.

Problem: Passive or Aggressive Communication Styles
Solution: Become Assertive

Among the three major communication styles—aggressive, passive, assertive—the one that conveys a message in the clearest, most productive way is the assertive style. The other two, while commonly used, throw the communication out of balance. An aggressive communicator often denies the receiver a chance to respond, while a passive communicator may have trouble getting the message out. Assertive behavior strikes a balance between aggression and passivity. If you can be an assertive communicator, you will be more likely to get your message across while assuring that others have a chance to speak as well. Table 10-3 compares some characteristics of each kind of communicator.

Aggressive communicators focus primarily on their own needs. They can become angry and impatient when those needs are not immediately satisfied. In order to become more assertive, aggressive communicators might try to take time to think before speaking, avoid ordering people around, use "I" statements, and focus on listening to what the other person has to say.

Passive communicators deny themselves the power that aggressive people grab. They focus almost exclusively on the needs of others instead of on their own needs, experiencing frustration and tension that remains unexpressed. In order to become more assertive, passive communicators might try to acknowledge anger or hurt more often, speak up when they feel strongly about something, realize that they have a right to make requests, and know that their ideas and feelings are as important as anyone else's.

Communication Success Strategies

The following strategies can help improve your communication.

Think before you speak. Spoken too soon, ideas can come out sounding nothing like you intended them to. Taking time to think, or even rehearsing mentally, can help you choose the best combination of words. Think it through and get it right the first time.

TERMS
Assertive Able to declare and affirm one's own opinions while respecting the rights of others to do the same.

AGGRESSIVE	PASSIVE	ASSERTIVE
Loud, heated arguing	Concealing one's own feelings	Expressing feelings without being nasty or overbearing
Physically violent encounters	Denying one's own anger	Acknowledging emotions but staying open to discussion
Blaming, name-calling, and verbal insults	Feeling that one has no right to express anger	Expressing self and giving others the chance to express themselves equally
Walking out of arguments before they are resolved	Avoiding arguments	Using "I" statements to defuse arguments
Being demanding: "Do this"	Being noncommittal: "You don't have to do this unless you really want to . . ."	Asking and giving reasons: "I would appreciate it if you would do this, and here's why . . ."

TABLE 10-3

Aggressive, passive, and assertive styles.

Don't withhold your message for too long. One danger of holding back is that a problem or negative feeling may become worse. Speaking promptly has two benefits: (1) you solve the problem sooner, and (2) you are more likely to focus on the problem at hand than to spill over into other issues.

Communicate in a variety of ways, and be sensitive to cultural differences. Remember that words, gestures, and tones mean different things to different people.

Be clear, precise, and to the point. Say exactly what you need to say. Link your ideas to clear examples, avoiding any extra information that can distract.

Communication is extremely important for building and maintaining personal relationships. Explore the role those relationships play in who you are.

HOW DO YOUR PERSONAL RELATIONSHIPS DEFINE YOU?

The relationships you have with friends, family members, and significant others often take center stage. Jobs and schooling can come and go, but you rely on the people with whom you share your life.

In addition to being part of your life, the people around you help to define who you are. Since birth, you have learned by taking in information from verbal and nonverbal language. The chain of learning stretches back through time, each link formed by an exchange of information between people. Those with whom you live, play, study, and work are primary sources of ideas, beliefs, and ways of living. You grow and change as you have new experiences, evaluate them, and decide what to learn from them.

These influential relationships can affect other areas of your life. You have probably experienced conflict that caused you to be unable to sleep, eat, or get any work done. On the other hand, a successful relationship can have positive effects on your life, increasing your success at work or at school. The ability to form relationships is a sign of psychological health.[7] Relationships are central to a caring response in the nursing practice. Following are some strategies for improving your personal relationships.

Relationship Strategies

If you can feel good about your personal relationships, other areas of your life will benefit. Here are some suggestions.

Make personal relationships a high priority. Nurture the ones you have and be open to developing new ones. Life is meant to be shared. In some marriage ceremonies, the bride and groom share a cup of wine that symbolizes life. One of the reasons for this tradition is to double the sweetness of life by tasting it together, and another is to cut the bitterness in half by sharing it. Any personal relationship can benefit from the experience of this kind of sharing.

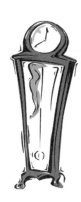

Invest time. You devote time to education, work, and the other priorities in your life. Relationships need the same investment. They are like plants in a garden, needing nourishment to grow and thrive. Your attention provides that nourishment. In addition, spending time with people you like can relieve everyday stress and strain. When you make time for others, everyone benefits.

Spend time with people you respect and admire. Life is too short to hang out with people who bring you down, encourage you to participate in activities you don't approve of, or behave in ways that upset you. Develop relationships with people whom you respect, whose choices you admire, and who inspire you to be all that you can be. This doesn't mean that you have to agree with everything that others do. For example, you may disagree with a friend who lets his child watch a lot of TV. However, you may severely disapprove of someone who disciplines a child violently, and you may choose to end your association with that person.

Work through tensions. Negative feelings can multiply when left unspoken. Unexpressed feelings about other issues may cause you to become disproportionately angry over a small issue. A small annoyance over dishes in the sink can turn into a gigantic fight about everything under the sun. Get to the root of the problem. Discuss it, deal with it, and move on.

Refuse to tolerate violence. It isn't easy to face the problem of violence or to leave a violent relationship. People may tolerate violence out of a belief that it will end, a desire to keep their families together, a self-esteem so low that they believe they deserve what they get, or a fear that trying to leave may lead to greater violence. No level of violence is acceptable. Someone who behaves violently toward you cannot possibly have your best interests at heart. If you find that you are either an aggressor or a victim, do your best to get help.

Show appreciation. In this fast-moving world, people don't thank each other often enough. If you think of something positive, say it. Thank someone for a service, express your affection with a smile. A little positive reinforcement goes a long way toward nurturing a relationship.

If you want a friend, be a friend. The Golden Rule, "Do unto others as you would have them do unto you," never goes out of style. If you treat a friend with the kind of loyalty and support that you appreciate yourself, you are more likely to receive the same in return.

Take risks. It can be frightening to reveal your deepest dreams and frustrations, to devote yourself to a friend, or to fall in love. You can choose not to reveal yourself or give yourself to a friendship at all. However, giving is what feeds a relationship, bringing satisfaction and growth. If you take the plunge, you risk disappointment and heartbreak, but you stand to gain the incredible benefits of companionship, which for most people outweigh the risks.

Keep personal problems in their place. Solve personal problems with the people directly involved and no one else. If at all possible, try not to bring your emotions into class or work. Doing so may hurt your performance while doing nothing to help your problem. If you are overwhelmed by a personal problem, try to address it before you go to class or work. If it's impossible to address it at that time, at least make a plan that you can carry out later. Making some step toward resolving the problem will help you concentrate on other things.

If it doesn't work out, find ways to cope. Everyone experiences strain and breakups in intimate relationships, friendships, and family ties. Be kind to yourself and use coping strategies that help you move on. Some people need lots of time alone; others need to spend time with their friends and family. Some seek more formal counseling. Some people throw their energy into a project, a job, a class, a new workout regimen, or anything else that will take their mind off what hurts. Some just need to cry it out and be miserable for a while. Some write in a journal or write letters to the person that they never mail. Do what's right for you, and believe that sooner or later you can emerge from the experience stronger and with new perspective.

Now and again, your personal relationships will experience conflict. Following are ideas for how to deal with conflict and criticism in a productive and positive way.

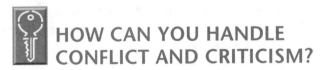

HOW CAN YOU HANDLE CONFLICT AND CRITICISM?

Conflict and criticism, as unpleasant as they can often be, are natural elements in the dynamic of getting along with others. It's normal to want to avoid people or situations that cause distress. However, if you can face your fears and think through them critically, you can gain valuable insight into human nature—your own and that of others. You may be able to make important changes in your life based on what you learn. In nursing school these issues will arise. Your nursing education allows you to learn by practicing in real clinical situations. You will be supported and criticized by your instructors to help you become a safe nurse above all else.

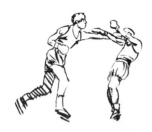

Conflict Strategies

Conflicts both large and small arise when there is a clash of ideas or interests. You may have small conflicts with a housemate over food left out overnight, a door left unlocked, or a bill that needs paying. On the other end of the spectrum, you might encounter major conflicts with your partner about finances, with an instructor about a failing grade, or with a person who treats you unfairly because of your race, gender, age, or ethnic origin.

Conflict can create anger and frustration, shutting down communication. The two most destructive tendencies are to avoid the conflict altogether (a passive tactic) or to let it escalate into a blowout fight (an aggressive tendency). Avoidance doesn't make the problem go away—in fact, it will probably worsen. If you tend to be passive, assert yourself by acknowledging and expressing your feelings as soon as you can put them into words. On the other hand, a shouting match gives no one an opportunity or desire to listen. If you tend to be aggressive, give yourself time to cool down before you address a conflict. Try to express what you feel without letting your emotions explode.

If calmly and intelligently handled, conflict can shed light on new ideas and help to strengthen bonds between those involved. The primary keys to conflict resolution are calm communication and critical-thinking skills. Think through any conflict using what you know about problem solving.

Identify and analyze the problem. Determine the severity of the problem by looking at its effects on everyone involved. Then, find and analyze the causes of the problem.

Brainstorm possible solutions. Consider as many angles as you can, without judgment. Explore what ideas you can come up with from what you or others have done in a similar situation.

Explore each solution. Evaluate the positive and negative effects of each solution. Why might each work, or not work, or work partially? What would take into account everyone's needs? What would cause the least stress? Make sure everyone has a chance to express an opinion.

Choose, carry out, and evaluate the solution you decide is best. When you have implemented your choice, evaluate its effects. Decide whether you feel it was a good choice.

One more hint: Use "I" statements. Focus on the effect the problem has had on you rather than focusing on someone who caused it. Show that you are taking responsibility for your role in the exchange.

Dealing with Criticism and Feedback

No one gets everything right all the time. People use constructive criticism and feedback to communicate what went wrong and to suggest improvements. Consider any criticism carefully. If you always interpret criticism as a threat, you will close yourself off from learning. Even if you eventually decide that you disagree, you can still learn from exploring the possibility. Know that you are strong enough to embrace criticism and become a better person because of it.

Criticism can be either constructive or unconstructive. Criticism is considered constructive when it is offered supportively and contains useful suggestions for improvement. On the other hand, *unconstructive* criticism focuses on what went wrong, doesn't offer alternatives or help, and is often delivered in a negative or harsh manner. Whereas constructive criticism can promote a sense of hope for improvement in the future, unconstructive criticism can create tension, bad feelings, and defensiveness.

Any criticism can be offered constructively or unconstructively. Consider a case where someone has continually been late to work. A supervisor can offer criticism in either of these ways:

Feedback
Evaluative or
corrective
information
about an action
or process.

Constructive
Promoting
improvement or
development.

Constructive: The clinical instructor talks privately with the nursing student. "I've noticed that you have been late to clinicals often. Other people are expecting you to be on time. Is there a problem that is keeping you from being on time? Is it something that I or someone else can help you with?"

Unconstructive: The clinical instructor watches the nursing student slip into clinicals late. The instructor says, in front of other nurses and students, "Nice to see you could make it. If you can't start getting here on time, I might have to give you a failing grade."

If you can learn to give constructive criticism and deal with whatever criticism comes your way from others, you will improve your relationships and your productivity. When offered constructively and carefully considered, criticism can bring about important changes.

Giving Constructive Criticism

"Do not use a hatchet to remove a fly from your friend's forehead."

CHINESE PROVERB

When you offer criticism, use the following steps to communicate clearly and effectively:

1. *Criticize the behavior rather than the person.* In addition, make sure the behavior you intend to criticize is changeable. Chronic lateness can be changed; a physical inability to perform a task cannot.

2. *Define specifically the behavior you want to change.* Try not to drag any side issues into the conversation.

3. *Balance criticism with positive words.* Alternate critical comments with praise in other areas.

4. *Stay calm and be brief.* Avoid threats, ultimatums, or accusations. Use "I" messages; choose positive, nonthreatening words, so the person knows that your intentions are positive.

5. *Explain the effects caused by the behavior that warrants the criticism.* Help the person understand why a change needs to happen, and talk about options in detail. Compare and contrast the effects of the current behavior with the effects of a potential change.

6. *Offer help in changing the behavior.* Lead by example.

Receiving Criticism

When you find yourself on the receiving end of criticism, use these coping techniques:

1. *Listen to the criticism before you speak up.* Resist the desire to defend yourself until you've heard all the details. Decide if the criticism is offered in a constructive or unconstructive manner.

2. *Think the criticism through critically.* Evaluate it carefully. While some criticism may come from a desire to help, other comments may have less honorable origins. People often criticize others out of jealousy, anger, frustration, or displaced feelings. In cases like those, it is best (though not always easy) to let the criticism wash right over you.

3. *If it is unconstructive, you may not want to respond at that moment.* Uncontructive criticism can inspire anger that might be destructive to express. Wait until you cool down and think about the criticism to see if there is anything important hiding under how it was presented. Then, tell the person that you see the value of the criticism, but also communicate to him or her how the delivery of the criticism made you feel. If he or she is willing to talk in a more constructive manner, continue with the following steps below. If not, your best bet may be to consider the case closed and move on.

4. *If it is constructive, ask for suggestions of how to change the criticized behavior.* You could ask, "How would you handle this if you were in my place?"

5. *Before the conversation ends, summarize the criticism and your response to it.* Repeat it back to the person who offered it. Make sure both of you understand the situation in the same way.

6. *If you feel that the criticism is valid, plan a specific strategy for correcting the behavior.* Think over what you might learn from changing your behavior. If you don't agree with the criticism even after the whole conversation, explain your behavior from your point of view.

Remember that the most important feedback you will receive in school is from your instructors, and the most important on-the-job feedback will come from your supervisors, more experienced peers, and occasionally clients. Making a special effort to take in this feedback and consider it carefully will help you learn many important lessons. Even when the criticism is not warranted, the way you respond is important. Furthermore, knowing how to handle conflict and criticism will help you define your role and communicate with others when you work in groups.

 ## WHAT ROLE DO YOU PLAY IN GROUPS?

Group interaction is an important part of your educational, personal, and working life. With a team project at work or a cooperative learning exercise in school, for example, being able to work well together is necessary in order to accomplish a goal.

The two major roles in the group experience are those of *participant* and *leader*. Any group needs both in order to function successfully. Become aware of the role you tend to play when relating to others. Try different roles to help you decide where you can be most effective. The following strategies (from *Contemporary Business Communication*, by Louis E. Boone, David L. Kurtz, and Judy R. Block) are linked to either participating or leading.[8]

Being an Effective Participant

Some people are happiest when participating in group activities that someone else leads and designs. They don't feel comfortable in a position of control or having the power to set the tone for the group as a whole. They trust others to make those decisions, preferring to help things run smoothly by taking on an assigned role in the project and seeing it through. Participators need to remember that they are "part owners" of the process. Each team member has a responsibility for, and a stake in, the outcome. The following strategies will help a participant to be effective.

Participation Strategies

Get involved. If a decision you don't like is made by a group of which you are a member and you stayed uninvolved in the decision, you have no one to blame but yourself for not speaking up. Put some energy into your participation and let people know your views. You are as important a team member as anyone else, and your views are likewise valuable.

Be organized. When you participate with the group as a whole, or with any of the team members, stay focused and organized. The more organized your ideas are, the more people will listen, take them into consideration, and be willing to try them.

Be willing to discuss. Everyone has an equal right to express his or her ideas. Even as you enthusiastically present your opinions, be willing to consider those of others. Keep an open mind and think critically about other ideas before you assume they won't work. If a discussion heats up, take a break or let a more neutral group member mediate.

Keep your word. Make a difference by doing what you say you're going to do. Let people know what you have accomplished. If you bring little or nothing to the process, your team may feel as if you weigh them down.

Focus on ideas, not people. One of the easiest ways to start an argument is for participants to attack group members themselves instead of discussing their ideas. Separate the person from the idea, and keep the idea in focus.

Play fairly. Give everyone a chance to participate. Be respectful of other people's ideas. Don't dominate the discussion or try to control or manipulate others.

Being an Effective Leader

Some people prefer to initiate the action, make decisions, and control how things proceed. They have ideas they want to put into practice and enjoy explaining them to others. They are comfortable giving direction to people and guiding group outcomes. Leaders often have a big-picture perspective; it allows them to see how all of the different aspects of a group project can come together. In any group setting, the following strategies will help a leader succeed.

Leadership Strategies

Define and limit projects. One of the biggest ways to waste time and energy is to assume that a group will know its purpose and will limit tasks on its own. A group needs a leader who can define the purpose of the gathering and limit tasks so the group doesn't take on too much. Some common purposes are giving/exchanging information, brainstorming, making a decision, delegating tasks, or collaborating on a project.

Map out who will perform which tasks. A group functions best when everyone has a particular contribution to make. You don't often choose who you work with—in school, at work, or in your family—but you can help different personalities work together by exploring who can do what best. Give people specific responsibilities, and trust that they will do their jobs.

Set the agenda. The leader is responsible for establishing and communicating the goal of the project and how it will proceed. Without a plan, it's easy to get off track. Having a written agenda to which group members can refer is helpful. A good leader invites advice from others when determining group direction.

Focus progress. Even when everyone knows the plan, it's still natural to wander off the topic. The leader should try to rein in the discussion when necessary, doing his or her best to keep everyone to the topic at hand. When challenges arise midstream, the leader may need to help the team change direction.

Set the tone. Different group members bring different attitudes and mental states to a gathering. Setting a positive tone helps to bring the group together and motivate people to peak performance. When a leader values diversity in ideas and backgrounds and sets a tone of fairness, respect, and encouragement, group members may feel more comfortable contributing their ideas.

Evaluate results. The leader should determine whether the team is accomplishing its goals. If the team is not moving ahead, the leader needs to make changes and decisions.

If you don't believe you fit into the traditional definition of a leader, remember that there are other ways to lead that don't involve taking charge of a group. You can lead others by setting an honorable example in your actions, choices, or words. You can lead by putting forth an idea that takes a group in a new direction. You can lead by being the kind of person whom others would like to be.

It takes the equal participation of all group members to achieve a goal. Whatever role works best for you, know that your contribution is essential. You may even play different roles with different groups, such as if you were a participator at school and a leader in a self-help group. Finally, stay aware of group dynamics; they can shift quickly and move you into a new position you may or may not like. If you don't feel comfortable, speak up. The happier each group member is, the more effectively the group as a whole will function.

Kente

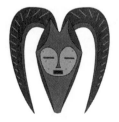

The African word *kente* means "that which will not tear under any condition." *Kente* cloth is worn by men and women in African countries such as Ghana, Ivory Coast, and Togo. There are many brightly colored patterns of *kente*, each beautiful, unique, and special.

Think of how this concept applies to being human. Like the cloth, all people are unique, with brilliant and subdued aspects. Despite any mistreatment or misunderstanding by the people you encounter in your life, you need to work to remain strong so that you don't tear and give way to disrespectful behavior. This strength can help you to endure, stand up against any injustice, and fight peacefully but relentlessly for the rights of all people.

Applications   **Chapter 10**

KEY INTO YOUR LIFE
Opportunities to Apply What You Learn

 Diversity Discovery

Express your own personal diversity. Describe yourself in response to the following questions.

What ethnic background(s) do you have? _____

_____

_____

_____

Name one or more facts about you that someone wouldn't know from simply looking at you. _____

_____

_____

_____

Name two values or beliefs that govern how you live, what you pursue, and/or with whom you associate. _____

_____

_____

_____

What other characteristics or choices define your uniqueness? _____

_____

_____

_____

Now, join with a partner in your class. Try to choose someone you don't know well. Your goal is to communicate what you have written to your partner, and for your partner to communicate to you in the same way. Spend ten minutes talking together, and take notes on what the other person says. At the end of that period, join together as a class. Each person will describe his or her partner to the class.

What did you learn about your partner that surprised you? _____

_____

_____

_____

What did you learn that went against any assumptions you may have made about that person based on his or her appearance, background, or behavior?

_____

_____

_____

Has this exercise changed the way you see this person or other people? Why or why not? _____

_____

_____

_____

10.2 *Your Communication Style*

Look back at the four styles on p. 263: Intuitor, Thinker, Feeler, and Senser. Which describes you the best? Rank the four styles, listing first the one that fits most, and listing last the one that fits least.

1. _____

2. _____

3. _____

4. _____

Of the two styles that best fit you, which one has more positive effects on your ability to communicate? What are those effects? _____

_____

_____

_____

Which style has more negative effects? What are they? _____

_____

_____

_____

To determine whether you are primarily passive, aggressive, or assertive, read the following sentences and circle the ones that sound like something you would say to a peer. _____

_____

_____

_____

1. Get me the keys.
2. Would you mind if I stepped out just for a second?
3. Don't slam the door.
4. I'd appreciate it if you would have this done by two o'clock.
5. I think maybe it needs a little work just at the end, but I'm not sure.
6. Please take this back to the library.
7. You will have a good time if you join us.
8. Your loss.
9. I don't know, if you think so. I'll try it.
10. Let me know what you want me to do.
11. Turn it this way and see what happens.
12. We'll try both our ideas and see what works best.
13. I want it on my desk by the end of the day.
14. Just do what I told you.
15. If this isn't how you wanted it to look, I can change it. Just tell me and I'll do it.

Aggressive communicators would be likely to use sentences 1, 3, 8, 13, and 14. Passive communicators would probably opt for sentences 2, 5, 9, 10, and 15. Assertive communicators would probably choose sentences 4, 6, 7, 11, and 12.

In which category did you choose the most sentences? _____

If you scored as an assertive communicator, you are on the right track. If you scored in the aggressive or passive categories, analyze your style. What are the effects? Give an example in your own life of the effects of your style.

_____

_____

_____

Turn back to pp. 266–267 to review suggestions for aggressive or passive communicators. What can you do to improve your skills?

_____

_____

_____

_____

10.3 *Problem Solving Close to Home*

Divide into small groups of two to five students. Assign one group member to take notes. Discuss the following questions, one by one:

1. What are the three largest problems my school faces with regard to how people get along with and accept others?
2. What could my school do to deal with the three problems listed above?
3. What can each individual student do to deal with the three problems listed above? (Talk about what you specifically feel that you can do.)

When you are finished, gather as a class. Each group should share their responses with the class. Observe the variety of problems and solutions. Notice whether more than one group came up with one or more of the same problems. You may want to assign one person in the class to gather all of the responses together. That person, together with your instructor, could put these responses into an organized document that you can share with the upper-level administrators at your school.

KEY TO SELF-EXPRESSION
Discovery Through Journal Writing

To record your thoughts, use a separate journal or the lined page at the end of the chapter.

New Perspective[9]

Imagine that you have no choice but to change either your gender (male/female) or your racial/ethnic/religious group. Which would you change, and why? What do you anticipate would be the positive and negative effects of the change—in your social life, in your family life, on the job, at school? How would what you know and experience before the change affect how you would behave after the change?

Journal

Name _____ Date _____

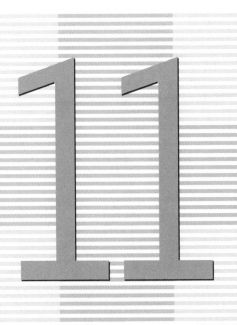

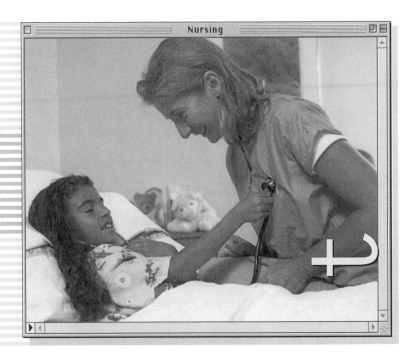

Nursing

Managing Career and Money

Reality Resources

More students than ever need to work while attending school. In addition to working, many have families and other important commitments. Any one of these can make going to school to pursue a career a complicated endeavor. Managing, or balancing, all your priorities is obviously difficult even though you know, in the long run, your efforts to obtain a degree in nursing will be worthwhile.

In this chapter you will find answers to questions such as how to plan a career while making sure it is the one you really want to pursue; how to earn the money necessary to do it; and, especially, how to still have some time for yourself and family.

Then you will explore how to bring in money with financial aid and how to manage the money you have. Managing your resources and investigating your career can help you develop skills and insights that will serve you throughout your life.

In this chapter, you will explore answers to the following questions:

- How can you plan your career?
- How can you juggle work and school?
- What should you know about financial aid?
- How can strategic planning help you manage money?
- How can you create a budget that works?

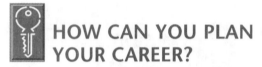

HOW CAN YOU PLAN YOUR CAREER?

College is an ideal time to investigate careers, because so many different resources are available to you. Students are in all different stages of thought when it comes to careers. You may have already had a career for years and are looking for a change. You may have been set on a particular career but are now thinking of nursing. Regardless of your starting point, now is the time to make progress.

Even outside this particular chapter, everything you read and work on in this book is geared toward college and workplace success. As you work on the exercises, you think critically, become a team player, hone writing skills, and develop long-term planning, all of which prepare you to thrive in your nursing career as well as in your studies.

Define a Career Path

Aiming for a job in a particular career, such as nursing, requires planning the steps to get you there. Whether these steps take months or years, they help you focus your energies on your goal. Defining your career path involves investigating yourself, exploring other potential careers, and building knowledge and experience. This process will help you be more certain if nursing is really what you choose to pursue.

Investigate

When you explored your learning style in Chapter 3, evaluated your ideal note-taking system in Chapter 7, or looked at how you relate to others in Chapter 10, you were building self-knowledge. Gather everything that you know about yourself, from this class or from any of your other life experiences, and investigate. What do you know or do best? Out of jobs you've had, what did you like and not like to do? How would you describe your personality? And finally, what kinds of careers make the best use of everything you are?

Don't feel as though you should automatically know what you want to do. Most students who have not been in the workplace don't know what career they want to pursue. Students who have been working often return to school to explore other careers that they might prefer. More and more, people are changing careers many times in their lives instead of sticking with one choice. This discovery is a lifelong process.

The potential for change applies to nursing majors as well. If you've already declared a nursing major and decide later that you don't like it, remember it is good to discover that fact about yourself before you put in a great deal of time and energy.

Explore Potential Careers

Your school's career center is an important resource in your investigation of career opportunities. The career center may offer job listings, occupation lists, assessments of skills and personality types, questionnaires to help you pinpoint career areas that may suit you, informational material about different career areas, and material about various companies. The people who work at the center can help you sort through the material.

Look at Table 11-1 for some of the kinds of questions you might ask as you talk to people, such as instructors, relatives, and fellow students, about careers or investigate materials. Use your critical-thinking skills to broaden your question-asking beyond just what tasks you perform for any given job. Many other factors will be important to you.

| TABLE 11-1 | Critical thinking questions for career investigation. |

What can I do in this area that I like/am good at?	Do I respect the company and/or the industry?
What are the educational requirements (certificates or degrees, courses)?	Do companies in this industry generally accommodate special needs (child care, sick days, flex time, or working at home)?
What skills are necessary?	Can I belong to a union?
What wage or salary is normal for an entry-level position, and what benefits can I expect?	Are there opportunities in this industry within a reasonable distance from where I live?
What kinds of personalities are best suited to this kind of work?	What other expectations are there beyond the regular workday (travel, overtime, etc.)?
What are the prospects for moving up to higher-level positions?	Do I prefer a service or manufacturing industry?

Within every career field, a wide array of job possibilities exists that you might not see right away. For example, the medical and health care worlds involve more than doctors and nurses. Emergency medical technicians respond to emergencies, administrators run hospitals, researchers test new drugs, lab technicians administer specific procedures such as X-rays, pharmacists administer prescriptions, retirement community employees work with the elderly, and more.

Within each job, there is also a variety of tasks and skills that often go beyond what you know. You may know that an instructor teaches, but you may not see that instructors also often write, research, study, create course outlines, create strategy with other instructors, give presentations, and counsel. Push past your first impression of any career and explore what else it entails. Expand your choices as much as you can using thorough investigation and an open mind.

Build Knowledge and Experience

Having knowledge and experience specific to the career area you want to pursue will be valuable on the job hunt. Courses, internships, jobs, and volunteering are four great ways to build both (see also Chapter 2).

Courses. When you narrow your career exploration to a couple of areas that interest you, look through your school course catalog and take a course or two in those fields. How you react to these courses will give you important clues as to how you feel about the area in general. Be careful to evaluate your experience based on how you feel about the subject matter and not other factors. Think critically. If you didn't like a course, what was the cause: an instructor you didn't like, a time of day when you tend to lose energy, or truly a lack of interest in the material?

> **TERMS**
>
> **Internships**
> A temporary work program in which a student can gain supervised practical experience in a particular professional field.

Internships. An internship may or may not offer pay. While this may be a financial drawback, the experience you can gather and contacts you can make may be worth the work. Many internships take place during the summer, but some part-time internships are also available during the school year. Agencies and organizations that offer internships are looking for people who will work hard in exchange for experience you can't get in the classroom.

Absorb all the knowledge you can while working as an intern. If you discover a career worth pursuing, you'll have the internship experience behind you when you go job hunting. Internships are one of the best ways to show a prospective employer some "real world" experience and initiative.

Jobs. No matter what you do for money while you are in college, whether it is in your area of interest or not, you may discover career opportunities that appeal to you. Someone who takes a night-shift nursing assistant job to make extra cash might discover an interest in health sciences research. Someone who answers phones for a newspaper company might be drawn into health sciences writing. Stay aware of the possibilities around you.

Volunteering. Offering your services in the community or at your school can introduce you to career areas and increase your experience. Some schools have programs that can help you find opportunities to work as an aid on campus or volunteer off campus. Recently, certain schools have even begun listing volunteer activities on student transcripts. Find out what services your school offers. Volunteer activities are important to note on your resume. Many health care facilities seek candidates who have shown commitment through volunteering.

Lin is an example of how volunteering to work with and observe a health professional can help clarify career goals. Lin wanted to be a doctor like the one who served her community. One summer between her freshman and sophomore years of college Lin decided to work with the local doctor as a volunteer. As she observed him visiting patients in the county hospital, she became clearer about what a career as a physician involved. She also noticed what the RNs were doing and that they spent much more time with the patients than the doctor: time spent teaching, counseling, and giving various types of care. From her experience, Lin realized that the kind of work she wanted to do was more like that of an RN. When she returned to school in the fall she changed her major from pre-med to pre-nursing.

Map Out Your Strategy

After you've gathered enough information to define your career goals, plan strategically to achieve them. Make a career time line that illustrates the steps toward your goal, as shown in Figure 11-1. Mark years and half-year points (and months for the first year), and write in the steps where you think they should take place. If your plan is five years long, indicate what you plan to do by the fourth, third, and second years, and then the first year, including a six-month goal and a one-month goal for that first year. Set goals that establish who you will talk to, what courses you will take, what skills you will work on, what jobs or internships you will investigate, and any other research you need to do. Your path may change, of course—use your time line as a guide rather than as a rigid plan.

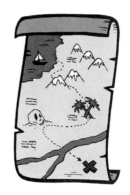

Know What Employers Want

Certain basic skills will make you an excellent job candidate no matter what career you decide to pursue. Employers look for particular skills and qualities that signify an efficient and effective employee. You can continue to develop these skills as you work in current and future jobs—and you will, if you always strive to improve.

Communication skills. Being able to listen well and express yourself in writing and speaking is a key to workplace success. Much can be accomplished through efficient, open communication. Being able to adjust to different communication styles is an important factor.

Problem solving. Any job will present problems that need to be solved. An employee who knows how to assess any situation and apply the problem-solving process to it will stand out.

FIGURE 11-1

Career time line.

1 month —— Enter community college on part-time schedule
3 months ——
6 months —— Meet with advisor to discuss desired major
            and required courses

1 year ——

        —— Declare major in nursing science

2 years —— Switch to full-time class schedule

3 years —— Graduate with associate's degree

        —— Transfer to 4-year college

4 years —— Work part-time in extended care facility

5 years —— Student internship at Cardiac Rehabilitation Clinic.

        —— Graduate with bachelor's degree in nursing science

6 years —— Get a job at Cardiac Rehabilitation Clinic and
            prepare to apply to graduate school

Decision making. Decisions large and small are made in every workplace every day. Knowing how to think through and make decisions will help you in any job.

Teamwork. It is a rare workplace that has only one employee, and even then, that person will interact with different kinds of people on the phone or through a computer. The importance of being able to work well with others cannot be overemphasized. If there is a weak link in any team, the whole company suffers.

Multicultural communication. The workplace is becoming increasingly diverse. The more you can work well with people different from yourself and open your mind to their points of view, the more valuable an employee you will be. If you are bilingual, you have a clear advantage.

Leadership. The ability to influence others in a positive way will earn you respect and keep you in line for promotions. Taking the lead will often command attention.

Creativity. When you can see the big picture as well as the details and can let your mind come up with unexpected new concepts and plans, you will bring valuable suggestions to your workplace.

Commitment. You will encounter many difficult situations at work. The ability to continue to work hard through such situations is extremely impor-

"For just a second his spirit and mine lived in that silence together. For just one moment I knew all the warmth and joy his spirit had ever given."

ECHO HERON, RN

tant. In addition, if you introduce a new and creative idea, you can gain support for it through having a strong commitment to it yourself.

Values and integrity. Your personal values and integrity will help guide everything you do. In your actions and decisions, consider what you value and what you believe is right.

These skills appear throughout this book, and they are as much a part of your school success as they are of your work success. The more you develop them now, the more employable and promotable you will prove yourself to be. You may already use them on the job if you are a student who works, which we will discuss next.

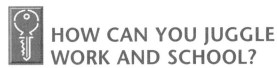

HOW CAN YOU JUGGLE WORK AND SCHOOL?

What you are studying today can prepare you to find a job, when you graduate, that suits your abilities and brings in enough money to support your needs and lifestyle choices. In the meantime, though, you can make work a part of your student life in order to make money, explore a career, and/or increase your future employability through contacts or resume building.

As the cost of education continues to rise, more and more students are working and taking classes at the same time. During the school year approximately 79 percent of undergraduates work while in school. Most student workers 23 years of age or younger work part-time jobs. Of students over the age of 23, a majority work full-time jobs.[1]

Being an employed student isn't for everyone. Adding a job to the list of demands on your time and energy may create problems if it sharply reduces study time or family time. However, many people want to work and many need to work in order to pay for school. Ask yourself important questions about why or why not to work. Weigh the potential positive and negative effects of working. From those answers you can make a choice that you feel benefits you most.

Effects of Working While in School

Working while in school has many different positive and negative effects, depending on the situation. Evaluate any job opportunity by looking at these effects. Many nursing programs offer part-time status for working students, or others who can't balance a full-time school schedule with the rest of their life. Following are some that might come into play.

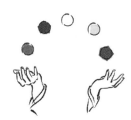

Potential Positive Effects

Money earned. A job can provide crucial income to pay for rent, transportation, food, and important bills. It may even help you put some savings away in order to create a financial cushion.

General and career-specific experience. Important learning comes from hands-on work. Your education "in the trenches" can complement your classroom experience. Even if you don't work in your chosen field, you can improve universal skills such as teamwork and communication.

Being able to keep a job you currently hold. If you leave a job temporarily, your company might not be able to hold your position open until you come back. Consider adjusting your responsibilities or hours while still holding down your job.

Keeping busy. Work can provide a stimulating break from studying. In fact, working up to fifteen hours a week may actually enhance academic performance, because working students often manage their time more efficiently and may gain confidence from their successes in the workplace. Working on campus may help you manage your time and connect to your school experience.

Potential Negative Effects

Time commitment. A nonworking student splits their time between academic and personal life, but a working student must add a third, time-consuming factor. More responsibilities and less time to fulfill them demand more efficient time management. Many schools recommend that students work a maximum of twenty hours a week while taking a full course load.

Adjusting priorities. The priority level of your job may vary. For a student who depends on the income, work may take priority over study time. Evaluate priorities carefully. Realize that you may have to reduce social activities, exercise at home, cut back on nonacademic activities, or lighten your course load in order to maintain a job and still get studying done. Your job is important, but if you are also committed to school, earning a good GPA may be just as crucial.

Shifting gears. Unless your job meshes with your classroom curriculum, it may take some effort to shift gears mentally as you move back and forth between academia and the workplace. Each environment has its own set of people, responsibilities, joys, and problems. Establish mental boundaries that can help you shake off academic stress while at work, and vice versa.

If you consider the positive and negative effects and decide that working will benefit you, you should establish what you need in a job (see Table 11-2).

Sources of Job Information

Many different routes can lead to satisfying jobs. Use your school's career planning and placement office, networking skills, classified ads, employment agencies, and on-line services to help you explore.

Your School's Career Planning and Placement Offices

Generally, the career planning and placement office deals with post-graduation job placements, while the student employment office, along with the financial aid office, has more information about working while in school. At

TABLE 11-2	What you may need in a job.

NEED	DESCRIPTION
Salary/wage level	Consider how much money you need to make month by month and yearly. You may need to make a certain amount for the year as a whole, but you may need to earn more of that total amount during the months when you are paying tuition. Consider also the amount that justifies taking the time to work. If a job pays well but takes extra hours that should go toward studying or classes, it might not be worth it. Take time to compare the positive effects with the negative effects of any job's pay structure.
Time of day	When you can work depends on your school schedule. For example, if you take classes Monday, Tuesday, and Thursday during the day, you could look for a job with weekend or evening hours. If you attend evening classes, a daytime job could work fine.
Hours per week (part-time vs. full-time)	If you take classes part-time, you may choose to work a full-time job. If you are a full-time student, it may be best to work part-time. Balance your priorities so that you can accomplish your schoolwork and still make the money you need.
Duties performed	If you want hands-on experience in your chosen field, narrow your search to jobs that can provide it. On the other hand, if a regular paycheck is your priority, you might not care as much about what you do. Consider if there is anything you absolutely hate to do. Working somewhere and/or doing something that makes you miserable may not be worth any amount of money.
Location	Weigh the effects of how long it takes to get to a job against what you are getting out of it, and decide whether it is worth your while. A job at or near your school may give unparalleled convenience. When you know you can get to work quickly, you can schedule your day more tightly and get more done.
Flexibility	Even if your classes are at regular times, you might have other projects and meetings at various times. Do you need a job that offers flexibility, allowing you to shift your working time when you have to attend to an academic or family responsibility that takes priority? Choose according to the flexibility you require.
Affiliation with school or financial aid program	Some financial aid packages, especially if they involve funds from your school, can require you to take work at the school or a federal organization. In that case you would have to choose among the opportunities offered.
Accommodation of special needs (Americans with Disabilities Act)	If you have a hearing or vision impairment, reduced mobility, or other special needs, colleges, universities, and employers must accommodate them.

either location you might find general workplace information, listings of job opportunities, sign-ups for interviews, and contact information for companies. The career office may hold frequent informational sessions on different topics. Your school may also sponsor job or career fairs that give you a chance to explore job opportunities.

Many students, because they don't seek job information until they're about to graduate, miss out on much of what the career office can do. Don't wait until the last minute. Start exploring your school's career office early in your university life. The people and resources there can help you at every stage of your career and job exploration process.

Networking

Networking
The exchange of information and/ or services among individuals, groups, or institutions.

Contact
A person who serves as a carrier or source of information.

Networking is one of the most important job-hunting strategies. With each person you get to know, you build your network and tap into someone else's. Imagine a giant think link connecting you to a web of people just a couple of phone calls away. Of course, not everyone with whom you network will come through for you. Keep in contact with as many people as possible in the hope that someone will. You never know who that person might be.

With whom can you network? Friends and family members may know of jobs or other people who can help you. At your school, instructors, administrators, or counselors may give you job or contact information. Attend professional conferences by contacting the on-campus club or state chapter. Some schools even have opportunities for students to interact with alumni. Look to your present and past work experience for more leads. Employers or coworkers may know someone who needs new employees. A former employer might even hire you back with similar or adjusted hours, if you left on good terms.

The contacts with whom you network aren't just sources of job opportunities. They are people with whom you can develop lasting, valuable relationships. They may be willing to talk to you about how to get established, the challenges on the job, what they do each day, how much you can expect to make, or any other questions you have similar to those in Table 11-1. Thank your contacts for their help and don't forget them. Networking is a two-way street. Even as you receive help, be ready to extend yourself to others who may need help and advice from you.

Classified Ads

Some of the best job listings are in daily or periodic newspapers. Most papers print help wanted sections in each issue, organized according to career field categories. At the beginning of most help wanted sections you will find an index that tells you the categories and on what pages they begin in the listings. Individual ads describe the kind of position available and will give a telephone number or post office box for you to contact. Some ads will include additional information such as job requirements, a contact person, and the salary or wages offered.

You can run your own classified ads if you have a skill you want to advertise. Many college students make extra cash by doing specific tasks for campus employees or other students, such as typing, editing, cleaning, tutoring, or baby-sitting. You may want to advertise your particular job skills in your school or local paper.

On-Line Services

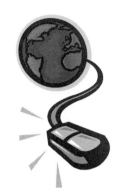

The Internet is growing as a source of job listings. Through it you can access job search databases such as the Career Placement Registry and U. S. Employment Opportunities. Websites such as CareerPath.com and CareerMosaic list all kinds of positions. Individual associations and companies may also post job listings and descriptions, often as part of their World Wide Web pages. For example, the American Nursing Association includes job openings on its web page.

Employment Agencies

Employment agencies are organizations that help people find work. Most employment agencies will put you through a screening process that consists of an interview and one or more tests in your area of expertise. For example, someone looking for secretarial work may take a word-processing test and a spelling test, while someone looking for accounting work may take accounting and math tests. If you pass the tests and interview well, they will try to place you in a job.

Most employment agencies specialize in particular career or skill areas, such as accounting, medicine, legal, computer operation, graphic arts, child care, and food services. Agencies may place job seekers in either part-time or full-time employment. Many agencies also place people in temporary jobs, which can work well for students who are available from time to time. Such agencies may have you call in whenever you are free and will see if anything is available that day or week.

Employment agencies are a great way to hook into job networks. However, they usually require a fee that either you or the employer has to pay. Investigate any agency before signing on. See if your school's career counselors know anything about the agency, or if any fellow students have used it successfully. Ask questions so that you know as much as possible about how the agency operates.

Making a Strategic Job Search Plan

When you have gathered information on the jobs you want, formulate a plan for pursuing them. Organize your approach according to what you need to do and how much time you have to devote to your search. Do you plan to make three phone calls per day? Will you fill out three job applications a week for a month? Keep a record—on 3-by-5-inch cards, a computer file, or in a notebook—of the following:

- People you contact
- Companies to which you apply
- Jobs you rule out (for example, jobs that become unavailable or which you find out don't suit your needs)

■ Response from your communications (phone calls to you, interviews, written communications) and the information on whomever contacted you (names, titles, times, and dates)

Keeping accurate records will enable you to both chart your progress and maintain a clear picture of the process. You never know when information might come in handy again. If you don't get a job now, another one could open up at the same company in a couple of months. In that case, well-kept records would enable you to contact key personnel quickly and efficiently. See Figure 11-2 for a sample file card.

Your Resume and Interview

Information on resumes and interviews fills many books. Therefore, your best bet is to consult some that will go into more detail, such as *The Resume Kit*, by Richard Beatty, or *Job Interviews for Dummies* by Joyce Lain Kennedy (don't be insulted by the title; it has lots of terrific information).

The following basic tips can get you started on giving yourself the best possible chance at a job.

Resume. Your resume should always be typed or printed on a computer. Design your resume neatly, using an acceptable format (books or your career office can show you some standard formats). Proofread it for errors, and have someone else proofread it as well. Type or print it on a heavier bond paper than is used for ordinary copies. Use only white or off-white paper and black ink.

Interview. Pay attention to your appearance. Be clean, neat, and appropriately dressed. Don't forget to choose a nice pair of shoes—people notice. Bring an extra copy of your resume with you, and any other materials that you want to show the interviewer, even if you have already sent a copy ahead of

---

FIGURE 11-2

Sample file card.

Job/company: Child-care worker at Morningside Day Care

Contact: Sally Wheeler, Morningside Day Care, 17 Parkside Road, Silver Spring, MD 20910

Phone/fax/e-mail: (301) 555-3353 phone, (301) 555-3354 fax, no e-mail

Communication: Saw ad in paper, sent resume and cover letter on October 7

Response: Call from Sally to set up interview

Interview on Oct. 15 at 2 p.m., seemed to get a positive response, she said she would contact me again by the end of the week

Follow-up: Sent thank-you note on October 16

time. Avoid chewing gum or smoking. Offer a confident handshake. Make eye contact. Show your integrity by speaking honestly about yourself. After the interview is over, no matter what the outcome, send a formal but pleasant thank-you note right away as a follow-up.

Earning the money you need is hard, especially if you work part-time in order to have time for school. Financial aid can take some of the burden off your shoulders. If you can gather one or more loans, grants, or scholarships, they may help make up for what you don't have time to earn.

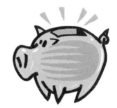

 ## WHAT SHOULD YOU KNOW ABOUT FINANCIAL AID?

Seeking help from various sources of financial aid has become a way of life for much of the student population. Education is an important but often expensive investment. The cost for a year's full-time tuition only (not including room and board) ranges from $900 to $15,000, with the national average hovering around $2,100 for public institutions and well over $11,000 for private ones.[2] Not many people can pay for tuition in full without aid. In fact, according to the data, over 41 percent of students enrolled received some kind of aid,[3] and that number almost certainly continues to increase along with rising tuition costs.

Most sources of financial aid don't seek out recipients. Take the initiative to learn how you (or you and your parents, if they currently help to support you) can finance your education. Find the people on campus who can help you with your finances. Do some research to find out what's available, weigh the pros and cons of each option, and decide what would work best for you. Try to apply as early as you can. The types of financial aid available to you are loans, grants, scholarships, and professional organizations.

Student Loans

A loan is given to you by a person, bank, or other lending agency, usually to put toward a specific purchase. You, as the recipient of the loan, then must pay back the amount of the loan, plus interest, in regular payments that stretch over a particular period of time. Interest is the fee that you pay for the privilege of using money that belongs to someone else.

Making a Loan Application

What happens when you apply for a loan?

1. *The loaning agency must approve you.* You may be asked about what you and any other family members earn, how much savings you have, your credit history, anything you own that is of substantial value (a home or business), and your history of payment on any previous loans.

2. *An interest charge will be set.* Interest can range from 5 percent to over 20 percent, depending on the loan and the economy. Variable-interest loans shift charges as the economy strengthens or weakens. Fixed-rate loans have one interest rate that remains constant.

3. *The loaning agency will establish a payment plan.* Most loan payments are made monthly or quarterly (four times per year). The payment amount depends on the total amount of the loan, how much you can comfortably pay per month, and the length of the repayment period.

Types of Student Loans

The federal government administers or oversees most student loans. To receive aid from any federal program, you must be a citizen or eligible noncitizen and be enrolled in a program of study that the government has determined is eligible. Individual states may differ in their aid programs. Check with your campus financial aid office to find out details about your state and your school in particular.

Following are the main student loan programs to which you can apply if you are eligible. Amounts vary according to individual circumstances. Contact your school or federal student aid office for further information. In most cases, the amount is limited to the cost of your education minus any other financial aid you are receiving. All the information on federal loans and grants comes from the 2000–2001 *Student Guide to Financial Aid*, published by the U. S. Department of Education.[4] See page 295 for information on how to obtain a copy of the guide.

Perkins Loans. Carrying a low, fixed rate of interest, these loans are available to those with exceptional financial need (need is determined by a government-determined formula that indicates how large a contribution toward your education your family should be able to make). Schools issue these loans from their own allotment of federal education funds. After you graduate, you have a "grace period" (up to nine months, depending on whether you were a part-time or full-time student) before you have to begin repaying your loan in monthly installments.

Stafford Loans. Students enrolled in school at least half-time may apply for a Stafford Loan. Exceptional need is not required. However, students who can prove exceptional need may qualify for a "subsidized" Stafford Loan, for which the government pays your interest until you begin repayment. There are two types of Stafford Loans. A Direct Stafford Loan comes from government funds, and an FFEL Stafford Loan comes from a bank or credit union participating in the FFEL (Federal Family Education Loan) program. The type available to you depends on your school's financial aid program. You begin to repay a Stafford Loan six months after you graduate, leave school, or drop below half-time enrollment.

Plus Loans. Your parents can apply for a Plus Loan if they currently claim you as a dependent and if you are enrolled at least half-time. They must also undergo a credit check in order to be eligible, although the loans are not based on income. If they do not pass the credit check, they may be able to sponsor the loan through a relative or friend who does pass. Interest is variable; the loans are available from either the government or banks and credit unions. Your parents will have to begin repayment sixty days after they receive the last loan payment; there is no grace period.

Grants and Scholarships

Both grants and scholarships require no repayment, and therefore give your finances a terrific boost. Grants, funded by the government, are awarded to students who show financial need. Scholarships are awarded to students who show talent or ability in the area specified by the scholarship. They may be financed by government or private organizations, schools, or individuals.

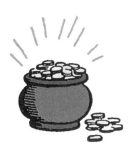

Federal Grant Programs

Pell Grants. These grants are need-based. The Department of Education uses a standard formula to evaluate the financial information you report on your application, and determines your eligibility from that "score" (called an EFC, or Expected Family Contribution, number). You must also be an undergraduate student who has earned no other degrees to be eligible. The Pell Grant serves as a foundation of aid to which you may add other aid sources, and the amount of the grant varies according to the cost of your education and your EFC. Pell Grants require no repayment.

FSEOG (Federal Supplemental Educational Opportunity Grants). Administered by the financial aid administrator at participating schools, FSEOG eligibility depends on need. Whereas the government guarantees that every student eligible for a Pell Grant will receive one, each school receives a limited amount of federal funds for FSEOGs, and once it's gone, it's gone. Schools set their own application deadlines. Apply early. No repayment is required.

Work-Study Program. Although you work in exchange for the aid, work-study is considered a grant because a limited number of positions are available. This program is need-based and encourages community service work or work related in some way to your course of study. You will earn at least the federal minimum wage and will be paid hourly. Jobs can be on-campus (usually for your school) or off-campus (often with a nonprofit organization or a local, state, or federal public agency). Find out who is in charge of the work-study program on your campus.

There is much more to say about these financial aid opportunities than can be touched on here. Many other important details about federal grants and loans are available in The 2000–2001 *Student Guide to Financial Aid.* You might find this information at your school's financial aid office, or you can request it by mail, phone, or on-line service:

Address:	Federal Student Aid Information Center P. O. Box 84 Washington, D. C. 20044
Phone:	1-800-4-FED-AID (1-800-433-3243) *TDD for the hearing-impaired:* 1-800-730-8913
Internet address:	www.ed.gov/prog_info/SFA/StudentGuide

For financial aid specifically for undergraduate and graduate nursing students, contact the Department of Health and Human Services (DHHS). Also, *Peterson's Guide to Nursing Programs* has information on schools *and* financial aid. This guide is found in library bookstores, or by calling 1-800-338-3282.

Scholarships

Scholarships are given for different kinds of abilities and talents. Some reward academic achievement. Some reward exceptional abilities in sports or the arts. Some reward citizenship or leadership. Certain scholarships are sponsored by federal agencies. If you display exceptional ability and are disabled, female, of an ethnic background classified as culturally diverse (such as African-American or American Indian), or a child of someone who draws benefits from a state agency (such as a POW or MIA), you might find scholarship opportunities geared toward you.

All kinds of organizations offer scholarships. You may receive scholarships from individual departments at your school or your school's independent scholarship funds, local organizations such as the Rotary Club, or privately operated aid foundations. Labor unions and companies may offer scholarship opportunities for children of their employees. Membership groups such as scouting organizations or the Y might offer scholarships, and religious organizations such as the Knights of Columbus or the Council of Jewish Federations might be another source. Most local nursing organizations offer scholarships to nursing students after you have completed a term in nursing school.

Researching Grants and Scholarships

It can take work to locate scholarships and work-study programs because many of them aren't widely advertised. Ask at your school's financial aid office. Visit your library or bookstore and look in the sections on College or Financial Aid. Guides to funding sources, such as Richard Black's *The Complete Family Guide to College Financial Aid*, catalog thousands of organizations and help you find what fits you. Check out on-line scholarship search services. Use common sense and time management when applying for aid— fill out the application as neatly as possible and send it in on time or even early. In addition, be wary of scholarship scam artists who ask you to pay a fee up front for them to find aid for you.

No matter where your money comes from—financial aid or paychecks from one or more jobs—you can take steps to help it stretch as far as it can go. The next sections concentrate on developing a philosophy about your money and budgeting effectively. Using those skills, you can more efficiently cover your expenses and still have some left over for savings and fun.

 ## HOW CAN STRATEGIC PLANNING HELP YOU MANAGE MONEY?

So you work hard to earn your wages and study hard to hold on to your grants and loans. What do you do with that money? Popular culture tells you to buy. You are surrounded by commercials, magazine ads, and notices in the mail that tell you how wonderful you'll feel if you indulge in some serious spending. On the other hand, there are some definite advantages to not taking that advice. Making some short-term sacrifices in order to save money can help you a great deal in the long run.

Short-Term Sacrifices Can Create Long-Term Gains

When you think about your money, take your values and your ability to plan strategically into account. Ask yourself what goals you value most and what steps you will have to take over time to achieve those goals. You are already planning ahead by being in school and committing to paying for tuition. You may be scrimping now, but you are planning for a career that may reward you with job security and financial stability. Sometimes the most important goals are also the ones that require a long-term commitment. If you can make that commitment, the reward will be worth the short-term sacrifices.

"It is thrifty to prepare today for the wants of tomorrow."

AESOP

Table 11-3 shows some potential effects of spending. Some effects are negative, some positive, and some more positive than others. Evaluate which

TABLE 11-3 Potential effects of spending.

OPTION	POTENTIAL SHORT-TERM EFFECTS	POTENTIAL LONG-TERM EFFECTS
Purchase new sound system	High-quality sound	If paid on credit, a credit card debt, with finance charges, that requires monthly payment; if paid in cash, a loss of benefits that could have come from saving that money
Reduce or pay off credit card debt	Less money for day-to-day expenses; reduction of monthly bills	Improved credit rating and credit history; increased ability to be approved for loans and mortgages; less money charged in interest and fees
Take a week's vacation	Fun and relaxation; stress reduction	Credit card debt or less money saved for future needs
Invest in mutual fund	Less money on hand; more money earning interest	More money earned, due to an interest rate higher than banks can offer
Buy a car	Transportation and independence; gas, maintenance, parking charges	Debt in the form of a car loan; monthly payments for a few years; gradual decrease in car value
Pay health insurance bills	Health insurance coverage; a tighter monthly budget	The safety and security of knowing that your health and the health of your family are protected
Invest in your family business	Commitment to family; less money to spend on extras	Involvement in a family business that can earn you money and provide solid employment for you and other family members
Put money toward tuition	Having to scrimp while in school due to less money on hand; fewer loans and debts	Less money to pay off later in student loans, which means less money charged in interest; more freedom to spend your money on getting settled after you graduate; shorter period of debt

you would prefer in the long run. You may find that the pleasure luxuries provide isn't worth the stress created by debt.

Critical thinking is the key to smart money planning. Impulsive spending usually happens when you don't take time to think through your decision before you buy. To use your hard-earned money to your greatest benefit, take time to think critically about your finances. First, establish your needs, and be honest about what you truly need and what you just want. Second, brainstorm available options of what to do with your money; evaluate the positive and negative effects of each. Third, choose an option and carry it out. Finally, evaluate the result.

Develop a Financial Philosophy

You can develop your own personal philosophy about spending, saving, and planning. Following are a couple of strategies that you might want to incorporate into that philosophy.

Live beneath your means. Spend less than you make. This strategy helps you create savings, no matter how much or how little. Any amount of savings will give you a buffer zone that can help with emergencies or bigger expenditures. Sometimes your basic needs will cost more than you make, in which case living beneath your means becomes very difficult. If you find, however, that extras are putting your spending over your earnings, cut back.

Pay yourself. After you pay your monthly bills, put whatever you can save from your monthly earnings in a savings account. Paying yourself helps you store money in your savings where it can grow.

HOW CAN YOU CREATE A BUDGET THAT WORKS?

TERMS

Budgeting
Making a plan for the coordination of resources and expenditures; setting goals with regards to money.

Every time you have some money in your pocket and have to figure out whether it will pay for what you want at that moment, you are budgeting your money. It takes some thought and energy to budget efficiently. The more money you can save each month, the more you will thank yourself later when you need it. Consider your resources (money coming in) and expenditures (money flowing out). A smart budget adjusts the money flow for the best possible chance that what comes in will be more than what goes out. Smart budgeting is a worthwhile investment in your future.

The Art of Budgeting

Budgeting involves following a few basic steps in order. These steps are: determining how much money you make, determining how much money you spend, subtracting the second number (what you spend) from the first number (what you make), evaluating the result, and making decisions about how to adjust your spending or earning based on that result. Budgeting regularly

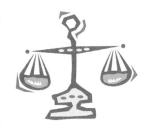

is easiest. Use a specified time frame, such as a week or month. Most people budget on a month-by-month basis.

Determine How Much You Will Make

Do this by adding up all your money receipts from the month. If you currently have a regular full-time or part-time job, add your pay stubs. If you have received any financial aid, loan funding, or scholarship money, determine how much of that you can allow for each month's income and add it to your total. For example, if you received a $1,200 grant for the year, each month would have an income of $100. Be sure when you are figuring your income, to use the amounts that remain *after* taxes have been taken out.

Figure Out How Much You Spend

You may or may not have a handle on your spending. Many people don't take the time to keep track. If you have never before paid much attention to how you spend money, examine your spending patterns. Over a month's time, record expenditures in a small notebook or on a piece of paper on a home bulletin board. You don't have to list everything down to the penny. Just indicate expenditures over five dollars, making sure to count smaller expenditures if they are frequent (a bus pass for a month, soda or newspaper purchases per week). In your list, include an estimate of the following:

- Rent/mortgage/school room fees
- Tuition or educational loan payments (divide your annual total by 12 to arrive at a monthly figure)
- Books, lab fees, and other educational expenses
- Regular bills (heat, gas, electric, phone, car payment, water)
- Credit card or other payments on credit
- Food, clothing, toiletries, and household supplies
- Child care
- Entertainment and related items (eating out, books and publications, movies)
- Health, auto, and home/renters' insurance
- Transportation and auto expenses

Subtract what you spend from what you make. Ideally, you will have a positive number. You may end up with a negative number, however, especially if you haven't made a habit of keeping track of your spending. This indicates that you are spending more than you make, which over a long period of time can create a nasty debt.

Evaluate the Result

After you arrive at your number, determine what it tells you. If you have a positive number, decide how to save it if you can. If you end up with a negative number, ask yourself questions about what is causing the deficit—where you are spending too much or earning too little. Of course, surprise expenses during some months may cause you to spend more than usual, such as if you have to replace your refrigerator, pay equipment fees for a particular course, or have an emergency medical procedure. However, when a negative number comes up for what seems to be a typical month, you may need to adjust your budget over the long term.

Make Decisions About How to Adjust Spending or Earning

Looking at what may cause you to overspend, brainstorm possible solutions that address those causes. Solutions can involve either increasing resources or decreasing spending. To deal with spending, prioritize your expenditures and trim the ones you really don't need to make. Do you eat out too much? Can you live without cable, a beeper, a cellular phone? Be smart. Cut out unaffordable extras. As for resources, investigate ways to take in more money. Taking a part-time job, hunting down scholarships or grants, or increasing hours at a current job may help.

A Sample Budget

Table 11-4 shows a sample budget of an unmarried student living with two other students. It will give you an idea of how to budget (all expenditures are general estimates, based on averages).

To make up the $190 that this student went over budget, he can adjust his spending. He could rent movies or check them out of the library instead of going to the theater. He could socialize with friends at someone's apartment instead of paying high prices and tips at a bar or restaurant. Instead of buying CDs and tapes, he could borrow them. He could also shop for specials and bargains in the grocery store or go to a warehouse supermarket to stock up on staples at discount prices. He could make his lunch instead of buying it and walk instead of taking public transportation.

TABLE 11-4

A student's sample budget.

Part-time salary: $10 an hour, 20 hours a week. $10 \times 20 = \$200$ a week, $\times$ 4 1/3 weeks (one month) = $866. Student loan from school's financial aid office: $2,000 divided by 12 months = $166. Total income per month: $1,032.

MONTHLY EXPENDITURES	AMOUNT
Tuition ($6500 per year)	$ 542
Public transportation	$ 90
Phone	$ 40
Food	$ 130
Medical insurance	$ 120
Rent (including utilities)	$ 200
Entertainment/miscellaneous	$ 100
Total spending	$1222

$1032 (income) – $1222 (spending) = $–190 ($190 over budget)

Not everyone likes the work involved in keeping a budget. While linear, factual, reflective, and verbal learners may take to it more easily, active, holistic, theoretical, and visual learners may resist the structure and detail (see Chapter 3). Visual learners may want to create a budget chart like the one shown in the example or construct a think link that shows the connections between all the month's expenditures. Use images to clarify ideas, such as picturing a bathtub you are filling that is draining at the same time. Use strategies that make budgeting more tangible, such as dumping all of your receipts into a big jar and tallying them at the end of the month. Even if you have to force yourself to do it, you will discover that budgeting can reduce stress and help you take control of your finances and your life.

Savings Strategies

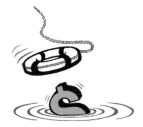

You can save money and still enjoy life. Make your fun less expensive and environmentally friendly—or save up for a while to splurge on a really special occasion. Here are some suggestions for saving a little bit of money here and there. Small amounts can add up to big savings after a while.

- Attend bargain movies.
- When safe for the fabric, hand-wash items you ordinarily dry-clean, or don't buy items that need dry-cleaning in the first place.
- Check movies, CDs, tapes, and books out of your library.
- Make popcorn instead of buying bags of chips.
- Walk or bike instead of paying for public transportation or driving.
- If you have storage space, buy detergent, paper products, toiletries, and other staples in bulk.
- Shop in secondhand stores.
- Keep your possessions neat, clean, and properly maintained—they will last longer.
- Take advantage of weekly supermarket specials, and bring coupons when you shop.
- Reuse grocery bags for food storage and garbage instead of buying bags.
- Return bottles and cans for deposits if you live in a state that accepts them.
- Trade clothing with friends and barter services (plumbing for baby-sitting, for example).
- Buy display models of appliances or electronics (stereo equipment, TVs, VCRs).
- Take your lunch instead of buying it.
- Find a low-rate long-distance calling plan, use e-mail, or write letters.
- Save on heat by dressing warmly and using blankets; save on air conditioning by using fans.
- Have potluck parties; ask people to bring dinner foods or munchies.

ERIKA SELLEKAERTS

Senior, University of Pennsylvania,
Philadelphia, Pennsylvania

I'm a single mother with a special needs child. Recently I graduated from Central Michigan University with a BSN and have recently entered graduate school at the University of Pennsylvania. I worked as a cake decorator at a bakery to pay for the moving costs, and all along I've borrowed money through school loans so that I could afford an education. It's been difficult to work, attend school, and be a mom, but I know nursing is what I want to do with my life.

I knew the University of Pennsylvania was a private school, but I still wasn't prepared for the shock of receiving my first bill. Instead of panicking, I sat down and wrote a letter to the administrative office and explained that my success as a student was already fragile because of being a single parent. I also explained how much I wanted to become an advanced practice nurse and that I plan to specialize in pediatric oncology. Thankfully, this effort paid off because I was awarded a grant. But that's only half the battle because I have to pay for housing. I qualified for a work study program, which paid $7.00 an hour but I had to pay $5.00 an hour for child care. You can't live on $2.00 an hour.

My graduate program requires that students work for nine months as a staff nurse before they can start clinicals. I would 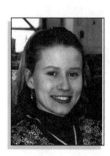 look for a staff nurse job right away; my daughter must have hip surgery. I'll be her personal nurse for six weeks, so I can't start work until she's well enough to go back to school. In the meantime, I'm working part-time as a research assistant in an outpatient oncology clinic where I study the late effects of cancer. Needless to say, I'm on a very tight budget.

In spite of the grant, the job and my determination to succeed, I continue to feel burdened about managing my finances. Even if I get a job right out of graduate school, I'll probably have to work nights, because often nurses must earn the day shifts. Working nights means I'll have to pay someone to take care of my daughter. Of course, I can try to get a job at an outpatient clinic with daytime hours, but I've heard those don't pay as well as hospital nursing positions. On top of all this, I'll have student loans to pay off. Sometimes I wonder if I'll ever get out of debt. How can I create a financial plan so that my daughter and I have a secure future?

DR. ROY ANN SHERROD

Assistant to the President, Professor of Nursing,
The University of Alabama, Tuscaloosa, Alabama

First, let me congratulate you for achieving so much already. At my campus, we frequently see college students in terribly stressful predicaments like yours. The good news is you have many options. Networking is one of these options. I suggest that you intentionally network to help provide for your various needs: 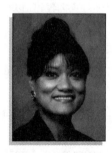 assistance with child care; emotional and spiritual support; and financial backing.

With so much going on in your life, you need the support of caring relationships. Cultivating adult companionship, so that you are interacting with people other than your child, can help you feel more connected to your new residence. Furthermore, we all need nurturing and replenishing, and close relationships can provide that.

There are many areas of funding and support for you to consider. One that is often overlooked by students is the local church. Churches often have scholarship programs for members and nonmembers of their congregations. Some churches also provide ministries for single parents, as well as other spiritually enriching outlets.

Professional nursing associations, such as the national association of nurse practitioners, usually offer scholarships and loans. The American Nurses Association is a good place to start your search because they offer several programs, especially for nurses that are seeking advanced degrees. Check with local associations first because they can provide information and contacts for support, both locally and nationally.

Another potential funding source is health care institutions, such as hospitals and clinics. They may present conditional scholarship programs that pay your tuition and some expenses, if you agree to work for them for a period of time upon graduation. Of course, if you decide you don't want to work for them, you must pay the money back.

There are also local women's groups that offer scholarships, and they do not limit themselves to one professional area.

I applaud the letter you wrote to the administrator at your school. Now, make an appointment with a counselor in the student services office within your graduate program. These people are aware of sources of funding that are specific to nurses, whereas your financial aid counselor might not be.

To help make ends meets, you might want to consider a roommate. You can arrange for this person to share housing expenses and/or barter some of the rent in exchange for child care. A roommate might also help you feel more supported than living alone. Obviously, you would want to be very careful about whom you choose, especially since you have a daughter.

With regard to your graduate program requirement of working nine months, investigate what is meant by that time frame. How many hours per week does that translate into? Their definition of "nine months" may not be as unmanageable as it sounds. In addition, many universities have student counseling centers to help you cope with the stress you're feeling. Perhaps you would find that useful as well.

Add your own suggestions here!

_____

_____

_____

_____

_____

You can also maximize savings and minimize spending by using credit cards wisely.

Managing Credit Cards

Most credit comes in the form of a powerful little plastic card. Credit card companies often solicit students on campus or through the mail. When choosing a card, pay attention to the *annual fee* and *interest rates*, the two ways in which a credit card company makes money from you. Some cards have no annual fee; others may charge a flat rate of $10 to $70 per year. Interest rates can be fixed or variable. A variable rate of 12 percent may shoot up to 18 percent when the economy slows down. You might be better off with a mid-range fixed rate that will always stay the same.

Following are some potential effects of using credit.

Positive Effects

Establishing a good credit history. If you use your credit card moderately and pay your bills on time, you will make a positive impression on your creditors. Your *credit history* (the record of your credit use, including positive actions such as paying on time and negative actions such as going over your credit limit) and *credit rating* (the score you are given based on your history) can make or break your ability to take out a loan or mortgage. How promptly you make loan payments and pay mortgage and utility bills affects your credit rating as well. Certain companies track your credit history and give you a credit rating. Banks or potential employers will contact these companies to see if you are a good credit risk.

Emergencies. Few people carry enough cash to handle unexpected expenses. Your credit card can help you in emergency situations such as when your car needs to be towed or your bike gets a flat.

Record of purchases. Credit card statements give you a monthly record of purchases made, where they were made, and exactly how much was paid. Using your credit card for purchases that you want to track, such as work expenses, can help you keep records for tax purposes.

Negative Effects

Credit can be addictive. Credit can be like a drug, seeming fun because the pain of paying is put off until later. If you get hooked, though, you can wind up thousands of dollars in debt to creditors. The high interest will enlarge your debt; your credit rating may fall, potentially hurting your eligibility for loans and mortgages; and you may lose your credit cards altogether.

Credit spending can be hard to monitor. Paying by credit can seem so easy that you don't realize how much you are spending. When the bill comes at the end of the month, the total can hit you hard.

You are taking out a high-interest loan. Buying on credit is similar to taking out a loan—you are using money with the promise to pay it back. Loan rates, however, especially on fixed-interest loans, are often much lower than the 11 to 23 percent on credit card debt. Fifteen percent interest per year on a credit card debt averaging $2000 is approximately $300; 5 percent interest per year on a loan in the same amount is $100.

Bad credit ratings can haunt you. Any time you are late with a payment, default on a payment, or in any way misuse your card, a record of that occurrence will be entered on your credit history, lowering your credit rating. If a prospective employer or loan officer discovers a low rating, you will seem less trustworthy and may lose the chance at a job or a loan.

Managing Credit Card Debt

There are ways to manage credit card debt so that it doesn't get worse. Stay in control by having only one or two cards and paying bills regularly and on time. Try to pay in full each month. If you can't, at least pay the minimum. Make as much of a dent in the bill as you can.

If you get into trouble, three steps will help you deal with the situation. First, *admit* that you made a mistake, even though you may be embarrassed. Then, *address* the problem immediately and honestly in order to minimize the damages. Call the bank or credit card company to talk to someone about the problem. They may draw up a payment plan that allows you to pay your debt gradually, in amounts that your budget can manage. Creditors would rather accept small payments than nothing at all.

Finally, *prevent* this problem from happening again. Figure out what got you into trouble and take steps to avoid it in the future if you can. Some financial disasters, such as medical emergencies, may be beyond your control.

TERMS

Creditors
People to whom debts are owed, usually money.

"Put not your trust in money, but put your money in trust."

OLIVER WENDELL HOLMES

Overspending on luxuries, however, is something you have the power to avoid. Make a habit of balancing your checkbook. Cut up a credit card or two if you have too many. Don't let a high credit limit tempt you to spend. Pay every month, even if you pay only the minimum. If you work to clean up your act, your credit history will gradually clean up as well.

Sacrifici

In Italy, parents often use the term *sacrifici*, meaning "sacrifices," to refer to tough choices that they make in order to improve the lives of their children and family members. They may sacrifice a larger home so that they can afford to pay for their children's sports and after-school activities. They may sacrifice a higher-paying job so that they can live close to where they work. They give up something in exchange for something else that they have decided is more important to them.

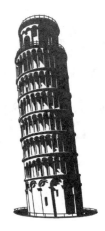

Think of the concept of *sacrifici* as you analyze the sacrifices you can make in order to get out of debt, reach your savings goals, and prepare for a career that you find satisfying. Many of the short-term sacrifices you are making today will help you do and have what you want in the future. Keep that notion as a light to guide you through the ups and downs of student life.

Applications   Chapter 11

KEY INTO YOUR LIFE
Opportunities to Apply What You Learn

 Mentors

First, consider the people you go to with problems and questions, people whom you trust and with whom you share a lot of yourself. Name up to three—don't fill the list unless you can really think of three people you trust.

1. _____
2. _____
3. _____

Evaluate your list. With which of those people do you feel you could have a mentoring relationship? Name up to two; for each, name two steps you can take to invest even further in your relationship.

1. _____

_____

2. _____

_____

 Your Job Priorities

What kind of a job could you manage while you're in school? How would you want a job to benefit you? Discuss your requirements in each of the following areas.

Salary/wage level _____

Time of day _____

Hours per week (part-time vs. full-time) _____

Duties _____

Location _____

Flexibility_____

Affiliation with school or financial aid program _____

What kind of job might fit all or most of your requirements? List two possibilities here.

1. _____

2. _____

 Savings Brainstorm

As a class, brainstorm areas that require financial management (such as funding an education, running a household, or putting savings away for the future) and write them on the board. Divide into small groups. Each group should choose one area to discuss (make sure all areas are chosen). In your group, brainstorm strategies that can help with the area you have chosen. Think of savings ideas, ways to control spending, ways to earn more money, and any other methods of relieving financial stress. Agree on a list of possible ideas for your area, and share it with the class.

KEY TO SELF-EXPRESSION
Discovery Through Journal Writing

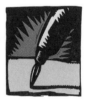

To record your thoughts, use a separate journal or the lined page at the end of the chapter.

Credit Cards

Describe how you use credit cards. Are you conservative, overindulgent, or in between? Do you pay on time, and do you pay the full balance of the card, or not? How does using a credit card make you feel—powerful, excited, apprehensive, or nervous? For what sort of purchases do you use credit cards? If you would like to change how you use credit, discuss any changes you want to make and how they would help you.

Name _____ Date _____

12

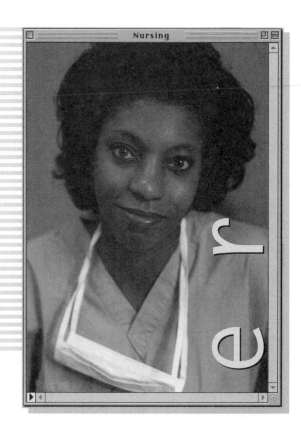

Nursing

Moving Ahead

Building a Smart Future

The end of one path can be the beginning of another. For example, graduation is often referred to as commencement, because the end of your student career is the beginning or renewal of your life as a working citizen. As you come to the end of your work in this course, you have built up a wealth of knowledge. Now you have more power to make decisions about what directions you want your studies, your career, and your personal growth to take.

This chapter will explore how to manage the constant change you will encounter. Developing your flexibility will enable you to adjust goals, make the most of successes, and work through failures. You will consider what is important about giving back to your community and continuing to learn throughout your life. Finally, you will revisit your personal mission, exploring how to revise it as you encounter changes in the future.

In this chapter, you will explore answers to the following questions:

- What are some of the big questions in nursing today?

- How can you live with change?

- What will help you handle success and failure?

- Why give back to the community and the world?

- Why is college just the beginning of lifelong learning?

- How can you live your mission?

WHAT ARE SOME OF THE BIG QUESTIONS IN NURSING TODAY?

Biotechnology and genetics are examples of the rapid changes occurring in the health sciences today. The Human Genome Project, an international effort launched in 1989, plans to map the entire human genome by the year 2005. But genetic innovations have been used in health care for years; examples include the production of insulin, human hemoglobin produced in pigs, and Factor IX for hemophilia in sheep's milk. Newer innovations include genetic disease treatment, or gene therapy, which places a fully functioning gene into cells to replace, or augment, the function of a defective gene. At this time gene therapy is primarily experimental, but that will soon change as techniques are improved and tested.

Questions about the use of new technology and discoveries arise in all areas of the health science. Genetics is a good example of how questions concern not only researchers but citizens as well. For instance, gene therapy that affects only somatic cells, body cells that are not involved in reproduction, will not affect future generations. On the other hand, gene therapy performed on germ cells, the cells of reproduction, alters the genes so that these changes are passed on to future generations. This raises many important questions concerning the desirability of permanently altering the human gene pool. Most geneticists currently agree that germ cell therapy is not advisable.

More recently, the use of stem cells from nonviable fetuses has been discussed. These cells have the possibility of regenerating human tissue. For example, experiments are being done with stem cells to see if they could be used in humans to grow arterial bypasses in the heart. If this works, many cardiac surgeries and invasive procedures would become unnecessary. This potential life- and cost-saving therapy raises ethical concerns for some people. Implications of research must be understood by researchers and nonresearchers or potentially breakthrough work may be overlooked and underfunded due to decisions based on uninformed reactions. Likewise, ethical issues must be equally considered.

Ethical Implications

As a nurse you will become familiar with ethical dilemmas. For instance, in genetics the ability to test for the predisposition to diseases may pose a risk to confidentiality and privacy. Discrimination based on genetic test results could be grounds for denial of employment or insurance, although the Americans with Disabilities Act may offer protection. People will need to be educated on test results and the possible consequences of releasing them.

The ability to perform gene therapy raises many ethical questions. "Disorder," "defect," "error," and "mutation" are words we often use when discussing genetic variations. They clearly imply failure. Will we become legally or morally bound to fix everything with gene therapy?

Genetics, along with many other areas of research, offers great opportunities to learn more about human physiology, disease, and the world around us. But this new knowledge must be thought about critically. It is vitally important that you, as a nursing major, take at least one ethics course.

Other questions nurses deal with in everyday practice include:

Emerging infectious diseases. How will their spread be curtailed? How are they best treated?

Proposed cuts in Medicare and Medicaid. Is it necessary to cut health benefits to the most vulnerable members of the population?

Safety issues such as gun control, protection of nurses from needle sticks, latex allergies, and workplace violence. Nursing and safety, along with nursing and care, are synonymous. How can nurses use this expertise to promote important legislation and education?

Life-and-death issues such as abortion, organ transplantation, assisted suicide or assisted dying, termination of life sustaining treatments, foods, or fluids. On a day-to-day, person-to-person basis, how are ethical decisions made that coincide with an individual's and society's values? Is it appropriate to keep a person alive at any cost? How are health care resources best used?

AIDS. Is research funding utilized to its fullest to battle the AIDS epidemic? What biases may interfere with research funding and care of AIDS patients?

Nursing's Agenda for Health Care Reform covers many of these issues and the full text can be found on the American Nurses Association's website: www.nursingworld.org/readroom/magenda.htm. The main points that nurses are promoting include the following:

Shifting the predominant focus on illness and cure to an orientation toward wellness and care. Millions of Americans lack access to even the most elementary services. Many people receive needed treatments too late because they live in areas, urban and rural, where service is inadequate. People come to the hospital with illnesses that are advanced and could have been better treated, and for less, if caught earlier using health promotion and prevention measures. A lack of preventative measures such as prenatal care means a high number of infant deaths each year. An unequal amount of health care funds are also used for expensive medical interventions that provide neither cure nor care.

Nurses, as caregivers in many different types of situations, are responsible for coordinating care, providing disease prevention and health promotion measures 24 hours a day. As members of the largest health care profession, nurses are acutely aware of the health system's shortcomings. Nurses strongly support access to services by all, keeping costs down, and most of all, ensuring quality.

Nurses also support managed care when it provides quality, access to effective treatments, cost containment, and case management. Case management is not the same as managed care, but part of it. Nurse case managers integrate and coordinate services to prevent overuse of hospitals, to keep people healthy, and to advocate for those in need.

> "Nothing causes as much destruction, misery, and death as obsession with a truth believed to be absolute. Every crime in history is the product of some fanaticism. Every massacre is performed in the name of virtue; in the name of legitimate nationalism, a true religion, a just ideology, the fight against Satan."
>
> FRANÇOIS JACOB

Something to Prove: Does the Truth Exist?

Ask yourself these questions: Is there an absolute truth? Who decides what is true and what is not true? Remember when you consider these questions that some people think there is evidence that the position of the stars at the time of their birth determines their future; others that the Christian Bible holds literal truths; and still others believe that women and girls do not need an education. How can you decide on the perplexing issues in nursing science? Can you decide what is the right thing for everyone?

Nursing Is Complex

Thinking about these tough questions, and others like them, will help you understand how nursing is also a philosophical, spiritual, social, and political pursuit. The more you understand these areas, along with science, the better off you'll be in planning and making decisions that affect you, your family, and your local and global communities. A thorough background in the sciences and in the liberal arts is a necessity in nursing and will help you in any career you choose. Big questions about truth and decisions based on values occur everywhere and they will occur throughout your lifetime.

Scientific Discoveries and Truth

Scientific discovery has been described as similar to peeling an onion. This analogy is based on the premise that there exists absolute truth and that each discovery removes a layer of the onion, bringing us one step closer to this truth. The assumption that a single truth exists is questioned by scientists who view scientific discovery not as seeking or finding an absolute truth but as adding to the body of knowledge about a subject. This body of knowledge then lends support to certain ideas, or hypotheses, creating theories. The more evidence there is for a theory, the stronger that theory is. Rarely are the words *truth* or *proof* used in nursing theories except in the context of philosophical or personal views and values.

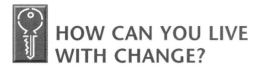

HOW CAN YOU LIVE WITH CHANGE?

Even the most carefully constructed plans can be turned upside down by change. In this section, you will explore some ways to make change a manageable part of your life by accepting the reality of change, maintaining flexibility, and adjusting your goals.

Accept the Reality of Change

As Russian-born author Isaac Asimov once said, "It is change, continuing change, inevitable change, that is the dominant factor in society today. No sensible decision can be made any longer without taking into account not only the world as it is, but the world as it will be."[5] Change is a sure thing.

Maintain Flexibility

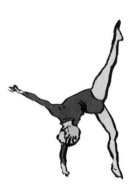

The fear of change is as inevitable as change itself. When you become comfortable with something, you tend to want it to stay the way it is, whether it is a relationship, a place you live, a job, a schedule, or the racial/cultural mix of people with whom you interact. Change may seem to have only negative effects, and consistency only positive effects. Think about your life right now. What do you wish would always stay the same? What changes have upset you and thrown you off balance?

You may have encountered any number of changes in your life to date, many of them unexpected. You may have experienced ups and downs in relationships, perhaps marriage or divorce. You may have changed schools, changed jobs, or moved to a new home. You may have shifted your course of study. You may have added to your family or lost family members. Financial shifts may have caused you to change the way you live. All of these changes, whether you perceive them as good or bad, cause a certain level of stress. They also cause a shift in your personal needs, which may lead to changing priorities.

Change Brings Different Needs

Your needs can change from day to day, year to year, and situation to situation. Although you may know about some changes ahead of time, such as when you plan to attend school or move in together with a partner, others may take you completely by surprise, such as losing a job, illness, or an unexpected pregnancy. Even the different times of year bring different needs, such as a need for extra cash around the holidays or a need for additional child care when your children are home for the summer.

Some changes that shift your needs will occur within a week or even a day. For example, an instructor may inform you that you have a quiz or extra assignment at the end of the week, or your supervisor at work may give you an additional goal for the week. During the course of a day, your daughter might tell you that she needs you to drive her somewhere that evening, or a friend may call and need your help with something that has come up suddenly. Table 12-1 below shows how the effects of certain changes can lead to new priorities.

Flexibility vs. Inflexibility

When change affects your needs, *flexibility* will help you shift your priorities so that you address those needs. You can react to change with either inflexibility or flexibility, each with its resulting effects.

Inflexibility. Not acknowledging a shift in needs can cause trouble. For example, if you lose your job and continue to spend as much money as you

---

TABLE 12-1	Change produces new priorities.

CHANGE	EFFECTS AND CHANGED NEEDS	NEW PRIORITIES
Lost job	Loss of income; need for others in your household to contribute more income	Job hunting; reduction in your spending; additional training or education in order to qualify for a different job
New job	Change in daily/weekly schedule; need for increased contribution of household help from others	Time and energy commitment to new job; maintaining confidence; learning new skills
Started school	Fewer hours for work, family, and personal time; responsibility for classwork; need to plan semesters ahead of time	Careful scheduling; making sure you have time to attend class and study adequately; strategic planning of classes and of career goals
Relationship/marriage	Responsibility toward your partner; merging of your schedules and perhaps your finances and belongings	Time and energy commitment to relationship
Breakup/divorce	Change in responsibility for any children; increased responsibility for your own finances; possibly a need to relocate; increased independence	Making time for yourself; gathering support from friends and family; securing your finances; making sure you have your own income
Bought car	Responsibility for monthly payment; responsibility for upkeep	Regular income so that you can make payments on time; time and money for upkeep
New baby	Increased parenting responsibility; need money to pay for baby or if you had to stop working; need help with other children	Child care; flexible employment; increased commitment from a partner or other supporter
New cultural environment (from new home, job, or school)	Exposure to unfamiliar people and traditions; tendency to keep to yourself	Learning about the culture with which you are now interacting; openness to new relationships

did before, ignoring your need to live more modestly, you can drive yourself into debt and make the situation worse. Or if you continue to spend little time with a partner who has expressed a need for more contact, you may lose your relationship.

Flexibility. Being flexible means acknowledging the change, examining your different needs, and addressing them in any way you can. As frightening as it can be, being flexible can help you move ahead. Discovering what change brings may help you uncover positive effects that you had no idea were there. For example, a painful breakup or divorce can lead you to discover greater capability and independence. A loss of a job can give you a chance to reevaluate your abilities and look for another job in an area that suits you better. An illness can give you perspective on what you truly value in life. In other words, a crisis can spur opportunity; you may learn that you want to adjust your goals in order to pursue that opportunity.

Sometimes you may need to resist for a while, until you are ready to face an important change. When you do decide you are ready, being flexible will help you cope with the negative effects and benefit from the positive effects.

Adjust Your Goals

Your changing life will often result in the need to adjust goals accordingly. Sometimes goals must change because they weren't appropriate in the first place. Some turn out to be unreachable; some may not pose enough of a challenge; others may be unhealthy for the person who set them or harmful to others.

Step One: Reevaluate

Before making adjustments in response to change, take time to *reevaluate* both your goals and your progress toward them.

Your goals. First, determine whether your goals still fit the person you have become in the past week, month, or year. Circumstances can change quickly. For example, an unexpected pregnancy might cause a female student to rethink her educational goals.

Your progress. If you feel you haven't gotten far, determine whether the goal is out of your range or simply requires more stamina than you had anticipated. As you work toward any goal, you will experience alternating periods of progress and stagnation. Sticking with a tough goal may be the hardest thing you'll ever do, but the payoff may be worth it. Seek the support and perspective of a friend or counselor as you evaluate your progress.

Step Two: Modify

If after your best efforts it becomes clear that a goal is out of reach, *modifying* your goal may bring success. Perhaps the goal doesn't suit you. For example, an active, interpersonal learner might become frustrated while pursuing a detail-oriented, sedentary career such as computer engineering.

"Risk! Risk anything! Care no more for the opinion of others, for those voices. Do the hardest thing on earth for you. Act for yourself. Face the truth."

KATHERINE MANSFIELD

Based on your reevaluation, you can modify a goal in two ways:

1. Adjust the existing goal. To adjust a goal, change one or more aspects that define that goal—for example, the time frame, the due dates, or the specifics of the expectations. For example, a woman with an unexpected pregnancy could adjust her educational due date, taking an extra year or two to complete her course work. She could also adjust the time frame, taking classes at night if she had to care for her child during the day.

2. Replace it with a different, more compatible goal. If you find that you just can't handle a particular goal, try to find another that makes more sense for you at this time. For example, a couple who wants to buy a home but just can't afford it can choose to work toward the goal of making improvements to their current living space. Because you and your circumstances never stop changing, your goals should keep up with those changes.

Being open to adjusting your goals will help you manage both failure and success along the way.

 ## WHAT WILL HELP YOU HANDLE SUCCESS AND FAILURE?

The perfect, trouble-free life is only a myth. The most wonderful, challenging, fulfilling life is full of problems and difficult decisions. If you want to handle the bumps and bruises without losing yourself, you should prepare to encounter setbacks along with your successes.

Dealing with Failure

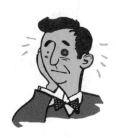

Things don't always go the way you want them to go. Sometimes you may come up against obstacles that are difficult to overcome. Sometimes you will let yourself down or disappoint others. You may make mistakes or lose your motivation. All people do, no matter who they are or how smart or accomplished they may be. What is important is how you choose to deal with what goes wrong. If you can arrive at reasonable definitions of failure and success, accept failure as part of being human, and examine failure so that you can learn from it, you will have the confidence to pick yourself up and keep improving.

Measuring Failure and Success

Most people measure failure by comparing where they are to where they believe they should be. Since individual circumstances vary widely, so do definitions of failure. What you consider a failure may seem like a positive step for someone else. Here are some examples:

- Imagine that your native language is Spanish. You have learned to speak English well, but you still have trouble writing it. Making writing mistakes may seem like failure to you, but to a recent immigrant from the Dominican Republic who knows limited English, your command of the language will seem like a success story.

- If two people apply for internships, one may see failure as receiving some offers but not the favorite one, while someone who was turned down may see any offer as a success.

- Having a job that doesn't pay you as much as you want may seem like a failure, but to someone who is having trouble finding any job, your job is a definite success.

Accepting Failure

No one escapes failure, no matter how hard he or she may try (or how successful he or she may be at hiding mistakes). The most successful people and organizations have experienced failures and mistakes. For example, the producers of the film *Waterworld* spent over $140 million on a film that made only a fraction of that cost at the box office. America Online miscalculated customer use and offered a flat rate per month, resulting in thousands of customers' having trouble logging on to the service. Many an otherwise successful individual has had a problematic relationship, a substance abuse problem, or a failing grade in a course.

You have choices when deciding how to view a failure or mistake. You can pretend it never happened, blame it on someone or something else, blame yourself, or forgive yourself.

Pretending it didn't happen. Avoiding the pain of dealing with a failure can deny you valuable lessons and could even create more serious problems. HIV is one example of this idea. Imagine that a person has unprotected sex with a potentially HIV-infected partner and then denies it ever happened. If that person later discovers that he or she has contracted HIV from the first partner, the deadly virus may have been passed on to any subsequent partners.

Blaming others. Putting the responsibility on someone else stifles opportunities to learn and grow. For example, imagine that an unprepared and inappropriately dressed person interviews for a job and is not hired. If he or she decides without clear evidence that the interviewer is biased, the interviewee won't learn to improve preparation or interview strategies. Evaluate causes carefully and try not to assign blame.

Blaming yourself. Getting angry at yourself for failing, or believing that you should be perfect, can only result in your feeling incapable of success and perhaps becoming afraid to try. Negative self-talk can become self-fulfilling and will hinder your growth as a nursing professional.

Forgiving yourself. This is by far the best way to cope. First, although you should always strive for your best, don't expect perfection of yourself or anyone else. Expect that you will do the best that you can within the circumstances of your life. Just getting through another day as a student, employee, and/or parent is an important success. Second, forgive yourself when you fail. Your value as a human being does not diminish when you make

"There are three great forms of service open to American nurses today...We must have nurses for teachers... We must have nurses for our wounded men in France...and we must maintain our home defense."
MARY BEARD, RN, 1918

a mistake. Forgiving yourself will give you more strength to learn from the experience, move on, and try again.

Once you are able to approach failure and mistakes in a productive way, you can explore what you can learn from them.

Learning from Failure

Learning from your failures and mistakes involves reflecting and thinking critically through what happened. The first step is to evaluate what happened and decide if it was within your control. It could have had nothing to do with you at all. You could have failed to win a job because someone else with equal qualifications was in line for it ahead of you. A family crisis that disrupted your sleep could have affected your studying, resulting in a failing grade on a test. These are unfortunate circumstances, but they are not failures. On the other hand, something you did or didn't do may have contributed to the failure.

If you decide that you have made a mistake, your next steps are to analyze the causes and effects of what happened, make any improvements that you can, and decide how to change your action or approach in the future.

For example, imagine that after a long night of studying, you forgot your part-time work-study commitment the next day.

Analyze causes and effects. *Causes:* Your exhaustion and your concern about your test caused you to forget to check on your work schedule. *Effects:* Because you weren't there, a crucial curriculum project wasn't completed. An entire class and instructor who needed the project have been affected by your mistake.

Make any possible improvements on the situation. Apologize to the instructor and see if there is still a chance to finish up part of the work that day.

Make changes for the future. You could set a goal to note your work schedule regularly in your date book—maybe in a bright color—and to check it more often. You could also arrange your future study schedule so that you will be less exhausted.

Think about the people you consider exceptionally successful. They didn't rise to the top without taking risks and making their share of mistakes. They have built much of their success upon their willingness to recognize and learn from their shortfalls. You too can benefit from staying open to this kind of active, demanding, hard-won education. Learning involves change and growth. Let what you learn from falling short of your goals inspire new and better ideas.

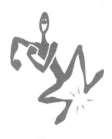

Think Positively About Failure

When you feel you have failed, how can you boost your outlook?

Stay aware of the fact that you are a capable, valuable person. People often react to failure by becoming convinced that they are incapable and incompetent. Fight that tendency by reminding yourself of your successes, focusing your energy on your best abilities, and knowing that you have the strength to try again. Realize that your failure isn't a setback as long as you learn from it and rededicate yourself to excellence. Remember that the energy you might expend on talking down to yourself would be better spent on trying again and moving ahead.

Share your thoughts and disappointment with others. Everybody fails. Trading stories will help you realize you're not alone. People refrain from talking about failures out of embarrassment, often feeling as though no one else could have made as big a mistake as they did. When you open up, though, you may be surprised to hear others exchange stories that rival your own. Be careful not to get caught in a destructive cycle of complaining. Instead, focus on the kind of creative energy that can help you find ways to learn from your failures.

Look on the bright side. At worst, you at least have learned a lesson that will help you avoid similar situations in the future. At best, there may be some positive results of what happened. If your romance flounders, the extra study time you suddenly have may help you boost your grades. If you fail a class, you may discover that you need to focus on a different subject that suits you better. What you learn from a failure may, in an unexpected way, bring you around to where you want to be.

Dealing with Success

Success isn't reserved for the wealthy, famous people you see glamorized in magazines and newspapers. Success isn't money or fame; success is being who you want to be and doing what you want to do. Success is within your reach.

Pay attention to the small things when measuring success. You may not feel successful until you reach an important goal you have set for yourself. However, along the way each step is a success. When you are trying to drop a harmful habit, each time you stay on course is a success. When you are juggling work, school, and personal life, just coping with what every new day brings equals success. If you received a C on a paper and then earned a B on the next one, your advancement is successful.

Remember that success is a process. If you deny yourself the label of "success" until you reach the top of where you want to be, you will have a much harder time getting there. Just moving ahead toward improvement and growth, however fast or slow the movement, equals success.

Here are some techniques to handle your successes.

First, appreciate yourself. Take time to appreciate yourself for a job well done—whether it be a good grade, an important step in learning a new language, a job offer, a promotion or graduation, or a personal victory over substance abuse. Bask in the glow a bit. Everybody hears about his or her mistakes, but people don't praise themselves (or each other) enough when success happens. Praise can give you a terrific vote of confidence.

Take that confidence on the road. This victory can lead to others. Based on this success, you may be expected to prove to yourself and others that you are

ROBERT DARY

Senior, University of Kansas, Kansas City, Kansas

I'm an ex-police officer who served on the force for eight years in a suburb of Kansas City. One of my responsibilities at that time was to investigate car accidents. This meant some of my work hours were spent at the local hospital. I've also given CPR while on duty. Of course, I got great satisfaction from knowing I helped save someone's life. After I got hurt on the job, I began to think about pursuing a new career and nursing became the obvious choice for me.

What drives me to be a nurse is that I'm making a difference in the life of a patient. I feel very comfortable working in ICU because I can get to know the patient and their families. Having someone you love in ICU can be a very traumatic experience. I find it gratifying to interact with the patient's family. By explaining the purpose of medical procedures and how different hospital equipment works, I help them understand what's going on with the patient.

Working toward a bachelor's degree is a real stretch for me. I've been forced to think in more creative ways. Back when I was in high school, learning seemed less complicated. I memorized the facts and regurgitated what I knew. In nursing, learning requires more than memorization. There's so much material to absorb that I've needed to understand how each component relates to the whole. I know

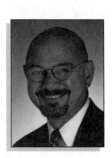

I'll need to continue learning long after graduation. Advances in technology cause procedures to change, and I'm also interested in learning more about pathophysiological processes. The idea of continuing to re-educate myself excites me.

Thinking about my future also raises another core issue of nursing. I'm deeply concerned about some of the ethical situations that affect a nurse, specifically, quality of life. I've seen patients come out of ICU who were on feeding tubes, and they are still ventilator dependent. Their survival depends on the machine. Sometimes I think technology takes away the natural process of dying, and I wonder if in my future career I'll be setting up some of my patients for poorer quality of life. Other than my brief exposure to Hospice, I've seen very little educational material that addresses death and dying. Can you offer suggestions for helping me come to terms with these tough issues as they relate to my future career?

DR. COURTNEY H. LYDER

Yale School of Nursing, New Haven, Connecticut

You raised very thoughtful issues about the profession of nursing. With regard to continuing

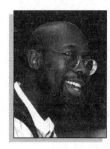

education, I think we have an inherent accountability both to our patients and to their families to expand our knowledge and clinical skills. Given the advances in health care technology, the methods by which we deliver nursing care could radically change, therefore, it is imperative that you keep up to date with the latest technology and effective care modalities based on nursing research.

One of the best things I ever did to continue my education was a brief study abroad program in England. In this course we compared the British system of psychiatric nursing care to the American model. This course gave me a different perspective, and I changed some of my nursing practices because of this experience. Sometimes the best learning isn't confined to the classroom; it happens experientially. Perhaps you can volunteer in a cultural setting different from what you are accustomed to or take a nontraditional course.

One of the most difficult challenges for critical care nurses is patients who are facing the end of life. You will definitely confront this issue again and again as a critical care nurse. Historically, the nursing profession has focused on maintaining or enhancing the quality of life for patients, as well as, helping the families adjust to the changes that chronic and acute illness brings. I can't point you to any one seminal piece of literature or strategy for grappling with this complex issue. However, I can tell you that coming to terms with dying patients is a process, as you move from being a novice to an expert. Several years ago I was an MICU nurse, and it became clear to me that I had to depend on the expertise of the senior nurses. I tapped their brains for help in dealing with my thoughts and feelings related to caring for patients with poor prognostic outcomes.

Palliative care is a type of nursing which deals with end-of-life issues, and the goal of your nursing care may change depending on whether the patient's condition is chronic or acute. There are courses you can take in palliative care which address death and dying. As you know, the goal of Hospice isn't cure, but to provide the best comfort for the patient. Nevertheless, you can have palliative care in the critical care area as well.

I have never felt more like a nurse than when I am helping a patient die peacefully. Nurses, unlike physicians, are with the patient around the clock. Being able to tell patients that you are there for them and that they will not die alone can help make death less frightening for them. My earlier experience as an MICU nurse taught me that death and dying were mechanical and technical processes. When I chose geriatric nursing, which is my current specialty, I began to see death as a more natural, even beautiful process. One of the wonderful things I've learned from caring for our elders is that they can teach us how to live.

capable of growth, of continuing your successes and building upon them. Show yourself and others that the confidence is well founded.

Stay sensitive to others. There could be people around you who may not have been so successful. Remember that you have been in their place, and they in yours, and the positions may change many times over in the future. Enjoy what you have, work to build on it and not to take it for granted, and support others as they need it.

Staying sensitive to others is an important goal always, whether you are feeling successful or less than successful. Giving what you can of your time, energy, and resources to the community and the world is part of being aware of what others need. Your contributions can help to bring success to others.

 ## WHY GIVE BACK TO THE COMMUNITY AND THE WORLD?

Everyday life is demanding. You can become so caught up in the issues of your own life that you neglect to look outside your immediate needs. However, from time to time you will realize that your mission extends beyond your personal life. You have spent time in this course working to improve yourself. Now that you've come so far, why not extend some of that energy and effort to the world outside? With all that you have to offer, you have the power to make positive differences in the lives of others. Every effort you make, no matter how small, improves the world.

Your Imprint on the World

As difficult as your life can sometimes seem, looking outside yourself and into the lives of others can help put everything in perspective. Sometimes you can evaluate your own hardships more reasonably when you look at them in light of what is happening elsewhere in the world. There are always many people in the world in great need. You have something to give to others. Making a lasting difference in the lives of others is something to be proud of and a nursing career can help you do just that!

Your perspective may change after working at a homeless shelter. Your appreciation of those close to you may increase after you spend time with cancer patients at the local hospice. Your perspective on your living situation may change after you help people improve their housing conditions by working for Habitat for Humanity.

If you could eavesdrop on someone *talking about you* to another person, what do you think you would hear? How would you like to hear yourself described? What you do for others makes an imprint that can have far more impact than you may imagine. Giving one person hope, comfort, or help can improve his or her ability to cope with life's changes. That person in turn may be able to offer help to someone else. As each person makes a contribution, a cycle of positive effects is generated. For example, Helen Keller, blind and deaf from the age of 2, was educated through the help of her teacher Annie Sullivan, and then spent much of her life lecturing to raise money for the teaching of the blind and deaf. Another example is Betty Ford, who was helped in her struggle with alcoholism and founded the Betty Ford Center to help others with addiction problems.

How can you make a difference? Many schools are realizing the importance of community involvement and have appointed committees to find and organize volunteering opportunities. Make some kind of volunteering activity a priority on your schedule. Join a group from your school that tutors at a school. Organize a group of students to clean, repair, or entertain at a nursing home or shelter. Look for what's available to you or create opportunities on your own. Table 12-2 lists organizations that provide volunteering opportunities; you might also look into more local efforts or private clearinghouses that set up a number of different smaller projects.

Volunteerism is also getting a great deal of attention on the national level. The government has made an effort to stress the importance of community service as part of what it means to be a good citizen, and it provides support for that effort through AmeriCorps. AmeriCorps provides financial awards for education in return for community service work. If you work for AmeriCorps, you can use the funds you receive to pay current tuition expenses or repay student loans. You may work either before, during, or after your college education. You can find more information on AmeriCorps by contacting this organization: www.Americorps.org.

The Corporation for National and Community Service
1201 New York Avenue, NW
Washington, D. C. 20525
1-800-942-2677

Sometimes it's hard to find time when so many responsibilities compete for your attention. One solution is to combine activities. Get exercise while cleaning a park or bring the whole family to sing at a nursing home on a weekend afternoon. Whatever you do, your actions will have a ripple effect, creating a positive impact for those you help and those they encounter in turn. The strength often found in people surviving difficult circumstances can strengthen you as well.

Valuing Your Environment

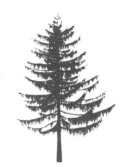

Your environment is your home. When you value it, you help to maintain a clean, safe, and healthy place to live. What you do every day has an impact on others around you and on the future. One famous slogan says that if you are not part of the solution, you are part of the problem. Every saved bottle, environmentally aware child, and reused bag is part of the solution. Take responsibility for what you can control—your own habits—and develop sound practices that contribute to the health of the environment.

Recycle anything that you can. What can be recycled varies with the system set up in your area. You may be able to recycle any combination of plastics, aluminum, glass, newspapers, and magazines. Products that make use of recycled materials are often more expensive, but if they are within your price range, try to reward the company's dedication by purchasing the products. Avoid buying products with lots of packaging and shop at a food store where you can refill your own containers.

Trade and reuse items. When your children have outgrown their crib, baby clothes, and toys, give away whatever is still usable. Give clothing you don't wear to others who can use it. Organizations like the Salvation Army may pick up used items in your neighborhood on certain days or when you make arrangements with them. Wrap presents in newspapers and decorate with markers. Use your imagination—there are many, many items that you can reuse all around you.

Respect the outdoors. Participate in maintaining a healthy environment. Use products that reduce chemical waste. Pick up after yourself. Through volunteering, voicing your opinion, or making monetary donations, support

AIDS-related organizations	Kiwanis/Knights of Columbus/ Lions Club/Rotary	**TABLE 12-2**
American Red Cross	Libraries	Organizations that can use your help.
Amnesty International	Meals on Wheels	
Audubon Society	Nursing homes	
Battered women shelters	Planned Parenthood	
Big Brothers and Big Sisters	Schools	
Churches, synagogues, temples, and affiliated organizations such as the YMCA/YWCA or YMHA/YWHA	Scouting organizations	
Educational support organizations	Share Our Strength/other food donation organizations	
Environmental awareness/support organizations such as Greenpeace	Shelters and organizations supporting the homeless	
Hospitals	Sierra Club/World Wildlife Fund	
Hot lines		

the maintenance of parks and the preservation of natural undeveloped land. Be creative. One young woman planned a cleanup of a local lakeside area as the main group activity for the guests at her birthday party (she joined them, of course). Everyone benefits when each person takes responsibility for maintaining the fragile earth.

Remember that valuing yourself is the base for valuing all other things. Improving the earth is difficult unless you value yourself and think you deserve the best living environment possible. Valuing yourself will also help you understand why you deserve to enjoy the benefits of learning throughout your life.

 ## WHY IS COLLEGE JUST THE BEGINNING OF LIFELONG LEARNING?

Although it may sometimes feel more like a burden, being a student is a golden opportunity. As a student, you are able to focus on learning for a period of time, and your school focuses on you in return, helping you gain access to knowledge, resources, and experiences. Take advantage of the academic atmosphere by developing a habit of seeking out new learning opportunities. That habit will encourage you to continue your learning long after you have graduated, even in the face of the pressures of everyday life.

Learning brings change, and change causes growth. As you change and the world changes, new knowledge and ideas continually emerge. Absorb them so that you can propel yourself into the future. Visualize yourself as a student of life who learns something new every single day.

Here are some lifelong learning strategies that can encourage you to continually ask questions and explore new ideas.

Investigate new interests. When information and events catch your attention, take your interest one step further and find out more. If you are fascinated by politics on television, find out if your school has political clubs that you can explore. If a friend of yours starts to take yoga, try out a class with him. If you really like one portion of a particular class, see if there are other classes that focus on that specific topic. Turn the regretful, "I wish I had tried that," into the purposeful, "I'm going to do it."

Read books, newspapers, magazines, and other writings. Reading opens a world of new perspectives. Check out what's on the bestseller list at your bookstore. Ask your friends about books that have changed their lives. Stay on top of current change in your community, your state, your country, and the world by reading newspapers and magazines. A newspaper that has a broad scope, such as *The New York Times* or *Washington Post*, can be an education in itself. Explore religious literature, family letters, and Internet news groups and web pages. Keep something with you to read for those moments when you have nothing to do.

Spend time with interesting people. When you meet someone new who inspires you and makes you think, keep in touch. Have a potluck dinner party and invite one person or couple from each corner of your life—your family, your work, your school, a club to which you belong, your neighborhood. Sometimes, meet for reasons beyond just being social. Start a book club, a home-repair group, a play-reading club, a hiking group, or an investing group. Get to know people of different cultures and perspectives. Learn something new from each other.

Pursue improvement in your studies and in your career. When at school, take classes outside of your major if you have time. After graduation, continue your education in nursing and in the realm of general knowledge. Stay on top of ideas, developments, structural changes, and new technology in your field by seeking out continuing education courses. Take single courses at a local college or community learning center. Most hospitals or health care agencies offer additional on-the-job training or will pay for their employees to take courses that will improve their knowledge and skills. If your company doesn't, you may want to set a small part of your income aside as a "learning budget." When you apply for jobs, you may want to ask about what kind of professional training or education the company offers or supports.

TERMS

Continuing education
Courses that students can take without having to be part of a degree program.

Nurture a spiritual life. You can find spirituality in many places. You don't have to regularly attend a house of worship to be spiritual, although that may be an important part of your spiritual life. "A spiritual life of some kind is absolutely necessary for psychological 'health,'" says psychologist and author Thomas Moore in his book *The Care of the Soul*. "We live in a time of deep division, in which mind is separated from body and spirituality is at odds with materialism."[1] The words *soul* and *spirituality* hold different meaning for each individual. Decide what they mean to you. Whether you discover them in music, organized religion, friendship, nature, cooking, sports, or anything else, making them a priority in your life will help you find a greater sense of balance and meaning.

Experience what others create. Art is "an adventure of the mind" (Eugene Ionesco, playwright); "a means of knowing the world" (Angela Carter, author); something that "does not reproduce the visible; rather, it makes visible" (Paul Klee, painter); "a lie that makes us realize truth" (Pablo Picasso, painter); a revealer of "our most secret self" (Jean-Luc Godard, filmmaker). Through art you can discover new ideas and shed new light on old ones. Explore all kinds of art and focus on any forms that hold your interest. Seek out whatever moves you—music, visual arts, theater, photography, dance, domestic arts, performance art, film and television, poetry, prose, and more.

Make your own creations. Bring out the creative artist in you. Take a class in drawing, in pottery, or in quilting. Learn to play an instrument that you have always wanted to master. Write poems for your favorite people or stories to read to your kids. Invent a recipe. Design and build a set of shelves for your home. Create a memoir of your life. You are a creative being. Express yourself, and learn more about yourself, through art.

Lifelong learning is the master key that unlocks every door you will encounter on your journey. If you keep it firmly in your hand, you will discover worlds of knowledge—and a place for yourself within them. Studies are also showing that lifelong learning may increase your lifespan.

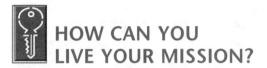

HOW CAN YOU LIVE YOUR MISSION?

As you learn and change, so may your life's mission. Whatever changes occur, your continued learning will give you a greater sense of security in your choices. Recall your mission statement from Chapter 4. Think about how it is changing as you learn and develop. It will continue to reflect your goals, values, and strengths if you live with integrity, roll with the changes that come your way, continue to observe the role models in your life, and work to achieve your personal best in all that you do.

Live With Integrity

Integrity
Adherence to a code of moral values; incorrupt-ibility, honesty.

You've spent a lot of time exploring who you are, how you learn, and what you value. Integrity is about being true to that picture you have drawn of yourself while also considering the needs of others. Living with integrity will bring you great personal and professional rewards.

Honesty and sincerity are at the heart of integrity. Many of the decisions you make and act upon in your life are based on your underlying sense of what is "the right thing to do." Having integrity puts that sense into day-to-day action.

The Marks of Integrity

A person of integrity lives by the following principles:

1. *Honest representation of yourself and your thoughts.* For example, you tell your partner when you are hurt over something that he or she did or didn't do.

2. *Sincerity in word and action.* You do what you say you will do. For example, you tell a coworker that you will finish a project when she has to leave early, and you follow through by completing the work.

3. *Consideration of the needs of others.* When making decisions, you take both your needs and the needs of others into account. You also avoid hurting others for the sake of your personal goals. For example, your sister cares for your elderly father in her home where he lives with her. You spend three nights a week with him so that she can take a course toward her degree.

The Benefits of Integrity

When you act with integrity, you earn trust and respect from yourself and from others. If people can trust you to be honest, to be sincere in what you say and do, and to consider the needs of others, they will be more likely to encourage you, support your goals, and reward your hard work. Integrity is a must for workplace success. To earn promotions, it helps to show that you have integrity in a variety of situations.

Think of situations in which a decision made with integrity has had a positive effect. Have you ever confessed to an instructor that your paper is late without a good excuse, only to find that despite your mistake you have earned the instructor's respect? Have extra efforts in the workplace ever helped you gain a promotion or a raise? Have your kindnesses toward a friend or spouse moved the relationship to a deeper level? When you decide to act with integrity, you can improve your life and the lives of others.

Most importantly, living with integrity helps you believe in yourself and in your ability to make good choices. A person of integrity isn't a perfect person but one who makes the effort to live according to values and principles, continually striving to learn from mistakes and to improve. Take responsibility for making the right moves, and you will follow your mission with strength and conviction.

> "And life is what we make it, always has been, always will be."
> GRANDMA MOSES

Roll with the Changes

Think again about yourself. How has your idea of where you want to be changed since you first opened this book? How has your self-image changed? What have you learned about your values, your goals, and your styles of communication and learning? Consider how your educational, professional, and personal goals have changed. As you continue to grow and develop, keep adjusting your goals to your changes and discoveries.

Stephen Covey says in *The Seven Habits of Highly Effective People*, "Change—real change—comes from the inside out. It doesn't come from hacking at the leaves of attitude and behavior with quick fix personality ethic techniques. It comes from striking at the root—the fabric of our thought, the fundamental essential paradigms which give definition to our character and create the lens through which we see the world."[2]

Examining yourself deeply in that way is a real risk. Most of all, it demands courage and strength of will. Questioning your established beliefs and facing the unknown are much more difficult than staying with how things are. When you have the courage to face the consequences of trying something unfamiliar, admitting failure, or challenging what you thought you knew, you open yourself to growth and learning opportunities. You can make your way through changes you never anticipated if you make the effort to live your mission—in whatever forms it takes as it changes—each day, each week, each month, and for years to come.

TERMS

Paradigm
An especially clear pattern or typical example.

Learn From Role Models

People often derive the highest level of motivation and inspiration from learning how others have struggled through the ups and downs of life and achieved their goals. Somehow, seeing how someone else went through difficult situations can give you hope for your own struggles. The positive effects of being true to one's self become more real when an actual person has earned them.

Learning about the lives of people who have achieved their own version of success can teach you what you can do in your own life. Bessie and Sadie Delany, sisters and accomplished African-American women born in the late 1800s, are two valuable role models. They took risks, becoming professionals in dentistry and teaching at a time when women and minorities were often denied both respect and opportunity. They worked hard to fight racial division and prejudice and taught others what they learned. They believed in their intelligence, beauty, and ability to give, and lived without regrets. Says Sadie in their *Book of Everyday Wisdom*, "If there's anything I've learned in all these years, it's that life is too good to waste a day. It's up to you to make it sweet."[3]

Aim for Your Personal Best

Your personal best is simply the best that you can do in any situation. It may not be the best you have ever done. It may include mistakes, for nothing significant is ever accomplished without making mistakes and taking risks. It may shift from situation to situation. As long as you aim to do your best, though, you are inviting growth and success.

Aim for your personal best in everything you do. As a lifelong learner, you will always have a new direction in which to grow and a new challenge to face. Seek constant improvement in your personal, educational, and professional life, knowing that you are capable of that improvement. Enjoy the richness of life by living each day to the fullest, developing your talents and potential into the achievement of your most valued goals.

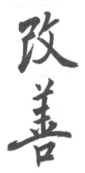

Kaizen is the Japanese word for "continual improvement." Striving for excellence, always finding ways to improve on what already exists, and believing that you can impact change are at the heart of the industrious Japanese spirit. The drive to improve who you are and what you do will help to provide the foundation of a successful future.

Think of this concept as you reflect on yourself, your goals, your lifelong education, your career, and your personal pursuits. Create excellence and quality by continually asking yourself, "How can I improve?" Living by *kaizen* will help you to be a respected friend and family member, a productive and valued employee, and a truly contributing member of society. You can change the world.

Applications   Chapter 12

KEY INTO YOUR LIFE
Opportunities to Apply What You Learn

 Questions in Nursing

Read the following article from *The American Nurse* (Nov./Dec. 1997), [4] and then answer the questions that follow.

LYING FOR CARE

A significant percentage of physicians participating in a nationwide survey indicated they'd be willing to use deception to obtain insurance coverage in certain cases, particularly when the severity of the patient's condition warrants such an approach.

In the survey, physicians were given six clinical vignettes and asked if they'd agree with a colleague's decision to deceive a third-party payer by providing inaccurate documentation to get a procedure done that otherwise would not be covered. In each scenario, the patient would be unable to pay for the treatment on her own.

In one scenario, a 55-year-old woman, homebound with occasional severe angina, wants a coronary bypass. Recently forced to switch insurance companies, she could only have the surgery for this preexisting condition if her chest pain is progressive, which it is not. About 58 percent of the 169 internists surveyed would support altering the facts of the case to her new insurance company to secure the procedure.

In another case, 47.5 percent of the respondents would approve lying to get intravenous pain medication and nutrition for a terminally ill woman who could only receive this "comfort care" if she had "recurring vomiting" and not just severe nausea after swallowing solids or liquids.

On the other hand, only 2.5 percent would sanction lying for a patient who wanted rhinoplasty because she is "sad about feeling less attractive with each passing year" by documenting that she has a deviated septum and problems breathing.

The survey results were published in the Oct. 25 *Archives of Internal Medicine* and released at a recent American Medical Association conference.

An earlier survey by the Kaiser Family Foundation also reported that many doctors—and nurses—say they have exaggerated a patient's condition to get coverage for them.

---

1. What ethical questions are raised? _____

_____

_____

_____

2. What legal questions are raised? _____

_____

_____

_____

3. What economic questions are raised? _____

_____

_____

_____

4. What is your personal reaction? _____

_____

_____

_____

5. As a person of science, what is your reaction? Is it different from your personal reaction and, if so, in what ways? _____

_____

_____

_____

Looking at Change, Failure, and Success

Life can go by so fast that you don't take time to evaluate what changes have taken place, what failures you could learn from, and what successes you have experienced. Take a moment now and answer the following questions for yourself.

What are the three biggest changes that have occurred in your life this year?

1. _____

2. _____

3. _____

Choose one that you feel you handled well. What shifts in priorities or goals did you make?

_____

_____

_____

_____

Choose one that you could have handled better. What happened? What do you think you should have done?

_____

_____

_____

_____

Now name a personal experience, occurring this year, that you would consider a failure. What happened?

_____

_____

_____

_____

How did you handle it—did you ignore it, blame it on someone else, or admit and explore it?

_____

_____

_____

_____

What did you learn from experiencing this failure?

_____

_____

_____

_____

Finally, describe a recent success of which you are the most proud.

_____

_____

_____

_____

How did this success give you confidence in other areas of your life?

_____

_____

_____

_____

12.3 Volunteering

Research community service opportunities. What are the organizations? What are their needs? Do any volunteer positions require an application, letters of reference, or background checks? List three possibilities for which you have an interest or a passion.

1. _____

2. _____

3. _____

Of these three, choose one that you feel you will have the time and ability to try next semester. Suggestions that don't take up too much time include spending an evening serving in a soup kitchen or driving for Meals on Wheels during a lunch or dinner shift. Name your choice here and tell why you selected it.

_____

_____

_____

_____

Research the suggestion you have chosen. Describe the activity. What is the time commitment? Is there any special training involved? Are there any problematic or difficult elements to this experience?

_____

_____

_____

_____

_____

_____

_____

_____

Lifelong Learning

Review the strategies for lifelong learning in this chapter. Which ones mean something to you? Which do you think you can do, or plan to do, in your life now and when you are out of school? Name them and briefly discuss the role they play in your life.

_____

_____

_____

_____

_____

KEY TO SELF-EXPRESSION
Discovery Through Journal Writing

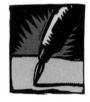

To record your thoughts, use a separate journal or the lined pages at the end of the chapter.

Ethical Questions

Take some time to write about questions you have concerning health care and technology discoveries and use.

Journal

Name _____ Date _____

Endnotes

Chapter 1

1. American Association of Colleges of Nursing, Education Center, *Your Nursing Career: A Look at the Facts, 1999,* www.aacn.nche.edu.education/Career.htm.

2. U.S. Department of Health and Human Services, Health Resources and Services Administration, Bureau of Health Professions, Division of Nursing, *The Registered Nurse Population, March 1996, Findings from The National Sample Survey of Registered Nurses.*

3. U.S. Department of Education, National Center for Education Statistics (NCES), *1996 Digest of Education Statistics,* Table 266 and Table 267.

4. Ibid., Table 266.

5. U.S. Department of Education, National Center for Education Statistics, *Nontraditional Undergraduates: Trends in Enrollment from 1986 to 1992 and Persistence and Attainment Among 1989–90 Beginning Post-Secondary Students,* NCES 97-578, by Laura J. Horn. Project Officer, Dennis Carroll (Washington, DC: U.S. Government Printing Office, 1996), 26.

6. NCES, *1996 Digest of Education Statistics,* Table 177.

7. U.S. Department of Education, National Center for Education Statistics, *The Condition of Education 1996,* NCES 96-304, by Thomas M. Smith (Washington, DC: U.S. Government Printing Office, 1996), 60–61.

8. American Association of Colleges of Nursing, Education Center, *Your Nursing Career: A Look at the Facts 1999* from website www.aacn.nche.edu.education/Career.htm.

9. Ibid.

10. Ibid.

11. Ibid.

12. American Association for Men in Nursing, *Purpose Statement,* 1996, from the website: www.aamn.org.

13. U.S. Department of Health and Human Services, Health Resources and Services Administration, Bureau of Health Professions, Division of Nursing. *The Registered Nurse Population, March 1996, Findings from The National Sample Survey of Registered Nurses.*

14. American Association of Colleges of Nursing, *Media Relations: Nursing Schools Lag Behind Rising Demand for RNs, AACN Survey Shows*, 1999, from Web site: www.aacn.nche.edu/Media/NewsRelease/enrl98wb.htm.

15. *Annual Wages of Nurses, Doctors, and Other Health Care Workers*, Occupational Employment Statistics, The Bureau of Labor Statistics, Dec. 23, 1999, from website http://stats.bls.gov/oes/national/oes32502.htm.

16. U.S. Department of Health and Human Services, Health Resources and Services Administration, Bureau of Health Professions, Division of Nursing, *The Registered Nurse Population, March 1996, Findings from The National Sample Survey of Registered Nurses.*

17. Ibid.

18. Ibid.

19. American Association of Colleges of Nursing, *Media Relations: Advanced Practice Nursing: Extending Primary Care's Reach*, 1999, from the website www.aacn. nche.edu/Media/NewsRelease/enrl98wb.htm.

20. Ibid.

21. Ibid.

22. Ibid.

23. *Lifeline to Future Leaders*, by Diane J. Mancino, EdD, RN, CAE NSNA, 1997–99 National Student Nurses' Association and International Thomson Publishing, from website www.nsna.org/Home/Faculty/Consultants.

24. Gonzaga University, *1997–1999 Catalog.* (Gonzaga University: Spokane, WA, 1997), 74.

Chapter 2

1. Mariah A. Taylor, The Clinic of Last Resort, *Reflections on Nursing Leadership*, Second quarter, 1999, 24–30.

2. Judith A. Huntington RN, MN, *The Washington Nurse, Nurse Shortage and Staffing Concerns Prompt Actions from Coast to Coast and Around the World*, Autumn 1999, 2224.

3. Ibid.

4. Ibid.

5. Ibid.

6. Ibid.

7. Ibid.

8. News: New Poll Shows Public Concern About Health Care, *Reflections on Nursing Leadership*, Fourth quarter, 1999, 39.

9. Ibid.

10. Fredrick May, Joan Kessner, and Victoria Champion. Attitudes, Values and Beliefs of the Public in Indiana Toward Nursing as a Career. *Study To Enhance Nursing Recruitment* (Indianapolis, IN: Sigma Theta Tau International, 1988), 7–12.

11. *Nursing Shortage Talking Points*, July, 1999. American Nurses Association, from website www.nursingworld.org/RNrealnews/Nurses'Toolkit.

12. Linda U. Krebs, Jamie Myers, Georgia Decker, Jan Kinzler, Pamela Asfahani, and Julie Jackson, The Oncology Nursing Image: Lifting the Mist, *Oncology Nursing Forum*, 23 (8), 1297–1304.

13. Bureau of Labor Statistics, *Occupational Outlook Handbook Home Page*, Theresa Cosca, Feb. 26, 1999. Registered Nurses Accessibility Information, www.bls.gov/oco/ocos083.htm.

14. Joanne Comi McCloskey and Helen Kennedy Grace, editors, *Current Issues in Nursing*, 5th ed. (St. Louis: Mosby, 1997); *Ambulatory Care Nursing: Concerns and Challenges*, Ida M. Androwich, Sheila A. Haas, 216–222.

15. Janet R. Katz, 1999, *Majoring in Nursing: From Prerequisites to Postgraduate and Beyond* (New York, Farrar, Straus and Giroux).

16. Joanne Comi McCloskey and Helen Kennedy Grace, editors, *Current Issues in Nursing*, 5th ed. (St. Louis: Mosby, 1997); Carole A. Gutt, *Recent Changes and Current Issues in Community Nursing*.

17. U.S. Department of Health and Human Services, Health Resources and Services Administration, Bureau of Health Professions, Division of Nursing, *The Registered Nurse Population, March 1996, Findings from The National Sample Survey of Registered Nurses*.

18. American Association of Colleges of Nursing, *Media Relations: Advanced Practice Nursing: Extending Primary Care's Reach*, 1999, from website www.aacn.nche.edu/Media/NewsRelease/enrl98wb.htm.

19. Joanne Comi McCloskey and Helen Kennedy Grace, editors, *Current Issues in Nursing*, 5th ed. (St. Louis: Mosby, 1997); Virginia M. Ohlson and Margretta Madden Styles, *International Nursing: The Role of the International Council of Nurses and The World Health Organization*, 403–411.

20. Ibid.

21. Bureau of Labor Statistics, *Occupational Outlook Handbook* Home Page, Theresa Cosca, Feb. 26, 1999, Registered Nurses Accessibility Information, http://stats/bls.gov/oco/ocos083.htm.

22. Ibid.

Chapter 3

1. *The Third International Mathematics and Science Study* (TIMSS), 1998, National Center for Education Statistics.

2. Richard W. Riley, Remarks to the Conference of American Mathematical Society and Mathematical Association of America: *The State of Mathematics Education: A Strong Foundation for the 21st Century*, January 8, 1998.

3. Barbara Soloman, North Carolina State University, Raleigh, NC.

4. Howard Gardner, *Multiple Intelligences: The Theory in Practice* (New York: HarperCollins, 1993), 5–49.

5. Joyce Bishop, Ph.D., Psychology Faculty, Golden West College, Huntington Beach, CA.

6. Felder, R., 1996, Matters of Style, ASEE Prism, 6(4), 18–23.

7. Felder, R., 1993, "Reaching the Second Tier: Learning and Teaching Styles in College Science Education," *Journal of College Science Teaching*, 23(5), 286–290.

8. Gardner, H., 1991, *The Unschooled Mind: How Children Think and How Schools Should Teach*.

9. Winter, E. *Seven Styles of Learning: Part 3*. Article's website address: www.bena.com/ewinters/articles.html.

Chapter 4

1. Paul R. Timm, Ph.D., *Successful Self Management: A Psychologically Sound Approach to Personal Effectiveness* (Los Altos, CA: Crisp Publications, 1987), 22–41.
2. Stephen Covey, *The Seven Habits of Highly Effective People* (New York: Simon and Schuster, 1989), 70–144, 309–318.

Chapter 5

1. Frank T. Lyman, Jr., Ph.D., Think-Pair-Share, Thinktrix, Thinklinks, and Weird Facts: An Interactive System for Cooperative Thinking, *Enhancing Thinking Through Cooperative Learning*, Neil Davidson and Toni Worsham, editors (New York: Teachers College Press, 1992), 169–181.
2. Roger von Oech, *A Kick in the Seat of the Pants* (New York: Harper & Row Publishers, 1986), 5–21.
3. R. M. Roberts, *Serendipity: Accidental Discoveries in Science* (New York: John Wiley & Sons, 1989), ix.
4. Ibid., 164.
5. Ibid., x.
6. Ibid., 51.
7. R. M. Roberts, *Serendipity*, x.
8. Dennis Coon, *Introduction to Psychology: Exploration and Application*, 6th ed. (St. Paul: West Publishing Company, 1992), 295.

Chapter 6

1. U. S. Department of Education, National Center for Education Statistics, *The Condition of Education 1996*, NCES 96-304, by Thomas M. Smith (Washington, DC: U. S. Government Printing Office, 1996), 84.
2. Sherwood Harris, *The New York Public Library Book of How and Where to Look It Up* (Upper Saddle River, NJ: Prentice Hall, 1991), 13.
3. George M. Usova, *Efficient Study Strategy Skills for Successful Learning* (Pacific Grove, CA: Brooks/Cole Publishing Company, 1989), 45.
4. Francis P. Robinson, *Effective Behavior* (New York: Harper & Row, 1941).
5. Sylvan Barnet and Hugo Bedau, *Critical Thinking, Reading, and Writing: A Brief Guide to Argument*, 2nd ed. (Boston: Bedford Books of St. Martin's Press, 1996), 15–21.
6. P. S. Fardy and F. G. Yanowitz, *Cardiac Rehabilitation, Adult Fitness, and Exercise Testing*, 3rd ed. (Baltimore: Williams & Wilkins, 1995), 246–247.
7. Teresa Audesirk and Gerald Audesirk, *Life on Earth* (Upper Saddle River, NJ: Prentice Hall, 1997), 55–56.

Chapter 7

1. Walter Pauk, *How to Study in College*, 5th ed. (Boston: Houghton Mifflin Company, 1993), 110–114.
2. Analysis based on Lynn Quitman Troyka, *Simon & Schuster Handbook for Writers* (Upper Saddle River, NJ: Prentice Hall, 1996), 22–23.

Chapter 8

1. Ralph G. Nichols, Do We Know How to Listen? Practical Helps in a Modern Age, *Speech Teacher* (March 1961), 118–124.

2. Ibid.

3. Herman Ebbinghaus, *Memory: A Contribution to Experimental Psychology*, trans. H. A. Ruger and C. E. Bussenius (New York: New York Teacher's College, Columbia University, 1885).

4. Many of the examples of objective questions used in this chapter are from Gary W. Piggrem, Test Item File for Charles G. Morris, *Understanding Psychology*, 3rd ed. (Upper Saddle River, NJ: Prentice Hall, 1996).

Chapter 9

1. Susan Beck, Breast and Prostate Cancer Pain, *Reflections on Nursing Leadership*, 1999, 20–28.

Chapter 10

1. Edith Warton, False Dawn, *Old New York* (New York: Simon and Schuster, 1951), 18–19.

2. Sheryl McCarthy, *Why Are The Heroes Always White?* (Kansas City: Andrews and McMeel, 1995), 188.

3. John Hockenberry, *Moving Violations* (New York: Hyperion, 1995), 78.

4. Tamera Trotter and Joycelyn Allen, *Talking Justice: 602 Ways to Build and Promote Racial Harmony* (Saratoga, CA: R & E Publishers, 1993), 51.

5. Sheryl McCarthy, *Why Are The Heroes?*, 137.

6. Deborah Tannen, *That's Not What I Meant: How Conversational Style Makes or Breaks Relationships* (New York: Ballantine, 1986), 3–15.

7. David W. Johnson and Frank P. Johnson, *Joining Together: Group Theory and Group Skills*, 6th ed. (Boston: Allyn and Bacon, 1997), 110.

8. Louis E. Boone, David L. Kurtz, and Judy R. Block, *Contemporary Business Communication* (Upper Saddle River, NJ: Prentice Hall, 1994), 49–54.

9. Adapted by Richard Bucher, Professor of Sociology, Baltimore City Community College, from Paula Rosenberg, William Paterson College of New Jersey.

Chapter 11

1. U. S. Department of Education, National Center for Education Statistics, *Profiles of Undergraduates Who Work: 1995–96*, NCES 98-084, by Laura J. Horn, Mark D. Premo, Andrew G. Malizio, Project Officer, and MPR Associates, Inc. (Washington, DC: U. S. Government Printing Office, May 1998), 15.

2. U. S. Department of Education, National Center for Education Statistics, *Digest of Education Statistics 1996*, NCES 96-133, by Thomas D. Snyder. Production Manager, Charlene M. Hoffman. Program Analyst, Claire M. Geddes (Washington, DC: U. S. Government Printing Office, 1996), 320–321.

3. Ibid., 324–325.

4. U. S. Department of Education, *The 2000–01 Student Guide to Financial Aid.*

Chapter 12

1. Thomas Moore, *The Care of the Soul* (New York: Harper Perennial, 1992), xi–xx.

2. Stephen Covey, *The Seven Habits of Highly Effective People* (New York: Simon & Schuster, 1989), 70–144, 309–318.

3. Sarah Delany and Elizabeth Delany with Amy Hill Hearth, *Book of Everyday Wisdom* (New York: Kodansha International, 1994), 123.

4. In Brief (Nov/Dec 1999). Lying for Care. *The American Nurse*, 10.

Index